"This excellent book is, in equal parts, fascinating and instructive! So much of our neuropsychological knowledge has emerged from the study of rare conditions and this book continues this vital tradition. By developing a deep understanding of a wide range of rare conditions, diagnostic challenges and controversial issues, we also improve our knowledge of how to manage conditions that are more common in clinical practice. I really enjoyed reading this book and thoroughly recommend it!"

Jon Evans, *Professor of Clinical Neuropsychology, University of Glasgow*

"This exceptional text is both groundbreaking and instructive. The detailed and clear presentation of rare cases accompanied by assessment findings, treatment protocols, theoretical implications and patient perspectives provides a roadmap for how to approach complex cases. The work of every clinician and researcher working to enhance the lives of individuals with challenging neurological conditions will be positively impacted by reading this volume and applying its concepts."

McKay Moore Sohlberg, PhD, *University of Oregon*

"An important text on the complexities of diagnosis in neuropsychology with fascinating case histories by leaders in the field."

Ian Robertson, *Global Brain Health Institute, Trinity College Dublin*

CW00763126

Rare Conditions, Diagnostic Challenges, and Controversies in Clinical Neuropsychology

This book highlights those rare, difficult to diagnose, or controversial cases in contemporary clinical neuropsychology. The evidence base relevant to this type of work is almost by definition insufficient to guide practice, but most clinicians will encounter such cases at some point in their careers. By documenting the experiences and learning of clinicians who have worked with cases that are 'out of the ordinary', the book addresses an important gap in the literature.

The book discusses 23 challenging and fascinating cases that fall outside what can be considered routine practice. Divided into three sections, the text begins by addressing rare and unusual conditions, defined as either conditions with a low incidence, or cases with an atypical presentation of a condition. It goes on to examine circumstances where an accurate diagnosis and/or coherent case formulation has been difficult to reach. The final section addresses controversial conditions in neuropsychology, including those where there is ongoing scientific debate, disagreement between important stakeholders, or an associated high-stakes decision. This text covers practice across lifespan and offers crucial information on specific conditions as well as implications for practice in rare disorders.

This book will be beneficial for clinical neuropsychologists and applied psychologists working with people with complex neurological conditions, along with individuals from medical, nursing, allied health, and social work backgrounds. It will further be of appeal to educators, researchers, and students of these professions and disciplines.

Dr Jessica Fish is a clinical psychologist and neuropsychologist. Trained at the universities of Exeter, Cambridge, and King's College London, she is a lecturer and researcher at the University of Glasgow, and works clinically at St George's Hospital, London. Her primary expertise is in acquired brain injury and neuropsychological rehabilitation.

Dr Shai Betteridge is Consultant Clinical Neuropsychologist and Chief Psychological Professions Officer at St George's University Hospitals NHS Foundation Trust, and a founder and director of Allied Neuro Therapy Ltd.

Her fields of expertise include neuropsychological rehabilitation, service development, quality improvement, and clinical excellence, spanning both public and private sectors.

Dr Barbara A. Wilson is a world-renowned clinical neuropsychologist. Now retired, Barbara has developed eight neuropsychological tests, written 32 books, and published more than 300 papers and chapters. Her main contributions are in ecologically valid assessment approaches, cognitive rehabilitation and errorless learning, the holistic model of rehabilitation, and disorders of consciousness.

Rare Conditions, Diagnostic Challenges, and Controversies in Clinical Neuropsychology

Out of the Ordinary

Edited by
Jessica Fish, Shai Betteridge,
and Barbara A. Wilson

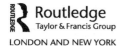
Routledge
Taylor & Francis Group

LONDON AND NEW YORK

Designed cover image: Getty Images

First published 2023
by Routledge
4 Park Square, Milton Park, Abingdon, Oxon OX14 4RN

and by Routledge
605 Third Avenue, New York, NY 10158

Routledge is an imprint of the Taylor & Francis Group, an informa business

British Library Cataloguing-in-Publication Data
A catalogue record for this book is available from the British Library

ISBN: 9781032132259 (hbk)
ISBN: 9781032132242 (pbk)
ISBN: 9781003228226 (ebk)

DOI: 10.4324/9781003228226

Typeset in Bembo
by codeMantra

This book is dedicated to the people featured in its chapters as patients or clients, along with their families. We recognise that this book represents a perspective on some of the most difficult life experiences and we thank you for allowing us to learn from you and to share this learning in the hope that we can help others in future.

Contents

Contributors

Dr Karen Addy, Salomons Institute for Applied Psychology, Canterbury Christ Church University, Tunbridge Wells. karen.addy@canterbury.ac.uk

Dr Joanna Atkinson, Deafness, Cognition and Language Research Centre, University College London. joanna.atkinson@ucl.ac.uk

Dr Shai Betteridge, Clinical Neuropsychology & Clinical Health Psychology, St George's University Hospitals NHS Foundation Trust, London; Allied Neuro Therapy, Egham, Surrey. shai.betteridge@stgeorges.nhs.uk

Dr Georgina Browne, Neuropsychology Department, Addenbrooke's Hospital, Cambridge. georgina.browne@addenbrookes.nhs.uk

Dr Laura Carroll, The Children's Trust, Tadworth.

Dr Enrique Childress, The Children's Trust, Tadworth.

Professor Rudi Coetzer, The Disabilities Trust, Silkwood Park, Wakefield; School of Human & Behavioural Sciences, Bangor University, Wales; Faulty of Medicine, Health & Life Science, Swansea University, Wales. Email: b.r.coetzer@bangor.ac.uk.

Dr Sal Connolly, The Royal Hospital for Neuro-disability, Putney, London; Connolly Neuro, Harley Street, London.

Dr Sarah Crawford, The Royal Hospital for Neuro-disability, Putney, London. scrawford@rhn.org.uk

Dr Michael Dilley, Brain & Mind Ltd, London; Kings College Hospital NHS Foundation Trust, London. Michael.Dilley@nhs.net

Louise Edwards, Independent Speech & Language Therapist, London.

Dr Sally Finnie, Department of Neuropsychology, Reading. Sally.Finnie@berkshire.nhs.uk

Dr Jessica Fish, School of Health & Wellbeing, University of Glasgow, Glasgow, UK; Clinical Neuropsychology & Clinical Health Psychology, St George's University Hospitals NHS Foundation Trust, London. jessica.fish@glasgow.ac.uk

Dr Fergus Gracey, Department of Clinical Psychology and Psychological Therapy, Norwich Medical School, University of East Anglia, Norwich. f.gracey@uea.ac.uk

Dr Andrew Hanrahan, The Royal Hospital for Neuro-disability, Putney, London.

Dr Catherine Harter, The Cambridge Centre for Paediatric Neuropsychological Rehabilitation (CCPNR), Cambridge and Peterborough NHS Foundation Trust. catherine.harter@nhs.net

Dr Jonathan Hinchliffe, The Royal Hospital for Neuro-disability, Putney, London; Cognisant Neuropsychology Ltd.

Dr Jenny Jim, The Children's Trust, Tadworth; University College London. jjim@thechildrenstrust.org.uk

Prof. Narinder Kapur, University College London; Imperial College NHS Trust, London. n.kapur@ucl.ac.uk

Dr Leigh Leppard, Lishman Neuropsychiatry Unit, South London and Maudsley NHS Trust, London. leigh@leppardpsychology.co.uk

Dr Valeria Lowing, The Children's Trust, Tadworth.

Prof. Sarah Mackenzie Ross, Research Department of Clinical, Educational & Health Psychology, University College London. s.mackenzie-ross@ucl.ac.uk

Dr Paolo Mantovani

Dr Ben Marram, Community Neurological Rehabilitation Service, Leeds Community Healthcare NHS Trust. benjamin.marram@nhs.net

Jwala Narayanan, Department of Neurology, Manipal Hospitals & Department of Neuropsychology, Annasawmy Mudaliar General Hospital. jwala.narayanan@gmail.com

Dr Elena Olgiati, The Royal Hospital for Neuro-disability, Putney, London; Imperial College London, Department of Brain Sciences.

Dr Louise Owen, The Children's Trust, Tadworth.

Dr Norman Poole, Department of Neuropsychiatry, St George's Hospital, South West London and St George's Mental Health NHS Trust.

Dr Priyanka Pradhan, St George's University Hospitals NHS Foundation Trust, London.

Dr Elizabeth Roberts, The Children's Trust, Tadworth.

Ms Alexandra E. Rose, Royal Hospital for Neuro-Disability, London; Mental Health & Wellbeing, School of Health & Wellbeing, University of Glasgow. arose@rhn.org.uk

Dr Stephanie Satariano, Evelina Children's Hospital, London; Child Psychology, London. stephanie@childpsychology.london

Dr Urvashi Shah, Department of Neurology, King Edward Memorial Hospital Mumbai, India. shahurvashi100@gmail.com

Dr Isabelle Sharples, The Children's Trust, Tadworth.

Dr Sonja Soeterik, Neurolink Psychology, London. dr.soeterik@neurolinkpsych.co.uk

Dr Victoria Teggart, Greater Manchester Mental Health NHS Foundation Trust, Manchester. viki.teggart@gmmh.nhs.uk

Darren Townsend-Handscomb, London.

Dr Roshni Vara, Evelina Children's Hospital, London.

Dr Barbara A. Wilson, Clinical Neuropsychology & Clinical Health Psychology, St George's University Hospitals NHS Foundation Trust, London; Allied Neuro Therapy, Egham, Surrey. barbara.wilson00@gmail.com

Prof. Andrew Worthington, Headwise, Birmingham; Faculty of Health, Medicine and Life Science, Swansea University, Swansea. aworthington@headwise.org.uk

Acknowledgements

We would first like to express our gratitude to the chapter authors for volunteering to contribute to this volume and for writing about their clinical work. Many of the chapters relate to complex and non-routine aspects of clinical practice which may have felt like a professional 'stretch', and that may not have reached a satisfactory conclusion. To conduct this work takes a great deal of creativity and resourcefulness as well as essential knowledge and experience. Writing about this work takes valuable time, effort, and perhaps the odd wrangle with one's inner critic. Sharing this work with others takes bravery and demonstrates a commitment to learning and development as individuals and beyond for our services and professional disciplines. Several authors demonstrated phenomenal patience when awaiting our feedback, and nonetheless responded swiftly to queries and requests for amendments. We thank you sincerely for all of this and hope that you are pleased with the finished product.

We would also like to thank our colleagues at the University of Glasgow, St George's University Hospitals NHS Foundation Trust, Allied Neuro Therapy Ltd, the Encephalitis Society, and the British Psychological Society Division of Neuropsychology for their support; in particular: Hamish McLeod, Jon Evans, Katherine Carpenter, Ingram Wright, Alexandra Rose, Gaby Parker, Juliet Lawson, and Tasneem Mohamed. We also acknowledge the late Mick Wilson for his support at the beginning of this project. His encouragement to write about our clinical neuropsychological practice will be an eternal inspiration to all of us.

Finally, we would like to thank Lucy Kennedy, Lakshay Gaba and the team at Routledge for their guidance, encouragement, insight, and patience throughout the process of producing this book.

1 Introduction

Rare conditions, diagnostic challenges, and controversies in clinical neuropsychology

Jessica Fish, Shai Betteridge, and Barbara A. Wilson

We have an admittedly entirely biased perspective that clinical neuropsychologists are ideally placed to work with people with rare disorders, to grapple with difficult diagnostic questions, and to engage with controversial topics within clinical neurosciences. The academic discipline of neuropsychology is founded on the study of rare cases; people with focal brain injuries whose specific cognitive impairments provided a wealth of information about the structure of the human mind and spawning more box-and-arrow diagrams than it would be feasible to count (for overviews see Marshall & Gurd, 2010; Vallar & Caputi, 2020; and the canon – Shallice, 1988). In contrast, training in clinical psychology provides a thorough grounding in the full range of mental health conditions as well as other areas of specialism, alongside psychological formulation and intervention from within a broad biopsychosocial framework (see British Psychological Society (BPS), 2019a). These disciplines converge in the profession of clinical neuropsychology, and the range of skills clinical neuropsychologists possess (see BPS, 2019b) applies extremely well to the care of people with complex neurological conditions. This is not to say that clinical neuropsychology is the only nor indeed the most important profession; the best care for people with complex neuro conditions undoubtedly arises from working in integrated systems and interdisciplinary teams towards shared goals – many hands making light work (e.g. Bernard et al., 2010; Wilson et al., 2009).

This book arose from discussions about various 'difficult' cases we and our colleagues have encountered in clinical practice. It is very important that we make clear from the outset that, when we refer to such cases, we do not mean that the *patients themselves* are difficult, rather we mean that the *circumstances of the cases* have been difficult. Many factors can contribute to such difficulties, and we have grouped these into three broad categories as follows:

1. **Rare and unusual conditions**. Within this, we include:

   a. Conditions that have a low incidence in the population, such as mitochondrial disorders, rare metabolic syndromes or prion diseases,

DOI: 10.4324/9781003228226-1

which outside the context of specialist services may be hard to recognise, poorly understood, and have inadequate provision; and

b. Cases with an atypical presentation of a condition, where the underlying condition may or may not be so rare. For example, in Chapter 3 a rare disconnection syndrome is found to result from a not-so-rare left posterior cerebral artery stroke. In Chapter 4, a case of the rare prion disease Creutzfeld-Jacob disease is identified presenting with the also rather rare Capgras delusion; and the cases in Chapter 6 who presented with the rare neuropsychological condition Balint's syndrome as a result of rare neurological manifestations of the not-so-rare systemic conditions dengue fever and Covid-19.

2. **Cases where an accurate diagnosis and/or coherent case formulation is difficult to reach**. The rare and/or atypical conditions in the first category may of course be difficult to formulate and diagnose, but a range of other circumstances may also complicate assessment, formulation, and diagnosis, for instance:

    a. The presence of comorbid conditions that 'muddy the waters' of what might otherwise be a clear-cut issue. The most striking example of this is in chapter 12, where a person's deafness overshadowed the identification of a brain injury for a period of decades.
    b. The limits of our current assessment tools. For example, where there is no standardised/stand-alone battery for identifying the condition, or if the tools that do exist are not accessible for reasons of disability, culture etc. (as illustrated in many of our chapters).
    c. Limits associated with the service provision. The commissioning arrangements of some services mean that access to tools, sources of data, other professionals, or time may be limited, making it difficult to obtain a full and clear overview of the case. Equally, the limits of our own experience and limits on access to supervision and consultation can lead to diagnostic difficulties.

3. **Cases that are controversial**. For example, where there is ongoing scientific debate about aspects of the condition, disagreement between professionals working with the case, differences in opinion between family members and professionals, or because the stakes are very high, such as in several medicolegal contexts.

We have used these approximate and far from mutually exclusive categories to structure our book. Though the term 'diagnosis' can be controversial, particularly in relation to psychiatric diagnoses (e.g. Johnstone, 2018), and though many neuropsychologists would consider their work as contributing towards rather than solely reaching a diagnosis, we have used it in the heading of Part 2 for a few reasons. First, we often use the term to refer to a previously established and well-documented medical condition, such as a particular type of stroke or other brain injury. At other times we use the term to refer to the identification of a specifically neuropsychological syndrome, such as Balint's syndrome. At other times we use the term essentially as a shorthand to refer to a sometimes lengthy and intricate process whereby a professional or team of professionals collaborate with the client and often numerous other stakeholders in order to reach a comprehensive understanding of a person's presentation, of which a diagnosis is one part of much broader, holistic, inter-disciplinary formulation. Indeed, we are active proponents of psychological and neuropsychological formulation, teaching on this topic on a number of training courses and also having published/presented on it (e.g. Wilson & Betteridge, 2019; Winegarder & Fish, 2017).

As a group of editors, we have considerable experience working on such cases. Barbara Wilson in particular has a longstanding interest in rare disorders. Wilson, Baddeley, and Young (1999) reported the case of LE, a 51-year-old sculptor with systemic lupus erythematosus, an autoimmune disorder associated with a range of cognitive impairments. LE showed only mild impairments on cognitive testing, and her subjective impressions of a more serious impairment that was impacting on her work were initially attributed to anxiety and a difficulty in adjusting to the mild reductions in ability from a previously higher level. However, LE was insistent that there was really something the matter with her memory and noted an observation whereby she had thought that two stained-glass windows were identical, when her husband pointed out that they were very different. This led to more detailed assessment of LE's visual short-term memory and, indeed, significant problems were identified. Cases such as this were followed by a series of papers documenting detailed assessment and intervention with people with rare conditions including people who had emerged from disorders of consciousness (e.g. Macniven et al., 2003; Wilson & Bainbridge, 2013; Wilson et al., 2005). The Routledge book series, *Survivor Stories: Life After Brain Injury*, documents further cases in detail, some entirely from the person's own perspective, others in collaboration with a professional or team of professionals.

In collaboration with Michael Perdices, Barbara Wilson co-edited a special issue of the journal *Neuropsychological Rehabilitation* on rare and unusual syndromes (Perdices & Wilson, 2018), which included cases of Alice in Wonderland syndrome, Alexander's disease, Diogenes syndrome, Brugada syndrome, co-occurring Sheehan's syndrome and sickle cell disease, and a case of a person with a brain injury who had experienced a highly unusual 'feral' period during childhood.

Jessica Fish has worked in a number of highly specialist services from early in her career, which sparked and maintained interests in rare conditions. Particularly influential periods included a training placement with people with very severe brain injury at the Royal Hospital for Neuro-Disability where a bespoke, hypothesis-driven approach to assessment and intervention was key. She later worked at Professor Mike Kopelman's Neuropsychiatry and

Memory Disorders Service and, as Professor Kopelman is a world-leading expert in memory disorders, people with rare conditions and unusual presentations were seen frequently and benefited from the combined clinical–academic and multidisciplinary service setting (see Kopelman & Crawford, 1996). Periods of work at the Oliver Zangwill Centre (OZC) and the Wolfson Neurorehabilitation Centre followed, affording the opportunity to work intensively with clients with interacting cognitive, emotional, and physical consequences of brain injury. During this time she joined the Professional Panel of the excellent charity, The Encephalitis Society, whose work over the last 20+ years has brought about huge improvements in the recognition and treatment of this rare group of disorders. While at the OZC, she co-wrote a paper published in the previously mentioned special issue of *Neuropsychological Rehabilitation* on rare and unusual syndromes (Fish & Forrester, 2018). This paper was notable for documenting the experience of confabulation from the patient's perspective, and for documenting an awareness-based intervention that drew on various transferable principles from other areas of practice but had seldom been noted in the confabulation literature. She has gone on to supervise research on this topic in an attempt to formalise some of the 'practice-based evidence' that clinicians hold yet does not seem to influence theory or practice to the extent that it might (Brooks et al., in prep.; Brooks, 2022), and it is hoped that this book will similarly support this endeavour.

Shai Betteridge's experience was what directly led to the development of the book. As head of a neuropsychology department within a busy regional neurosciences centre, 'rare', 'controversial', and 'difficult to diagnose' cases are encountered at what may seem like a paradoxically frequent rate. The idea for the book was conceived during a supervision discussion Barbara had with Shai. While discussing two current cases, firstly the case described in Chapter 10 by Rose and Dilley, and secondly a case where a person's memory disorder appeared inconsistent with the established theories of memory (e.g. evident learning during the day and complete lack of carryover to the following day after a night of sleep). The case was very similar to the one described by Smith et al. (2010) in which the patient presented with a memory profile that had been depicted in the fictional film *50 First Dates*. This case was understood to be a functional amnesia, primarily confirmed by the observed recovery in function following psychological intervention. However, Shai's case (described in Chapter 24) was not responding to psychological treatment in the way expected from the functional amnesia formulation. This led to the reformulation of the case in order to identify alternative treatment approaches. Further exploration of the organic hypotheses that might account for the client's presentation has revealed fascinating hypotheses that, if confirmed, could revolutionise our understanding of memory profiles. Barbara proposed that these cases ought to be published, as both challenged conventional views regarding memory profiles. We considered how much we were learning from these cases, especially in relation to the dangers of body–mind dualism driving the misguided search for differential diagnoses in patients with multimorbidity, and we knew that others would have similar experiences. Indeed, many people consider their 'on the job' learning far more influential in shaping their practice than the initial training (though of course this provides the essential foundations); so the idea for this book was born.

We wanted to compile this book to inspire our professional community to drive forward holistic models of body and mind through a comprehensive picture of contemporary practice in clinical neuropsychology in non-routine circumstances and less established areas of practice. We were confident that the contents would be of interest and reflect the discrepancies between the empirical literature, which often concerns single diagnoses, and clinical practice, where multimorbidity and especially comorbidity of physical and mental health conditions is common. Our objective was that reading this book might speed up the rate at which people develop competence in this kind of work. We therefore contacted our professional networks and included an open call for chapter proposals in the newsletter of our key professional body, the British Psychological Society (BPS) Division of Neuropsychology. The fact that our colleagues shared our vision and responded in abundance to the call for cases highlights how common diagnostic challenges and controversies are in clinical practice.

Naturally the majority of the chapter authors are neuropsychologists in the United Kingdom, but there are many chapters co-written with colleagues who have different professional backgrounds, reflecting the multi- and/or interdisciplinary settings in which many of us work and which, in our view, are crucial to providing integrated care. We are delighted that the chapters represent people from childhood to old age. There is also considerable variation in the service contexts from which these cases are drawn. Many are from the UK National Health Service (NHS), several are based on third sector charitable organisations, and there are also two chapters from colleagues in India. We think that, collectively, the chapters provide fascinating insights into how neuropsychological principles are applied and translated – across the lifespan, between different conditions, across the range of severity, over myriad service settings, as well as geographical boundaries.

We hope you enjoy reading the ensuing chapters and will be back with some concluding thoughts thereafter.

References

Bernard, S., Aspinal, F., Gridley, K., & Parker, G. (2010). Integrated services for people with long-term neurological conditions: Evaluation of the impact of the National Service Framework, Final Report, SPRU Working Paper No. SDO 2399, Social Policy Research Unit, University of York, York.

British Psychological Society (2019a). Standards for the accreditation of Doctoral programmes in clinical psychology. Leicester, BPS.

British Psychological Society (2019b). Standards for the accreditation of programmes in adult clinical neuropsychology. Leicester, BPS.

Brooks, E. (2022). Exploring the clinical management of confabulation within neuropsychology services. D Clin Psy thesis, University of Glasgow.

Brooks, E., Evans, J., & Fish, J. (in preparation). *The clinical management of confabulation in neuropsychology services: A practitioner survey and interview study.*

Fish, J., & Forrester, J. (2018). Developing awareness of confabulation through psychological formulation: A case report and first-person perspective. *Neuropsychological Rehabilitation, 28*(2), 277–292.

Johnstone, L. (2018). Psychological formulation as an alternative to psychiatric diagnosis. *Journal of Humanistic Psychology, 58*(1), 30–46.

Macniven, J. A., Poz, R., Bainbridge, K., Gracey, F., & Wilson, B. A. (2003). Emotional adjustment following cognitive recovery from 'persistent vegetative state': Psychological and personal perspectives. *Brain Injury, 17*(6), 525–533.

Kopelman, M., & Crawford, S. (1996). Not all memory clinics are dementia clinics. *Neuropsychological Rehabilitation, 6*(3), 187–202.

Macniven, J. A., Poz, R., Bainbridge, K., Gracey, F., & Wilson, B. A. (2003). Emotional adjustment following cognitive recovery from 'persistent vegetative state': Psychological and personal perspectives. *Brain Injury, 17*(6), 525–533.

Marshall, J. C., & Gurd, J. M. (2010). Neuropsychology: Past, present, and future. In J. Gurd & U. Kischka (Eds), *The handbook of clinical neuropsychology*, 2nd edn. Oxford: Oxford Academic, online edition. https://doi.org/10.1093/acprof:oso/9780199234110.003.01

Perdices, M., & Wilson, B. A. (2018). Introduction to the special issue on rare and unusual syndromes. *Neuropsychological Rehabilitation, 28*(2), 185–188.

Shallice, T. (1988). *From neuropsychology to mental structure.* Cambridge University Press.

Smith, C. N., Frascino, J. C., Kripke, D. L., McHugh, P. R., Treisman, G. J., & Squire, L. R. (2010). Losing memories overnight: A unique form of human amnesia. *Neuropsychologia, 48*(10), 2833–2840.

Vallar, G., & Caputi, N. (2020). The history of human neuropsychology. In S. Della Sala (Ed.), *Encyclopedia of behavioral neuroscience* (2nd ed.). Elsevier. https://doi.org/10.1016/B978-0-12-809324-5.23914-X

Wilson, B. A., Baddeley, A. D., & Young, A. W. (1999). L.E.: A person who lost her 'Mind's Eye'. *Neurocase, 5*, 119–127.

Wilson, B. A., & Bainbridge, K. (2013). Kate's story: Recovery takes time, so don't give up. In B. A. Wilson, J. Winegardner, & F. Ashworth (Eds.), *Life after brain injury* (pp. 68–80). Psychology Press.

Wilson, B. A., Berry, E., Gracey, F., Harrison, C., Stow, I., Macniven, J., ... & Young, A. W. (2005). Egocentric disorientation following bilateral parietal lobe damage. *Cortex, 41*(4), 547–554.

Wilson, B. A., & Betteridge, S. (2019). *Essentials of neuropsychological rehabilitation.* Guilford Publications.

Wilson, B. A., Gracey, F., Evans, J. J., & Bateman, A. (2009). *Neuropsychological rehabilitation: Theory, models, therapy and outcome.* Cambridge University Press.

Winegardner, J., & Fish, J. E. (2017, July). *A novel approach to interdisciplinary team assessment: Joining the dots.* Abstract of datablitz presentation at the World Federation of NeuroRehabilitation (WFNR) 14th annual conference on neuropsychological rehabilitation, Cape Town, South Africa.

Part 1

Rare and unusual conditions

2 Gas geyser syndrome in India

A tragic, preventable
neuropsychological morbidity

Urvashi Shah

Introduction

> *It often happens that the real tragedies of life occur in such an inartistic manner that
> they hurt us by their crude violence, their absolute incoherence, their absurd want
> of meaning, their entire lack of style.*
>
> (Oscar Wilde, *The Picture of Dorian Gray*,
> ed. J. Bistrow (2005), p. 78)

'Gas geyser syndrome' (GGS) is a known phenomenon to the medical fraternity in India. Although infrequent, cases are seen in emergency units and many physicians have become familiar with the history and pattern of symptom presentation. However, the diagnosis can still be confounding as many symptoms may be similar to those seen after exposure to other gases. Various published case reports have underscored the need for a careful history and review of imaging findings to reach a conclusive diagnosis (Anand et al., 2006; Correia et al., 2012; Mehta et al., 2016). Gas geyser syndrome has also been reported in other South Asian countries such as Pakistan (Quasim, 2017), Nepal (Bista et al., 2017), and BRICS countries (Brazil, Russia, India, China, and South Africa) (Sampson, 2017) where erratic electricity supply and the low cost of gas geysers makes them a popular choice.

In western countries, common causes of carbon monoxide (CO) toxicity are exhaust from engines, fire (smoke inhalation), and poorly installed furnaces. Flue-less (no duct/chimney) gas heaters are cheaper to run as compared to electric fires and are easy to install. In India, the commonest cause of CO poisoning is the use of faulty gas appliances for cooking in enclosed spaces, especially in the winter months (Sikary et al., 2017).

Gas geysers are connected to liquefied petroleum gas (LPG) cylinders. LPG contains C_3 and C_4 hydrocarbons and the gas contains butane and propane. The gas is heated by a gas burner and is delivered by an inlet pipe. When there is proper combustion, carbon dioxide and water are produced. As the gas heats and pressure is built up, the safety pressure valve in the unit discharges the pressure. An attractive feature of this geyser is that there is an instant and continuous supply of heated water and this appeals to people living in areas where there are frequent power cuts and harsh winters.

DOI: 10.4324/9781003228226-3

However, in many homes in India, there are small bathing spaces with poor cross-ventilation and in winter families tend to keep the windows shut, resulting in poorly ventilated bathrooms with insufficient oxygen. In these spaces, an incomplete combustion results in the formation of the toxic, lethal carbon monoxide gas.

Despite several media reports of death due to carbon monoxide poisoning after using a gas geyser, and case reports in the Indian medical literature, the gas geyser continues to be popular and there appears to be little or no awareness about the precautions that need to be taken while using this geyser.

There have been no guidelines about the safe use of gas geysers and it is only recently that in India a government gas agency has brought out a document listing recommendations for the proper installation of these geysers (Mahanagar Gas Limited, 2020).

CO is an odourless, colourless, tasteless, non-irritant gas that binds to the hemoglobin creating carboxyhemoglobin (COHb). Hemoglobin (Hb) has a very high affinity to bind with CO, almost 250 times higher than oxygen. COHb reduces the capacity of the blood to bind oxygen, thereby decreasing the oxygen transport mechanism and delivery of oxygen to the tissues, thus causing hypoxia. Additionally, the exposure to CO brings about mitochondrial inhibition and free radical generation resulting in ischemic and anoxic brain injury that causes the cognitive deficits (Rose et al., 2017). Certain organs such as the heart and the brain that have a greater requirement of oxygen are more vulnerable than other organ systems. The most common imaging findings are white matter hyperintensities and hippocampal damage (Weaver et al., 2015; Parkinson et al., 2002). The magnitude and spectrum of symptoms vary according to the degree of exposure-concentration of CO and duration of exposure. Several patients have been found in an unconscious state. Increasing concentrations of COHb, ranging from 10% to 60%, are associated with different presenting symptoms such as headaches and dizziness, altered mentation and cognitive deficits, and at higher percentages, to seizures, coma, or even death.

It has been suggested that even low level exposure, but of longer duration, can result in significant cognitive issues (Townsend & Maynard, 2002). Long-term problems (> 6 years) have been reported in a subgroup of patients suggesting irreversibility in some people (Weaver et al., 2008). The quality of life in these survivors is significantly impacted in the long term with persisting cognitive and mood issues (Pages et al., 2014). Depression and anxiety are common and occur independently of the severity of the poisoning (Chelsea et al., 2007).

In terms of management, the current recommendation, although not mandated, is either hyperbaric (HbO_2) or normobaric (NBO_2) oxygen as soon as possible (Wolf et al., 2008). A double blind, randomized trial for HbO_2 has shown that hyperbaric-oxygen within the first 24 hours has benefit on long-term cognitive outcomes (Weaver et al, 2002).

Case history

SJ, a 32-year-old, high functioning, young graduate in Fashion Design was working as an assistant store manager in a high fashion luxury store. She travelled with her fiancée and his family for a vacation to a mountain resort.

The next morning her fiancé and family went out early in the morning to visit a local temple. She stayed back and told them that she would join them later for breakfast. When she did not show up at the restaurant and was not answering her phone, her fiancé returned to the room to check on her and found her lying undressed and unconscious on the bathroom floor. The transfer to a city hospital took several hours and at admission, about 8 hours after the event, she was conscious but confused and disoriented and was unable to recognize the family members.

Investigations

Magnetic resonance imaging (MRI) revealed a bilateral symmetrical hyperintense signal in the hippocampus, lentiform nucleus, and cerebellum with restricted diffusion on diffusion images suggestive of toxic encephalopathy (Figure 2.1); COHb levels were 40%. An electroencephalogram (EEG) revealed intermittent generalized background slowing and the diagnosis noted in the hospital papers was (G92) toxic encephalopathy, which is a major complication and comorbidity (MCC) code.

Hospital medical management

Diagnosis of CO poisoning is made on the basis of three clinical criteria: symptom presentation, history of recent exposure, and increased levels of

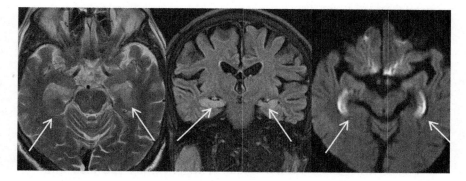

Figure 2.1 MR imaging showing bilateral symmetric T2/ FLAIR hyperintense signals in the hippocampal formation on axial and coronal FLAIR images respectively. Diffusion restriction also detected on the axial DW image

COHb. In SJ's case the diagnosis of gas geyser syndrome was made on the basis of her presenting history, imaging findings, and high levels of COHb. She was immediately referred for Hyperbaric Oxygen Therapy where she was placed in a special chamber to breathe 100% pure oxygen at high air pressure levels to oxygenate the blood and speed up tissue recovery after CO poisoning. The therapy used high pressure of 2.5–3 atmosphere absolute (ATA, the average atmospheric pressure exerted at sea level). She had three one-hour sessions over the week. She tolerated the same well except for developing tinnitus that lasted for a week.

Post discharge status

At discharge she continued to be confused about ongoing events and complained of forgetfulness and feeling that she was 'going crazy'. The family reported that she would forget what she had eaten, which family members had visited, and did not recognize the therapists who visited her daily. She was confused about why she was in hospital and repeatedly asked the same questions. She became irritable and agitated and after a psychiatry review she was started on a mood stabilizer. As the extreme forgetfulness persisted she was also started on a cholinesterase inhibitor.

At home, she was able to manage her self-care activities of daily living (ADL) but was unable to handle any household chores or return to work. The family was perplexed about the presentation of her forgetfulness. She appeared to have clear memories of her early childhood (school days), but patchy memories of the recent past (e.g. the engagement a year prior), and a complete inability to remember events that had transpired just an hour ago. Sensing that the family was becoming impatient with her confusion, she gradually began to withdraw and disengage from family activities.

Neuropsychological evaluation

SJ was referred for neuropsychological evaluation and rehabilitation planning three months after the event. She presented with significant distress and spoke of her forgetfulness, feeling disconnected and not being able to function beyond a simple repetitive routine. She reported anxiety about returning to work and diffidence about going out and participating in any activity. She had no personal memory of the gas geyser episode but was aware of the details based on what her family had shared. She reported feeling insecure about the prognosis and extent of recovery in the long term.

Her sister discussed the challenges of living with her and managing the mood issues and forgetfulness in daily life. Her behaviour appeared to be impacting the family dynamics and also her relationship with her fiancé and

Table 2.1 Test scores by cognitive domain

Domain	Test	Measure	Impaired	Borderline	Low average	Average	Above average/Superior
Speed of processing							
Attention	*Digit Symbol*	Total time				✓	
	Coloured Trails I	Total time		✓			
Memory							
Verbal memory	*Auditory Verbal Learning Test (AVLT)*	Total learning (5 trials)	✓				
		Immediate recall	✓				
		Delayed recall	✓				
		Recognition	✓				
		Percent retention	✓				
	Passages (Story Recall)	Immediate recall	✓				
		Delayed recall			✓		
Visual memory	*Visual Reproduction (WMS III)*	Immediate recall	✓				
		Delayed recall	✓				
		Recognition trial	✓				
	Complex Figure Test	Immediate recall	✓				
		Delayed recall		✓			
Executive function							
Working memory	*N-Back 1*	Hits		✓			
	N-Back 2	Errors		✓			
		Hits		✓			
		Errors		✓			
Verbal fluency	*Phonemic Fluency*	Average number of words		✓			
	Animal Fluency	Total number of words		✓			
Cognitive flexibility (Set shifting)	*Coloured Trails II*	Total time			✓		
Problem solving	*Tower of London*	Number of moves					✓✓
		Time taken					
Language							
Comprehension	*Token Test*						✓✓
Naming	*Boston Naming Test*						

his parents. She reported that her fiancé and his family were beginning to doubt her complaints and were wondering if she was being manipulative to gain attention.

SJ was evaluated on a standardized test protocol that was adapted, translated, and normed for the Indian population. The selected tests examined most of the pertinent cognitive domains and the scores were interpreted on the basis of the age and education-based normative data. As per the normative data, scores below the 15th percentile were interpreted as being in the impaired range. The 15th percentile represents 1 standard deviation below the normative data mean score for each test. This is used as the cut-off score for establishing impairment as per the normative data for the Indian population (Rao et al., 2004; see Table 2.1).

SJ's performance on the domain-specific tests revealed a profile of relatively well-preserved attention, executive functions, and language, but borderline functioning in the domains of working memory and processing speed.

The profile revealed significant memory impairment with scores for delayed recall in all the memory tests at zero after a delay of half an hour. She also had challenges with learning and immediate recall. She was unable to respond correctly even in the recognition trial and confessed that she was 'just guessing'. She was observed to be persistent and putting in her best effort, but struggling to remember, and asking for more time to recall. She was visibly distressed and frustrated with her inability to recall. Her performance across all the memory test trials were in the impaired range, suggesting a severe anterograde memory loss that correlated with the imaging findings of bilateral hippocampal damage. The performance on these tests appeared to be valid, as scores improved in the recognition, cued trial. In the delayed recall trial the score was zero, but in the recognition trial, she identified six words correctly and these were the same words that she had managed to learn during the encoding trials.

SJ had partial insight about the extent of her cognitive challenges and the details of her illness. The severe recent memory impairment had a devastating impact on her ability to function in daily life.

Mood profile

SJ was visibly disturbed and her family reported frequent crying spells and expressed distress regarding her inability to function in daily life. The score on hospital anxiety and depression scale (HADS) was 20 (0–7 = Normal, 8–10 = Borderline abnormal, 11–21 = Abnormal) indicating severe depression (Zigmond & Snaith, 1983). Additionally, the Millon Clinical personality Inventory MCMI III (Millon et al., 2006) was administered and the score of 88 on the severe syndrome scale suggested the presence of major depression. Her personality profile suggested a pattern of social inhibition, feelings of inadequacy, and very high dependency needs (Figure 2.2).

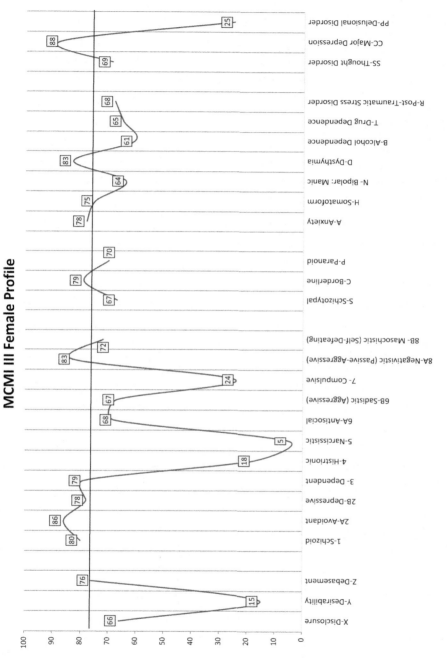

Figure 2.2 SJ's profile on the Millon Clinical Multiaxial Inventory (MCMI-III)'

Neuropsychological interventions

1. Case formulation

A session with SJ and the family helped delineate the goals and a case formulation based on a template (Evans, 2006, cited in Wilson & Gracey, 2009) helped to understand the multiple interacting factors that were impacting SJ's ability to function adequately in daily life (see Figure 2.3).

2. Rehabilitation program

SJ moved with her family to another city and underwent a focused rehabilitation programme. In India, very few centres offer multidisciplinary team services. Individual therapists work in private practice and coordinate with each other and the family to implement a programme. The family becomes the centre of the rehabilitation programme and their involvement and training is critical to achieve a holistic, home-based, family-centred programme (see Table 2.2 for details).

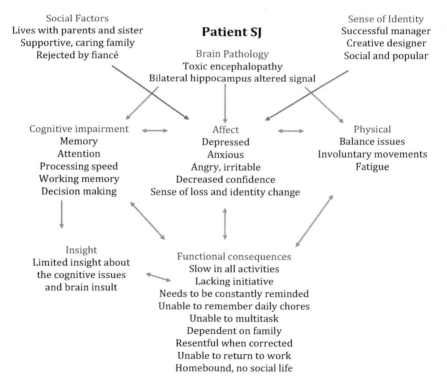

Figure 2.3 Case formulation

Table 2.2 Overview of rehabilitation programme

Recovery phases When	Goals (Family/SJ) Why	Clinic/Home Where	Interventions What	Professional/Family Who
Phase I Post acute Six months **Managing symptoms**	**Family goals** – Reduce confusion and agitation – Develop insight	Psychology clinic	– Family psycho-education – Individual counselling – Orientation log – Cognitive exercises	Clinical neuropsychologist
	– Establish simple daily routine	Home	– White board	
	Family and SJ's goals Reduce involuntary movements, tremors, and improve walking	Rehabilitation centre	Timetable of daily self-care activities and simple household chores Fine motor activities Balance training	Family Physical and occupational therapists
Phase II 2 years **Optimizing home and social activities**	**Family and SJ's goals** Managing memory issues (Repetitiveness, forgetting medications, names of people other than family members)	Home	Compensatory strategies – Diary writing (daily events) – Planner (Prospective appointments, chores) – Memory book (names and details of friends, colleagues, and relatives) – Pill box and phone reminders (medication, daily activities)	Family
	Addressing diffidence in engaging socially		Planned visits by colleagues, friends at home and weekend outings with family and friends	
	Building confidence for shopping or travelling		Supervised by sister, daily outings for shopping simple items in a neighbouring store. Visits to malls, movies	

(Continued)

Table 2.2 Continued

Recovery phases *When*	Goals (Family/SJ) *Why*	Clinic/Home *Where*	Interventions *What*	Professional/Family *Who*
Phase III *2 to 5 years* **Return to the community**	**Family and SJ's goals**			
	– Independent Travel	Home	Private taxis for shopping and classes	Family
	– Socialization	Home and community	– Hosting small groups of friends at home – Attending family events – Attending community cultural events	
	– Skill development	Professional classes	Joining art and music classes	Art and music teachers
	– Career planning, improving initiative, motivation, and self-confidence	Hospital clinic	Vocational guidance and counselling	Counselling psychologist
	– Mood management	Clinic	for mood, cognitive, and personality issues Addressing depression and anxiety	Psychiatrist

Phase I: For about a year SJ worked with a clinical neuropsychologist and physical and occupational therapist. A programme was initiated that involved cognitive exercises three times a week with the neuropsychologist, training for daily use of compensatory strategies (supervised diary writing, reminders) with her father, and functional home activities (cleaning and cooking), supervised by her mother and sister. Additionally, she underwent physiotherapy three times a week for improving fine motor activities (hand tremors) and balance (gait disturbances).

Phase II: The family had been counselled about the need to optimize functional abilities and prioritize social engagements. In this phase, the family worked on strengthening the compensatory memory strategies and planned the socialization opportunities to train her for greater independence and participation in the home and community.

Phase III: The family re-engaged with professionals to address SJ's persisting mood and social issues, and for guidance about pre-vocational training. This final phase is ongoing with the goal of encouraging her towards some form of paid work and reintegrating her in the community.

The rehabilitation programme was largely family driven and there were limited opportunities for professional inputs to learn and practice specific, beneficial memory strategies like errorless learning (Baddeley & Wilson, 1994). The emotional issues were challenging for the family. Emotional and behavioural issues after brain insult may be related to neurological, psychological, and psychosocial factors (Gianotti, 1993; Harvey et al., 2004). In SJ's case the persisting impairments in memory was a huge challenge. She found it difficult to accept her disability and felt dissatisfied despite making progress at all levels. She would compare her current state with her previous levels of functioning and feel hopeless. The loss of her old friends, colleagues and her fiancé was also emotionally distressing.

Outcome

Cognitive reassessment for tracking of changes was not done as SJ and her family relocated to another city and were unable to travel.

However, in a remote session, the family reported that in a recent evaluation by the local psychiatrist, the score on a screening tool (Montreal Cognitive Assessment MoCA; Nasreddine et al., 2005) was 18/30 (Normal ≥26/30). She had challenges with Visuospatial/Executive (clock drawing), Memory (delayed recall), Language (verbal fluency), Attention (serial subtractions), and Abstraction (similarities). The psychiatrist's note mentioned moderate severity of depression and anxiety symptoms and she had been prescribed a monoamine oxidase-A inhibitor (MAO-AI), escitalopram oxalate, and a cholinesterase inhibitor.

The family reported that she had improved significantly but they referred to her recovering abilities as a 'work in progress'. They reported persisting challenges that continued to disable her and marginalize her from optimal participation in life. Her fiancé had rejected her six months after the event. The family was anxious that in her current state, given the arranged marriage system in India, it would be challenging for her to find a life partner. They added that over the last five years, their sole focus was her care and the younger sister had decided to not marry so that she could support her parents to manage their financial and care burdens.

SJ reported that due to her persisting memory issues she was unsure about engaging in any conversations in social situations. She felt that if she repeated things people would judge her and so she either avoided social events or remained aloof in any gathering. She reported feelings of guilt about being a burden on her parents and her inability to repay them in any way for the numerous 'sacrifices' that they had made over the years. SJ felt that the positive aspect in her life was finding the Art and Music tutors who were working with her to enhance her natural skills. She was hopeful that she might be able to convert this learning into a career opportunity and teach art and music to schoolchildren.

At five years post the event SJ continued to have significant anterograde memory loss that interfered with her daily life functioning. She had learnt a number of compensatory strategies and was able to manage a simple daily routine. She had become independent in traveling by a private taxi to her classes but was still not confident using public transport. She had not been able to return to gainful employment and was largely homebound. There was limited socialization and she only had opportunities when there were family and community celebrations.

Learning points

Gas geyser syndrome raises several important issues.

- In low–middle income countries (LMICs), poor awareness of and lack of advocacy for preventable neuropsychological morbidity is a major concern. Several conditions can easily be prevented if there is awareness of simple measures and stringent legislation to ensure implementation of the safety guidelines.
- Even a brief exposure to CO can result in significant long-term neuropsychological morbidity.
- The damage to the brain in this condition may not be reversible and memory loss may persist long term, thereby impacting mood and self-confidence with the final quality of life outcomes remaining suboptimal.
- Often the cognitive deficits result in an invisible disability that is poorly understood by the family and community.
- Holistic neuropsychological rehabilitation may be needed to ameliorate the multidimensional challenges in daily functioning.
- In LMICs, there are very few centres offering multidisciplinary rehabilitation. Moreover, payment for rehabilitation services is out of the client's pocket. The challenges of lack of 'Accessibility, Availability, and

Affordability' marginalize the vast majority of the population from availing of professional services.

- The family becomes the centre of the rehabilitation effort. In cases like SJ that need long-term, continuing inputs, the role of the family becomes vital. However, there is a need for intermittent consultations and guidance by a multidisciplinary team to help steer the family in the right direction. It is this partnership between the family and the professionals in LMICs that needs to be strengthened and developed as a model for home-based, family-centred rehabilitation.

Conclusions

Carbon monoxide (CO) is one of the commonest environmental contaminants and is a 'silent killer' responsible for a large number of accidental poisoning cases in humans. Yet, there is a paucity of evidence-based literature on the medical therapies. Gas geyser syndrome (GGS) is an unusual example of CO poisoning that is difficult to diagnose and is controversial as it can be easily prevented. GGS occurs in LMICs and there is no neuropsychological data on the long-term neurocognitive and affective sequelae and rehabilitation interventions. The cognitive deficits due to GGS lead to a significant invisible disability that is poorly understood and remains largely unacknowledged and unaddressed. Public health advocacy – legislation about safety measures and prevention awareness – is still in its nascent stage in many LMICs. Conditions like gas geyser syndrome that cause irreversible damage need to be highlighted in all public health forums and the popular press so that the lives of many SJs in the world are not wantonly wasted.

References

Anand, R., Verma, A., & Jagmohan, P. (2006). Gas geyser: A preventable cause of carbon monoxide poisoning. *Indian Journal of Radiology and Imaging, 16*(1), 95–96.

Baddeley, A. D., & Wilson, B. A. (1994). When implicit learning fails: Amnesia and the problem of error elimination. *Neuropsychologia, 32*, 53–68.

Bista, B., Manandhar, D., Mishra, R., Shrestha, P., & Dhungel, A. (2017). Carbon monoxide poisoning due to gas water. *Janaki Medical College Journal of Medical Sciences, 5*(2), 56–59.

Chelsea, A., Chambers, Hopkins, R. O., Weaver, L. K., & Key, C. (2008). Cognitive and affective outcomes of more severe compared to less severe carbon monoxide poisoning. *Brain Injury, 22*(5), 387–395.

Correia, P., Agrawal, C., & Ranjan, R. (2012). Gas geyser syndrome: An important preventable cause of disabling neurological events. *Annals Indian Academy of Neurology, 15*, 245–248.

Bistrow, J. (Ed.). (2005). *The Picture of Dorian Gray.* In *The Complete Works of Oscar Wilde* (Vol. 3, p. 78). Oxford University Press.

Gainotti, G. (1993). Emotional and psychosocial problems after brain injury. *Neuropsychological Rehabilitation, 3*, 259–277.

Harvey, A., Watkins, E., Mansell, W., & Shafran, R. (2004). *Cognitive behavioural processes across psychological disorders.* Oxford University Press.

Mahanagar Gas Limited, Government of Maharashtra. (2020). Guidelines on installation of instantaneous water heaters (gas geysers) with natural gas for domestic use. www.mahanagargas.com/UploadAssets/UploadedFiles/_Guidelines_on_ Gas_Installation._9328a232da.pdf (accessed 26 September 2021).

Mehta, A., Mahale, R., John, A. A., Abbas, M. M., Javali, M., Acharya P., & Rangasetty, S. (2016). Odorless inhalant toxic encephalopathy in developing countries household: Gas geyser syndrome. *Journal of Neuroscience Rural Practice, 7,* 228–231.

Millon, T., Millon, C., Davis, R., & Grossman, S. (2006). *MCMI-III Manual* (3rd ed.). Pearson Education.

Nasreddine, Z. S., Phillips, N. A., Bédirian, V., Charbonneau, S., Whitehead, V., Collin, I.,... & Chertkow, H. (2005). The Montreal Cognitive Assessment, MoCA: A brief screening tool for mild cognitive impairment. *Journal of the American Geriatrics Society, 53*(4), 695–699.

Pages, B., Planton, M., Buys, S., Lemesle, B., Birmes, P., Barbeau, E. J., Maziero, S., Cordier, L., Cabot, C., Puel, M., Genestal, M., Chollet, F., & Pariente, J. (2014). Neuropsychological outcome after carbon monoxide exposure following a storm: A case-control study. *BMC neurology, 14,* 153. https://doi.org/10.1186/1471-2377-14-153

Parkinson, R. B., Hopkins, R. O., Cleavinger, H. B., Weaver, L. K., Victoroff, J., Foley, J. F., & Bigler, E. D. (2002). White matter hyperintensities and neuropsychological outcome following carbon monoxide poisoning. *Neurology, 58,* 1525–1532.

Quasim, M. (2017, January 9). Using gas geysers in bathrooms without safety measures can be risky. International. *The News,* Islamabad. www.thenews.com.pk/ print/177727-Using-gas-geysers-in-bathrooms-without-safety-measures-can-be-risky

Rao, S., Subbakrishna, D.K, & Gopukumar, K. (2004). *NIMHANS Neuropsychology Battery-2004 Manual.* National Institute of Mental Health and Neurosciences, Bangalore, India.

Rose, J. J., Wang, L., Xu, Q., McTiernan, C. F., Shiva, S., Tejero, J., & Gladwin, M. T. (2017). Carbon monoxide poisoning: Pathogenesis, management and future directions of therapy. *American Journal of Respiratory and Critical Care Medicine, 195*(5), 596–606.

Sampson, L. A. (2017). Commentary on the neurological findings associated with overexposure to liquefied petroleum gas. *Open Access Journal of Neurology and Neurosurgery, 4*(4), 1–2.

Sikary, A. K., Dixit, S., & Murty, O. P. (2017). Fatal carbon monoxide poisoning: A lesson from a retrospective study at All India Institute of Medical Sciences, New Delhi. *Journal of Family Medicine and Primary Care, 6*(4), 791–794.

Townsend, C. L., & Maynard, R. L. (2002). Effects on health of prolonged exposure to low concentrations of carbon monoxide. *Occupational and Environmental Medicine, 59*(10), 708–711. https://doi.org/10.1136/oem.59.10.708

Weaver, L. K., Hopkins, R. O., Chan, K. J., Churchill, S., Elliott, C. G., Clemmer, T. P., Orme, J. F., Jr, Thomas, F. O., & Morris, A. H. (2002). Hyperbaric oxygen for acute carbon monoxide poisoning. *The New England Journal of Medicine, 347*(14), 1057–1067. https://doi.org/10.1056/NEJMoa013121

Weaver, L. K., Hopkins, R.O., Churchill, S.K., & Deru, K. (2008). Neurological outcomes 6 years after acute carbon monoxide poisoning. *Undersea Hyperbaric Medicine, 35*, 258–259.

Weaver, L. K., Orrison, W. W., Deru, K., & McIntosh, J. (2015). Brain imaging abnormalities in carbon monoxide-poisoned patients with ongoing symptoms at least 6 months after poisoning. *Undersea Hyperbaric Medicine, 42*, 469–470.

Wilson, B., & Gracey, F. (2009). Towards a comprehensive model of neuropsychological rehabilitation. In B. A. Wilson, F., Gracey, J. Evans, & A. Bateman (Eds.), *Neuropsychological rehabilitation: Theory, models, therapy & outcome* (pp. 1–21). Cambridge University Press.

Wolf, S. J., Lavonas, E. J., Sloan, E. P., & Jagoda, A. S. (2008). American College of Emergency Physicians. Clinical policy: critical issues in the management of adult patients presenting to the emergency department with acute carbon monoxide poisoning. *Annals of Emergency Medicine, 51*, 138–152.

Zigmond, A.S., & Snaith, R. P. (1983). The hospital anxiety and depression scale. *Acta Psychiatrica Scandinavica, 67*, 361–370.

3 Disconnection syndrome and optic aphasia following left hemisphere posterior cerebral artery stroke

A deductive assessment approach

Joanna Atkinson

Introduction

I met 'June Robinson' early in my career in 2004, while I was a trainee clinical psychologist on placement with an older adult psychology team that provided input to the post-stroke rehabilitation services, which included a community speech and language team. 'June' is a pseudonym and she provided informed consent to share anonymised details in academic publications. This chapter is based on my write-up of her case at the time as part of my clinical training. It provides an example of customised assessment or detective work that may be necessary, particularly when detailed neuroimaging findings and full neuropsychological work-up are not available, as was commonplace in stroke services at that time but can also be true today. At the end of the chapter, I provide updated literature and how I would approach things differently now.

June was referred to the older adult service by the Speech and Language Therapy (SLT) team with a specific remit to try and make sense of her 'odd' aphasia presentation and to help both her and her husband to understand her difficulties in the context of friction in their relationship. She was a SLT community patient and had not received multidisciplinary rehabilitation or broader cognitive assessment. There were no reported cognitive or memory difficulties, and she had no obvious language difficulties during conversation that would indicate a dysfluent Broca's aphasia or a fluent Wernicke's aphasia, but she had an unusual pattern of anomic naming difficulties which appeared inconsistent and would be apparent only sometimes, such as when naming colours. I was asked to see her to do a brief piece of work to unpick what was going on.

I was approached by a speech and language therapist working in the community to assess June urgently, to try and make sense of her perplexing symptoms, because she and her husband had been arguing during her speech therapy sessions. Her husband was concerned about her ability to identify her medication correctly due to, what he termed 'colour-blindness'. June would get in a muddle when instructed to take 'the blue tablet' and would swallow the wrong-coloured tablet. This was a source of ongoing tension and

DOI: 10.4324/9781003228226-4

frequent outbursts between them and was limiting progress in speech therapy. The speech and language therapist wanted to know why June appeared to be misperceiving the colours of her medication and whether there was any visuoperceptual impairment that would explain this. She noted that although June did make some anomic errors in her speech, these were puzzling because they did not fit typical aphasic error profiles. The SLT requested a detailed psychological assessment of visuoperceptual and semantic difficulties in relation to her difficulties with colours. The speech and language therapy sessions were put on hold while the neuropsychology assessment took place.

The referral information noted that June had hemianopia with vision loss in the right visual field, and alexia without agraphia, which is a severely curtailed ability to read without any obvious difficulties with writing. The CT scan report at hospital admission following her stroke showed a zone of low density in the left occipital and posterior temporal lobes in keeping with a posterior cerebellar artery infarct. There was also a small cerebral spinal-fluid-filled structure in the right frontal region in keeping with an arachnoid cyst.

It was a fascinating opportunity for a trainee psychologist, and although my clinical placement did not have a particular focus on neuropsychology, my supervisor knew that I had a keen interest and that I had worked as an academic researcher developing new assessments for aphasia and apraxia in deaf people who use British Sign Language, which involved similar detective work and deductive thinking. Therefore, I was asked to investigate, with supervision from my supervisor, a neuropsychology practice group, and the neuropsychology team at the Burden Institute in Bristol. I relished the creativity and sleuth work of such a case.

Background literature

At the time, there was limited relevant literature. I used this to guide my initial formulation and hypotheses. Here, I summarise the information that I had recourse to, and in the discussion of findings, I provide an updated summary of new research from the 18 years since I worked with June.

Literature available in 2004

A search of the literature quickly revealed that individuals with colour anomia – which causes speech errors in using and understanding colour names – almost always also have alexia and right-field hemianopia, and do not have any primary impairment in colour vision or visual agnosia (De Renzi et al., 1987). Several authors attributed the co-occurrence of these impairments to a disconnection syndrome (e.g. Geschwind, 1972; Alaoui-Faris et al., 1994). The literature suggested that the likely lesion site for this constellation of symptoms was within the left occipital-temporal junction, and that there would be no direct damage to the colour processing areas of the occipital cortex. June's colour naming difficulties could be explained by damage to the neural pathway *between* the visual association cortex in the occipital lobes, and the perisylvian language area of the temporal lobes. The disconnection between the cortices resulted in a lack of direct access between visual and verbal representations of colours (Beauvois & Saillant, 1985). Furthermore, this disconnection syndrome would be expected to result in difficulties with other tasks that rely on information transfer between visual and verbal areas such as reading and producing or understanding language about things that you can *see* around you in your environment. Based on the literature, it was expected that June might also show signs of optic aphasia, which is a rare phenomenon where a person is unable to name visually presented objects but has no difficulty in naming the same objects when they hold them or hear the sound that they make. Interestingly, the literature suggested that one reason that this syndrome is so uncommon is that disconnection is required to prevent information transfer: (1) within the left hemisphere, and also, (2) between the left and right hemispheres. Coslett and Saffran (1991) stated that this cluster of impairments only occurred when there was additional damage to the splenium of the corpus callosum, which is the information highway between the two hemispheres, so the right hemisphere occipital region must also be disconnected from the left hemisphere language cortex (Binder & Mohr, 1992).

Optic aphasia results from a disconnection between visual perceptual analysis and the semantic knowledge that facilitates object naming (Martin, 1998). The idea of semantic involvement is supported by Chanoire et al. (1998) who observed that impairment is more striking when semantically similar objects have to be distinguished. Differences in visual complexity are thought to account for widely reported dissociations between naming categories of objects in optic aphasia (e.g. animates and inanimates) (Stewart et al., 1992). It seemed that semantic relatedness and visual relatedness are both contributory factors. In 2004, knowledge of the exact structure of the semantic system remained sketchy, but a gradual consensus was emerging in favour of an anatomically diffuse organisation, in which some routes can be damaged and others spared across different modalities. For example, pure optic aphasics would be able to name objects presented tactilely or aurally. However, direct damage to semantic stores, rather than just disconnection, will result in global naming errors across all modalities. Hart et al. (2002) stated that lesion studies consistently relate the posterior–superior temporal region and the bilateral temporo-occipital region with semantic processing, suggesting that June may be vulnerable to global semantic difficulties since she sustained damage to these areas.

Interestingly, residual semantic knowledge may be expressed through miming, which was thought to invoke right hemisphere regions. Gestures can facilitate word naming, suggesting that processing may be re-routed via the right hemisphere. Coslett and Saffran (1991) suggest that errors occur because semantic representations in the right hemisphere are less precise than left hemisphere representations. Furthermore, the gesture of people with optic aphasia is observed to incorporate only structural knowledge from visual analysis without semantic information about how the object is used (Riddoch & Humphreys, 1987). This might explain why gestures can be partially preserved in the face of visuo-semantic disconnection.

Case presentation

June was a 78-year-old lady, who had a left hemisphere stroke in the summer of 2003 whilst hanging out washing. Myocardial infarct and high blood pressure were noted in her medical records. She was admitted to a specialist stroke unit for 3 months. June experienced right-sided paresis and right visual field hemianopia as a result of the stroke. During inpatient assessment, she displayed significant word-finding problems but had fewer problems in spontaneous conversation. She was discharged from the hospital in the autumn and continued to receive weekly visits from the community speech and language therapy team, who focused on the assessment of communication.

Information was collected from several sources: a retrospective search of clinical files; a discussion with the SLT; and a semi-structured clinical interview in which Mr and Mrs Robinson's concerns and priorities were gauged.

June lived with her husband and described her extended family as supportive. She reported feeling despondent and downhearted about her stroke and the loss of role this entailed. Her husband took over most of the domestic chores. She found this adjustment difficult, but the mood assessment did not show clinical levels of depression or anxiety.

June reported a profound post-stroke difficulty with reading following her stroke. SLT assessments confirmed alexia without agraphia. She could not see whole words or whole sentences at a time due to her hemianopia causing blindness in her right visual field. She was able to recognise individual letters with few errors but could not use whole-word reading strategies. She could use audition to recognise words formed from letters spoken aloud but was unable to use the visual channel unless she employed a laborious letter-by-letter reading strategy. June was previously an avid reader, reading approximately three books per week. She felt particularly disabled by her post-stroke inability to read.

June had word-finding difficulties, particularly in relation to naming objects or colours. Her difficulties were hard to detect in spontaneous conversation because her anomia only affected the ability to talk about things she was looking at. For example, she might ask her husband to close the curtains, but it would come out as, 'Close the door'. This caused arguments between them when he would correct her and could not understand why she was making mistakes with some words and not others. Her visual naming difficulties were more apparent when formally tested using pictorial stimuli or real objects when she would make semantic errors (such as bear for 'cat', or chair for 'table'). Her husband tried to help by pushing her until she could say the right word, even if he knew what she was trying to say. June said that this strategy left her feeling frustrated and inadequate. During my sessions, this was observed to be a source of some tension in the relationship and provoked arguments. At times she asked him to leave the room, due to comments about not trying hard enough. Mr and Mrs Robinson expressed a wish to better understand her cognitive difficulties so that she might be able to explain to others exactly what the problem was. They both felt confused by her extreme difficulty with specific things such as reading and colour naming but in the face of widely preserved language and visual function.

Neuropsychological formulation

The initial assessment provided information about post-stroke cognitive disabilities including colour anomia, alexia without agraphia, hemianopia, and semantic errors in word-finding. This distinct and unusual pattern of impairment was suggestive of a cortical disconnection syndrome caused by an infarct to the temporo-occipital junction. The scan data were consistent with this observation. In disconnection syndrome, different functional regions within the brain are cut off from one another and the individual will show difficulties with tasks that rely on an interaction between these areas. It was hypothesised that June would show the greatest difficulties with tasks that involve the transfer of information from visual areas (occipital lobes) to the language area in the temporal lobes, with preservation of functions that do not rely on the transfer of information between these areas. Further assessment was indicated:

- To test this hypothesis and establish whether her impairments arose from cortical disconnection syndrome or whether there was evidence for direct impairment of the visual, lexical, or semantic systems.
- To furnish Mr and Mrs Robinson, and those working with them, with a greater understanding of her cognitive problems and to inform coping strategies.

It was hoped that Mr Robinson would gain increased insight into the subtle nature of his wife's difficulties by observing her undergoing formal assessment. An indirect clinical objective was to provide validation of her difficulties and modelling of appropriate communication strategies, with the hope that it might decrease tension in their relationship.

Neuropsychological assessment

An in-depth assessment of colour anomia, visual perception, and semantic abilities took place over five sessions. Information was obtained from both standardised neuropsychological assessments and non-standard tests that were devised to investigate particular phenomena as they emerged.

Colour anomia

Colour processing was investigated at lexical, perceptual, and semantic levels to identify where the breakdown occurred.

Lexical

June had severe problems with naming colours and understanding colour names. When asked to point to colour targets among an array of nine basic colours she scored 4/9. She was able to name only 3/9 colours presented for naming.

Perceptual

There was no evidence of a primary impairment in colour vision. Performance on Ishihara's Test for Colour Blindness (1970) was at the test ceiling. This test involves identifying hidden numerals within a coloured plate made up of random dots of different colours and sizes. People with normal vision can clearly see the numerals but these are hard to see with deficient colour vision. June responded by tracing the numerals with her finger because her verbal responses were unreliable, as she made semantic errors with the names of the numbers. Her manual responses were accurate even when her verbal responses were incorrect. This suggested intact colour vision.

A range of colour-matching and sorting tasks were devised using paint charts. These sorting tasks were designed to be completed wholly using the visual modality and no verbal instructions or responses were required. This was to ensure as pure a test of her colour vision as possible because otherwise response artefacts would be caused by her visual anomia. The paint colour charts were cut up. June was able to sort into colour categories using various criteria such as colour, hue, or brightness. She made no errors during these tasks, suggesting that colour perception was preserved.

Semantic

Semantic knowledge about colours was assessed using colour association tasks. These were assessed separately for the verbal and visual modalities to ensure they were measuring the semantic knowledge accessed within each modality, and that the findings were not impacted by June's cross-modal aphasia. A verbal task involved responding to spoken questions such as, 'What colour would you associate with a banana?' The same concepts were presented non-verbally using line drawings. She was asked to colour these, using the correct coloured pencil. This was similar to a task described by McKee and Damasio (1979). The presentation was counterbalanced and split over separate sessions to reduce any practice/priming effects. For the verbal task, she scored 3/8 and for the non-verbal task 5/8, suggesting a disruption of semantic knowledge about colour for both modalities. Slightly better performance on the visual colouring task may have been influenced by the closed-set of only four colouring pencils to choose from.

To further examine colour semantic knowledge, an Erroneous Colour Association task similar to that described in Lezak (1995) was devised. Pictures showing correctly and incorrectly coloured line drawings were presented to June. Examples of these are shown in Figure 3.1. Correct items depicted the colour commonly associated with the object (e.g. red heart, yellow lemon, green frog, blue sky). Incorrect items showed the object in another colour (e.g., green heart, blue lemon, pink frog, yellow sky). June pointed to a tick or a cross according to whether she thought the drawings showed the commonly associated colour or not. This pointing response format avoided the need for a verbal response. She did better in this forced binary-choice task, scoring 12/16, which was above the chance level, which was 8/16, but the score is off-ceiling. This suggested limited or partial access to preserved colour association semantic knowledge when tested wholly within the visual modality. Her performance was poorer if testing relied on the transfer of information from the visual to the verbal modality or vice versa. For example, verbal presentation with a visual pointing response decreased performance to only 1/8. She also scored 1/8 for the opposite paradigm with visual presentation of the coloured object and verbal naming. This supports the notion of a disconnection between visual and language neural regions.

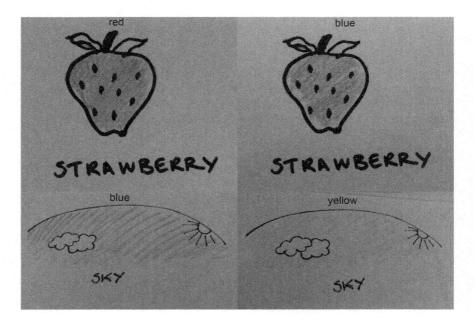

Figure 3.1 Examples of correctly and incorrectly coloured items from the erroneous colour association task

Note the images were shaded as follows: upper left quadrant red, upper right blue, lower left blue, and lower right yellow

Severe disruption of semantic colour knowledge remained even when tested purely within the verbal modality. June was unable to assign atypical exemplars to colour categories (e.g. burgundy→red, navy→blue) (4/16). Her difficulty with colours also extended to colour metaphors. She was asked, what colour is associated with being 'angry' (red) or 'envious' (green). She scored 1/7 showing disrupted colour metaphor knowledge. This suggests either that preserved connections between the visual and language areas are necessary for talking about colour metaphors or that the semantic system, specifically the colour association areas, has been directly disrupted.

Interestingly, June showed a dissociation between different types of colour knowledge. In striking contrast to impaired colour category and metaphor knowledge, she had preserved knowledge of symbolic colour associations. She scored 7/7 when asked what colour was associated with words such as, 'cold', 'go', 'vacant', and 'not allowed'. It is possible that symbol-colour associations are right-lateralised in the brain and colour name recall may be facilitated via right rather than left hemisphere association areas. Coslett and Saffran (1991) describe research indicating an right hemisphere role in non-literal and symbol processing, which might explain these findings. Alternatively, these types of associations often have functional meaning such as selecting a cold tap, a vacant toilet cubicle or avoiding danger, and may be processed differently by the left hemisphere semantic regions that are associated with behavioural actions.

Optic aphasia

In spontaneous conversation, June had few word-finding difficulties. Her speech was fluent although she showed some slowing in the amount of time it took to respond to a question. These verbal strengths lay in contrast with her performance on tests that used her vision to elicit a verbal response with pictures presented for naming. She scored 3/15 on the 15-item version of the Boston Naming Test indicating profound naming problems. Similarly, when presented with an object for visual naming she struggled (2/10), although she was able to provide a gesture for all items, which showed that she recognised the object and did not have visual agnosia.

Several subtests from the Birmingham Object Recognition Battery (Humphreys & Riddoch, 1994) confirmed that she had no visual agnosia or perceptual problems. All scores were within normal limits. These included: a test distinguishing real from unreal animals and objects (26/30), matching exemplars from the same class of object (18/18), ability to distinguish pairs of overlapping objects (10/10). She retained the ability to recognise, draw, and copy objects to command (e.g. a house, a flower, a dog, a teapot etc.).

The types of error that June made on naming tests were informative. People with optic aphasia typically make semantic errors rather than visual errors. The opposite pattern is true for people with visual agnosia (Farah, 2004). June did not make errors related to visual dimensions of objects that you would expect in associative agnosia. Instead, all her errors in both speech and gesture had semantic underpinnings, even when they share few visual features in common. The literature suggests that other ways to distinguish optic aphasia from visual agnosia include that they are able to recognise objects and indicate this via gesture, they can sort visual stimuli into categories showing access to visual semantic knowledge even if they cannot name them, and have no differences in performance for objects, photographs, or line drawings, to which people with agnosia show differential impairment (e.g. De Almeida Rodrigues et al., 2008).

The inability to name or describe visual stimuli with preserved visuoperception suggested that June had optic aphasia. However, although her naming difficulties were worse for the visual channel, she also showed impairment with naming auditory sounds (14/25). Furthermore, tactile presentation of objects did not facilitate improved naming after visual failures. Semantic cues did not aid retrieval in any modality, increasing the evidence for additional direct damage to a general semantic system.

Gestures were spontaneously produced during all the naming tasks, and these were observed to facilitate retrieval. Gesture comprehension was examined using a gesture-to-picture matching task (Atkinson et al., 2004). The correct picture must be indicated in response to a gesture from an array of four. Distractors include unrelated objects and an exemplar from the same object category, which is used and gestured differently (e.g. Target: hand drill, Distractors: electric drill/rifle/pistol). June scored 10/21, which was severely impaired relative to elderly controls (20/21). Her errors were almost entirely semantic in nature. For example, selecting the electric drill rather than the hand drill, which are used and gestured in very different ways but have the same function. This suggested that she was able to access semantic meaning about the object category but failed to maintain information about the surface form of gesture and precisely how the object is used when selecting the picture. This may represent a breakdown between semantic meanings about object–class and visual gestural representations. In a test of gesture production (ibid.) she was consistently able to produce a gesture (18/18); however, occasional semantic errors were observed (e.g. knife action in response to a spoon). Moreover, her gestures were formationally weak and, whilst understandable in context, appeared only to provide information about the visual properties of the object rather than how they were used. This is in keeping with Riddoch and Humphrey's (1987) claim that gesture will only be partially preserved if semantic access is denied. Thus, it appeared that June's semantic impairment extended beyond language since it affected gesture as well. The next step was to explore her semantic abilities in more detail.

Semantic impairment

June had semantic impairments that were not just cross–modal in nature but occurred within one modality. Semantic difficulties affecting the verbal domain were observed within June's spoken descriptions of verbally presented target words. Her errors included 'Apple is a vegetable' and 'skiing is done at sea'). Semantic knowledge tested wholly within the visual domain was also impaired. On the Pyramid and Palm Trees test (Howard & Patterson, 1992), which required the selection of the picture item semantically linked to a pictorial target, June showed severe impairment (21/27). The verbal version of this test which used printed words was not done due to her inability to read. In retrospect, it would have been useful to have administered this out loud using speech.

A category naming test was developed to look at differences in performance between specific semantic categories. For a cross-modal picture naming task, June was presented with ten line drawings for verbal naming within four categories. For a unimodal verbal naming task, June was asked to name the same items in response to semantic descriptions. The presentation was counterbalanced and split across sessions to reduce practice effects. The test was designed to be easy, with a low ceiling, familiar items, and within her vocabulary as established by previous speech and language therapy tests.

The results in Table 3.1 show greater impairment in the visual than verbal modality. Semantic impairment in the verbal modality was reduced to only three errors if colours are not included. This suggests that verbal semantic impairment was worse for categories that demand a visual representation to co-occur with linguistic conceptualisations (i.e. colours). June was most impaired when cross-modality semantic processing was required.

These findings suggest that there was impaired access to the general semantic system in addition to optic aphasia, which accounted for the fact that the visual modality was June's weakest channel but that she also had some word-finding and semantic difficulties with other sensory modalities including sounds, touch, and gesture.

Summary of findings

June displayed the hallmarks of a left posterior temporo-occipital disconnection syndrome including optic aphasia, colour anomia, and alexia. The

Table 3.1 June's performance on a custom uni- and cross-modal category naming task

	Verbal presentation (unimodal)	Visual presentation (cross-modal)
Animals	9	10
Clothes	10	6
Tools	8	5
Colours	5	2
TOTAL	**32/40**	**23/40**
Total without colours	27/30	21/30

hypothesis that she would show impairment on cross-modal tasks that rely on both visual and verbal abilities was confirmed. She showed no direct perceptual impairment and generally intact performance where a transfer of information across domains was not required. The exception to this was for semantic tasks and she showed semantic difficulties within all modalities, but this was most severe for cross-modal tasks that directly or indirectly required language about visual representations. A traditional disconnection model involving a disconnection between separate visual and verbal semantic areas would not account for all these findings; instead, these results suggest that there is impaired general semantic access, which is worse when cross-modal processing is required.

Treatment

The assessment process was part of the intervention. June's husband observed all sessions and gained a new understanding of her difficulties. A feedback session was held with Mr and Mrs Robinson. The findings were explained in lay terms using simple verbal explanations as the verbal medium is June's strongest. Additionally, simple picture diagrams were drawn as a reinforcer to explain, without words, wholly in the visual modality. The aim was to provide both June and her husband with an understanding of how her stroke caused a disconnection between the visual and language areas of her brain, which accounted for her unusual pattern of difficulties. Another aim was to empower both partners through knowledge and to give them the tools to explain to others (family and friends). This was particularly important since both partners felt that her problems were hidden and not immediately observable during interaction with her. Furthermore, the subtle nature of her problems, and variable ability depending on tiredness and stress levels, had previously led her husband to believe that she was not always trying hard enough. Discussion centred on appropriate ways of helping, and how to work as a team to get around difficulties rather than trying to tackle them head-on since it was likely that her colour naming and reading problems would persist. Taking the right medication was the issue that caused the biggest anxiety and friction, so we spent time understanding that June could perceive and identify the correctly coloured tablet but would get in a muddle if verbal instructions referred to their colour. We took photos of her different medications and pinned them to a timetable as a reminder to take the correct tablet at the correct time. We discussed how it was important to ensure that all the information about medication was provided in just one modality – in this case, the visual modality, as cross-modal information would be problematic. A report was sent with the neuropsychological formulation and recommendations to the speech and language therapy team, and June's aphasia rehabilitation was recommenced. An audiotape version of the letter was sent to June on account of her difficulty with reading. She was also introduced to 'Talking book' CDs as an alternative format to reading books.

Couple perspectives

Both partners stated that they felt relieved to receive an explanation of her difficulties; in particular, they were pleased to understand why hemianopia only affects one visual field. They both felt that the sessions had been 'stimulating and informative'. It was also observed that June stopped attributing her problems to her own 'dimness' or 'stupidity' in later sessions as she gained increasing awareness of why she failed certain tasks. They both noted an improvement in her mood as a result of this. Their relationship improved tangibly with fewer scathing comments and outbursts witnessed as sessions progressed. They reported that it had been very hard to readjust but were feeling more comfortable with each other and their renegotiated roles.

Discussion

This chapter describes my learning process during an evolving assessment that was led by patient and partner concerns and based on seeking to understand the nature of problematic symptoms. At the time I did not have specialist neuropsychology training or advanced neuroanatomical knowledge. It was a step-by-step deductive discovery process, often using bespoke assessment materials, some of which I had to draw myself, with consultation of the available literature after each session to inform the assessment plan for the next session. It was an iterative process with gradual learning, refinement, and new understanding as the assessment proceeded. It was time limited and clinically focused on the issues that most affected the patient and her relationship with her husband. In this respect, the approach differed from research data collection, which might have focused on greater exploration of how the semantic system is structured through category fluency tasks and exploration of semantic memory. The couple did not raise any concerns about executive function or behaviours that may have arisen from her right frontal arachnoid cyst, which it may have been useful to investigate, particularly as semantic function is also associated with the dorsolateral prefrontal cortex, especially knowledge about how to use tools, although this is more related to the left frontal hemisphere. If I were doing the same assessment now, I would have ensured that a general cognitive assessment to include posterior cognitive functions was completed and would hopefully have recourse to more detailed neuroimaging; however, an investigative approach would have still been required to pick up the very specific pattern of category impairments that might be missed by standard tests.

Updated literature since 2004

Since 2004, there have been significant research developments that alter what I would do in a similar case in future. I would pay greater attention to the role of her semantic abilities in her presentation. At the time, the idea of neural modularity with separate semantic systems for each sensory modality was still influential, and optic aphasia was largely attributed to a disconnection between distinct functional anatomical modules. Since then, theory has shifted from the notion of multiple separate semantic systems for each modality toward the notion of amodal semantic hubs within each hemisphere (e.g. Caramazza et al., 2006 review; Patterson et al., 2007). Optic aphasia is now characterised as involving broader semantic disruption, involving not only a disruption in the semantic interaction between visual and verbal areas (Kurland & Stokes, 2016) but also between verbal areas and other sensory modalities too, albeit to a less marked extent. Several studies have reported only *relatively* preserved semantic abilities in other sensory modalities in patients with optic aphasia following left Posterior Cortical Artery (PCA) strokes with damage to both the left temporo-occipital lobes and the left splenium. Kurland and Stokes (ibid.) described a case of impaired visual naming, with reduced ability to name from tactile input, a semantic error for naming sounds, and only relatively preserved ability to gesture, which was similar to June's presentation. Marsh and Hillis (2005) reported a similar case of hemianopia, optic aphasia, and alexia without agraphia following PCA stroke damage to the same area. There were impaired lexical and semantic representations from vision but also a milder deficit in accessing lexical representations in all other input modalities. They noted possible explanations for the inability to access a complete semantic lexical representation from vision (written words or pictures). Firstly, it could reflect reliance on the impoverished right hemisphere semantic system from an intact right occipitotemporal area. Secondly, partial access to the left hemisphere lexical-semantic system might still be possible through a damaged splenium. They argued for a partial access explanation because they noted improvement in reading words when presented with the correct picture or a semantically related picture, stating that it provided evidence that this allowed partial access to semantics and partial access to phonological reading areas, which in summation allowed the correct lexical name to be retrieved. Both these possibilities might explain why there were lesser impairments in other sensory modalities, because the pathways between different types of sensory input and the left hemisphere semantic system would be differently disrupted to different degrees. However, they do not account for the finding of semantic difficulties purely within the visual modality. Caramazza et al. (2006) describe subtle fine-grained semantic difficulties for harder visual semantic matching tasks in a person with optic aphasia. June was impaired on visual semantic matching on the Pyramid and Palm Trees test. This suggests that in optic aphasia the visual system has access to sufficient semantic information for visual recognition, but may not have complete access, and this is why there may be semantic errors on visual association tasks and within the gestural modality. The implication is that visual semantic processing is not wholly intact in optic aphasia. So, it represents more than just a disconnection but rather arises as part of a broader semantic deficit. This is supported by the preponderance of semantic naming errors in optic aphasia.

The most plausible interpretation of these findings is that they result from the failure to access a modality-independent semantic hub. Patterson, Nestor and Rogers (2007) proposed that the anterior temporal lobes (ATL) may underpin amodal semantic hubs within each brain hemisphere, citing supportive data from focal atrophy to the ATL in semantic dementia that affects conceptual knowledge in all sensory modalities (sound, vision, touch, reading, writing, drawing, gesture).

Damage to the left ATL can selectively impair semantic naming categories such as people, animals, or tools (Noppeney et al., 2007). June showed selective deficits for colours that affected both visual and verbal input modalities and for inanimates (clothes and tools), which were worse in response to visual input. She had a selectively preserved ability to name animals even when visually presented. There is ongoing debate about the phenomenon of category-specific semantic impairments disproportionately affecting a certain semantic category such as knowledge about colour, animate things, inanimate objects, or tools. These very specific semantic deficits are sometimes seen in optic aphasia (e.g. colour), herpes simplex virus encephalitis, or primary progressive aphasia (animates) (e.g. Noppeney et al., 2007; Henderson et al., 2021). This has led to debate in the literature about whether domains of conceptual knowledge are distinctly represented within the amodal hub, or whether category naming dissociations can be explained by attributes such as animals having more shared conceptual features meaning that they are tightly packed in semantic space, whereas non-animates may be organised more in terms of functional usage (Noppeney et al., 2007).

An alternative account is provided by ATL convergence theory that suggests that colour knowledge must be supported by representation in both the posterior temporal-occipital regions and the amodal semantic hub of the ATL which provides mapping with the lexical areas of the perisylvian cortex. This model was posited from the finding that people with ATL damage from semantic dementia show colour knowledge impairments in all modalities even though their posterior temporal-occipital lobes are intact (Rogers, Patterson & Graham, 2007). Interestingly, Siuda-Krzywicka et al. (2019) found relatively preserved naming of achromatic colours (white, grey, black) in a patient with selective colour anomia, hemianopia, and alexia after left PCA stroke, suggesting within-category interactions that are not yet fully understood. If I were repeating this assessment as part of a research study, I would dig further into these interactions and control for things like familiarity and frequency effects. For any clinical case as interesting and unusual as this one, it is a fine balance to ensure that the patient's needs are the main driver rather than academic curiosity and to recognise when the boundary between clinical practice and research may become blurred. This was a clinical case and that affected the assessment decisions.

Theoretical implications

It seems that June's pattern of impairments are best explained by damage that prevents intact visual input from her right hemisphere reaching the semantic and phonological systems of the left hemisphere. Not only is there damage to the connection between these areas, but there may also be a restriction in access to semantic knowledge relating to colours and inanimate things in the left hemisphere. The fact that knowledge about inanimate objects can still be accessed in the verbal domain, and that animals can be named in either modality suggests that there is no direct damage to amodal semantic representations about these concepts. A connectionist account with incomplete semantic access best explains these findings. The colour anomia is more severe and affects both modalities suggesting that there may be direct impairment to the colour association areas. Within the verbal domain, the dissociation between preserved verbal knowledge about colour symbols and impaired knowledge about colour metaphors for emotions suggests either differently distributed, possibly more right lateralised, semantic networks for colour symbols or differently disrupted neural connections with an amodal hub in the left hemisphere.

June's pattern of performance where objects cannot be named, or their use gestured, but visual attributes can be gestured may signify partial access to a modality-independent semantic system, or that the intact right anterior temporal lobe may provide coarser semantic information represented at a lower level rather than high-level abstract classifications provided by the left ATL (McMenamin et al. 2015).

The findings are not theoretically conclusive but add to a growing body of research about the nature of the human semantic system.

Transferable learning

Neuropsychologists often stick to familiar test batteries and norms but there are times when we should not be afraid to be more deductive and investigative in our approach if this has a clear clinical benefit for the patient. This can be an exciting way to work as a neuropsychologist and leads to discoveries that drive forward theoretical understanding particularly when working in poorly charted clinical territory with highly unusual cases.

References

Alaoui-Faris, M., Benbelaid, F., Alaoui, C., Tahiri, L., Jiddane, M., Amarti, A., & Chkili, T. (1994). Alexia without agraphia. *Revue Neurologie* (Paris), *150*(11), 771–775. https://pubmed.ncbi.nlm.nih.gov/7597370/

Atkinson, J. R., Marshall, J., Thacker, A., & Woll, B. (2004). Stroke in users of BSL: Investigating sign language impairments. In S. Austen & S. Crocker (Eds.), *Deafness in mind: Working psychologically with deaf people across the lifespan* (pp. 284–301). Whurr Publishers.

Beauvois, M. F., & Saillant, B. (1985). Optic aphasia for colours and colour agnosia: A distinction between visual and visuo-verbal impairments in the processing of colours. *Cognitive Neuropsychology, 2*(1), 1–48.

Binder, J. R., & Mohr, J. P. (1992). The topography of callosal reading pathways: A case-control analysis, *Brain, 115*, 1807–1826.

Caramazza, A., Hillis, A. E., Rapp, B. C., & Roman, J. C. (1990). The multiple semantics hypothesis: Multiple confusions? *Cognitive Neuropsychology, 7*, 161–190.

Caramazza, A., Mahon, & Bradford, Z. (2006). The organisation of conceptual knowledge in the brain: The future's past and some future directions. *Cognitive Neuropsychology, 23*(1), 13–38.

Chanoire, V., Ferreira, C. T., Demonet, J. F., Nespoulous, J. L., & Poncet, M. (1998). Optic aphasia with pure alexia: A mild form of visual associative agnosia? A case study. *Cortex, 34*, 437–448.

Coslett, H. B., & Saffran, E. M. (1991). Simultanagnosia: To see but not two see. *Brain, 114*, 1082–1107.

De Almeida Rodrigues, M., Adda, C. C., de Sousa, L. M. C., Scaff, M., & Miotto, E. C. (2008). Cognitive deficits associated with optic aphasia: Neurological contribution to differential diagnosis. *Dementia and Neuropsychologica, 2*(2), 151–154.

De Renzi, E., Zamborlin, A., & Crisi, G. (1987). The pattern of impairment associated with left posterior cerebral artery infarcts. *Brain, 100*(5), 1099–1116.

Farah, M. J. (2004). *Visual agnosia.* MIT Press.

Geschwind, N. (1972). Language and the brain. *Scientific American, 226*, 76–83.

Hart, J., Moo, L. R., Segal J. B., Adkins, E., & Kraut, M. A. (2002). Neural substrates of semantics. In A. Hillis (Ed.), *The handbook of adult language disorders*, Psychology Press.

Henderson, S. K., Dev, S. I., Ezzo, R., Quimby, M., Wong, B., Brickhouse, M., Hochberg, D., Touroutoglou, A. Dickerson, B. C., Cordella, C., & Collins, J. A. (2021). A category-selective semantic memory deficit for animate objects in semantic variant primary progressive aphasia. *Brain Communications, 3*(4). https://doi.org/10.1093/braincomms/fcab210

Howard, D., & Patterson, K. (1992). *Pyramids and Palm Trees: A test of semantic access from pictures and words.* Thames Valley Test Company.

Humphreys, H. W., & Riddoch, M. J. (1994). Birmingham Object Recognition Battery (BORB). Lawrence Erlbaum Associates.

Ishihara, S. (1970). *Test for colour blindness.* Kanehara Shippan.

Kurland, J., & Stokes, P. (2016). Contribution of neuroimaging to understanding the organisation of semantic representations in a case of optic aphasia. *Frontiers in Psychology, 7.* www.frontiersin.org/10.3389/conf.fpsyg.2016.68.00133/event_abstract

Lezak, M. D. (1995). *Neuropsychological assessment.* Oxford University Press.

Marsh, E., & Hillis, A. (2005). Cognitive and neural mechanisms underlying reading and naming: Evidence from letter-by-letter reading and optic aphasia. *Neurocase, 11*, 325–337.

Martin, G. N. (1998). *Human Neuropsychology.* Prentice Hall.

McKee J., & Damasio, A. R. (1979). Determinants of performance in colour anomia. *Brain and Language, 7*(1), 74–85.

McMenamin, B. W., Deason, R. G., Steele, V. R., Koutstaal, W., & Marsolek, C. J. (2015). Separability of abstract-category and specific-exemplar visual object subsystems: Evidence from fMRI pattern analysis. *Brain and Cognition, 93*, 54–63. https://doi.org/10.1016/j.bandc.2014.11.007

Noppeney, U., Patterson, K., Tyler, L. K., Moss, H., Stamatakis, E. A., Bright, P., Mummery, C., & Price C. J. (2007). Temporal lobe lesions and semantic impairment: A comparison of herpes simplex virus encephalitis and semantic dementia. *Brain: A Journal of Neurology, 130*(4), 1138–1147.

Patterson, K., Nestor, P. J., & Rogers, T. T. (2007). Where do you know what you know? The representation of semantic knowledge in the human brain. *Nature Reviews Neuroscience, 8*, 976–978.

Riddoch, M. J., & Humphreys, H. W. (1987). Visual object processing in optic aphasia: A case of semantic access agnosia. *Cognitive Neuropsychology, 4*, 131–185.

Rogers, T., Patterson, K., & Graham, K. (2007). Colour knowledge in semantic dementia: It is not all black and white. *Neuropsychologica, 45*(14), 3285–3298.

Siuda-Krzywicka, K., Witzel, C., Chabani, E., Taga, M., Coste, C., Cools, N., Ferrieux, S., Cohen, L., Malkinson, T. S., & Bartolomeo, P. (2019). Color categorization independent of color naming. *Cell Reports, 28*, 2471–2479.

Stewart, F., Parkin, A. J., & Hunkin, N. M. (1992). Naming impairments following recovery from herpes simplex encephalitis: Category-specific effects. *Quarterly Journal of Experimental Psychology, 44*, 261–284.

4 Creutzfeldt–Jakob disease presenting with Capgras syndrome

Narinder Kapur and Norman Poole

Introduction

Creutzfelt-Jakob disease (CJD) is a form of prion disease and is one of the more dramatic forms of dementia, presenting as it does with a rapidly progressive course and usually with a combination of marked cognitive impairment and prominent movement disorder. CJD, like other prion diseases, is characterised by vacuolation, astrocytosis, neuronal cell death, and accumulation of prions, which are insoluble forms of a naturally occurring intracellular protein. The insoluble form can be triggered by an exogenous protein (variant CJD), a random occurrence in a genetically prone individual (sporadic CJD), or a mutation that increases conversion to the insoluble form (familial CJD) (Lovestone, 2009).

The clinical presentation of CJD is varied with onset usually in the fifth or sixth decades, and it can frequently present a diagnostic challenge – Qi et al. (2020) found a misdiagnosis rate of 56% for sporadic CJD, and Baiardi et al. (2018) highlighted the wide range of unusual ways in which CJD can present in clinical settings. There is usually a prodrome involving non-specific symptoms such as fatigue, insomnia, mood disturbance, apathy, and behaviour changes. Psychiatric symptoms, including depression, hallucinations, confabulations, and delusions, are present over the first few months in around 80% of cases (Wall et al., 2005), so a primary psychiatric disorder is often suspected in the initial stages before the more typical cognitive, speech, and movement disturbances come to dominate the picture. A range of phenotypes has been described in CJD (Kapur et al., 2003; Caine et al., 2015). Thus, some patients may present with the visual variant of CJD – the so-called 'Hedenhain variant' (Kropp et al., 1999; Cooper et al., 2005) – which presents with blurred vision, visual field restriction, metamorphopsia, or cortical blindness along with marked executive dysfunction (Snowden et al., 2002), expressive dysphasia (Mandell et al., 1989), and hemi-spatial neglect (Hillis & Selnes, 1999).

Capgras' delusion of misidentification involves the erroneous belief that an imposter has replaced someone else, usually a close friend or relative of the sufferer. His original paper (Capgras & Reboul-Lachaux, 1923) described a patient who, after the deaths of two daughters and twin boys, became

DOI: 10.4324/9781003228226-5

convinced her sole surviving daughter had been abducted and replaced by an imposter. This imposter was replaced by yet another who in turn was also replaced, so that over the years she identified more than 2,000 doubles of her remaining daughter. The delusion also involved her husband, whom she believed had been murdered and another person set in his place, then came to incorporate the police and medical staff after she was eventually detained in hospital. Capgras initially suggested that the delusion arose because, 'some faces that she sees with their normal features, the memory of which is not altered in any way, are nevertheless no longer accompanied by [the] feeling of exclusive familiarity which determines direct perception, immediate recognition' (Capgras & Reboul-Lachaux, 1923, p. 128).

This is strikingly similar to modern accounts within the cognitive neuropsychiatric literature (Ellis & Young, 1990; Coltheart et al, 2010), which hypothesise a lesion in the visuo–affective pathway. Accordingly, an impaired autonomic response to familiar faces has been demonstrated. This represents a double-dissociation with prosopagnosia, in which the autonomic response is preserved in conjunction with a deficit in explicit recognition. Nevertheless, Capgras quickly performed a *volte-face* after falling under the spell of Freudian analysis and the next year he co-authored a case report with Carette (Capgrass & Carette, 1924) describing a young woman convinced her parents were imposters. This was portrayed as a solution to an erotic attachment to her father and psychodynamic theories dominated the field over the following decades until Gluckman (1968) described the Capgras delusion in a case with definite neurological disease. Since then, it has been described in numerous neurodegenerative conditions (Harciarek & Kertesz, 2008), including Parkinson's disease (Cannas et al., 2016), Lewy body dementia (Reimers et al., 2014), and Alzheimer's disease (Kaufman et al., 2014), somewhat undermining psychodynamic interpretations of the delusion. Indeed, a recent thorough review of all 255 cases reported in the English language (Pandis et al., 2019) found that 43% occurred in the context of neurological disease and this proportion was increasing over time. While psychiatric presentations of CJD have been well described (Wall et al., 2005), as well as one case of hallucinations and persecutory delusions (Javed et al., 2010), there has to our knowledge been no reported case of Capgras syndrome in CJD, and we present here the first such case.

Case presentation

The patient, Mrs X, a 74-year-old white Caucasian woman, had an unremarkable past medical and psychiatric history. She was a vegetarian, and her father and brother were reported to have suffered from Parkinson's disease. She initially presented to her general practitioner in early 2016 with symptoms of tremor, and she was concerned – in view of her family history – that she might have Parkinson's disease. A few months later, she developed symptoms of giving up pastimes such as doing crossword puzzles and reading, presumably as she found them challenging. She was then initially seen by a psychiatrist who referred her on to a neurologist. The neurologist initiated a series of investigations to come to a diagnosis, one of which was a formal neuropsychological assessment. She was therefore primarily seen in the neuropsychology clinic for diagnostic purposes. While being seen in the neuropsychology clinic, a magnetic resonance (MR) scan, but not an electroencephalography (EEG) or cerebrospinal fluid (CSF) analysis, had already been carried out, so CJD was considered to be one of the possible diagnoses, but there was still some uncertainty about this. Misidentification had been reported by the patient and by her family both to the neurologist and to the neuropsychologist, but a formal diagnosis of Capgras syndrome was only made after the neuropsychological assessment. When seen for neuropsychological assessment in December 2016, she reported her symptom of tremor in her hands, which she indicated had been present for a number of months. She also reported difficulty in concentrating when she tried to read, and that the words became jumbled on the page. She was aware of visual hallucinations whereby she would see people she knew getting into and out of a car.

When her husband was interviewed, he noted that his wife had some shaking of her hands during a holiday in March 2016. This tremor gradually worsened, but it appeared to be relieved by beta blockers started a few months later. Around September 2016, she began to have problems in concentration, in particular for activities such as reading. It was around this time that she also began to experience visual hallucinations. She would see people in a car when she looked out from her home, and on one occasion this involved seeing a woman sitting next to her husband in the car. For the preceding two months, he had found that she would misidentify him, and sometimes see him as an imposter for the 'real Peter' [not his real name for reasons of anonymity]. She would think that there were two versions of him at home, and on one occasion told him there was a woman waiting for a version of him at the top of the drive. She could at times misrecognise her daughter as being her sister, and also confused the sons by calling one by the other's name. She also misidentified the tops of her bannisters as small children.

She had an acute 'breakdown' episode around September 2016, when she was very tearful and fearful. In December 2016, she became lost while walking home, and was eventually found and taken home by the police. Her husband considered that she had become a little more forgetful than usual. Her clothes drawers became disorganised, and she would go to bed around 7pm. She stopped driving around four months before assessment after an incident in which she hit an object that was on the side of the road. Her husband did not report her having any symptoms such as loss of smell or taste sensation, sensory symptoms, or incontinence. He began to feel that he had to be with her 24 hours a day.

The patient's daughter also recounted that her mother might put on odd pairs of socks and would occasionally put her clothes on inside out. She would not know the day of the week. In the summer, she had numerous symptoms that entailed many investigations, as she was concerned that she had serious diseases such as cancer. She would sometimes think that her current home was not her real home, and that there was another house similar to her own.

MR brain imaging

An MRI scan was reported as showing high signal streak in the cortex on diffusion weighted imaging, a form of 'cortical ribbon' sign that is often found on diffusion weighted imaging in those with sporadic CJD (Figure 4.1). This was reported to be more prominent on the right side, and to be evident across all four lobes. EEG showed non-specific abnormalities, with generalised slowing. CSF analysis showed a positive real-time quaking induced conversion (RT-QuIC) test, although S100 and 14:33 levels were normal. A formal diagnosis of CJD, probably sporadic given the absence of a family history, her vegetarianism, and the cortical ribbon sign, was made by a consultant neurologist.

Neuropsychological assessment

During testing, the patient was very anxious on occasions, and this was sometimes accompanied by marked tremor in her hands. Her anxiety and occasional tremor placed some restrictions on the number and range of tests administered. She was disoriented regarding days of the week (said Monday when it was Wednesday), months (said January, when it was December), and year (gave 2017 instead of 2016).

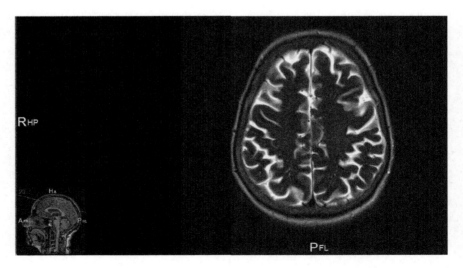

Figure 4.1 Axial MR scan showing cortical ribbon feature often seen in sporadic CJD

On a range of neuropsychological tests (Table 4.1), she had a moderate to marked visuoperceptual impairment, in the context of additional deficits on tests of attention, memory, and executive function. Thus, she had low scores on story recall, word list retention (with evidence of confabulation and intrusions in story and word list recall), digit span, faces and pictures recognition memory, copy of a complex figure (with 'closing-in' phenomenon), picture naming (with perceptual errors), semantic verbal fluency, digit symbol substitution, and visuospatial reasoning as evident on a spatial anticipation test of executive function. She had difficulty naming fragmented letters, identifying silhouette figures, and counting 3-D cubes. She performed within normal

Table 4.1 Neuropsychological score sheet

Test	Raw Score	Statistic Scores & Comments
Verbal Memory		
WMS IV Story Recall – Immediate ★	19 ★	Scaled Score = 6 ★
WMS IV Story Recall – Delayed ★★★	2 ★★★	Scaled Score=3 ★★★
WMS IV Story Recog – Delayed ★	14 ★	% ile = 3-9 ★
WMS III Word List Learning ★	17 ★	Scaled Score=5 ★
WMS III Word List Delayed Recall★★	0 ★★	Scaled Score=6 ★★
WMS III Word List Delayed Recog★	18 ★	Scaled Score=6 ★
WAIS III Digit Span ★	10 (F=4,B=3) ★	Scaled Score=6 ★
Nonverbal Memory		
Camden Recog Memory - Faces ★★	15/25 ★★	%ile = <5★★
Camden Topographical Memory ★★★	11/30 ★★★	% ile = <5 ★★★
Verbal Skills		
Test of Premorbid Functioning	24	Low-average
Graded Naming Test ★	12/30 ★	%ile=1-5 ★
Letter Fluency - FAS	25	%ile==20-30
Category Fluency – Animals ★★	9 ★★	% ile = < 10 ★★
Nonverbal skills		
Rey Figure - Copy ★★★	4 ★★★	%ile=<1 ★★★
VOSP Screening Test	19/20	Pass
VO SP Incomplete Letters ★	15/20 ★	Fail ★
VO SP Object Decision★★	11/20 ★★	Fail ★★
VOSP Number Location	08/10	Pass
VOSP Dot Counting	10/10	Pass
VO SP Cube Analysis ★★★	02/10 ★★★	Fail ★★★
WAIS-III Digit Symbol ★★★	9 ★★★	Scaled Score = 2★★★
Executive Functions		
Brixton Spatial Anticipation Test ★★	32 errors ★★	Moderate Impairment ★★

In relation to estimated premorbid cognitive functioning
★   = Mild Impairment
★★   = Moderate Impairment
★★★ = Marked Impairment

limits on tests of phonemic verbal fluency and basic visuoperceptual process-ing. She could produce meaningful movements to command, but her copy of hand postures, especially bimanual postures, was impaired. Informal testing for identification of famous faces was found to be largely intact.

At the time of the neuropsychological assessment, a formal diagnosis of CJD had not yet been made, and this diagnosis was fed back to the patient and her family at a later appointment in the neurology clinic after all other inves-tigations had been completed. The term 'Capgras syndrome' was not used in discussions with the patient or her family. Her family were, however, given some general advice on dealing with the symptoms of visual hallucinations and misidentification, this advice primarily revolving round the strategies of reassurance and distraction. In view of the rapid decline in the patient's con-dition, no other formal neuropsychological interventions were introduced. The patient had stopped driving a few months earlier, so this was no longer an issue. Her family had taken over domestic activities, such as cooking, so no specific rehabilitation input was considered appropriate to help her cope better at home.

Discussion

We have documented the first reported case of Capgras syndrome in CJD. Harciarek and Kertesz (2008) noted that Capgras syndrome could occur early in Alzheimer's disease and Lewy body dementia, both of which condi-tions are often accompanied by significant visuoperceptual and visuospatial impairments, as we found in our case. They also noted the frequent co-occurrence of reduplicative paramnesia with Capgras syndrome in neurode-generative conditions, something that was also evident in our case. Indeed, in the review by Pandis et al. (2019), Capgras delusion in neurological disease was more frequently associated with the spouse being duplicated, multiple people having imposters, and the presence of other misidentification syn-dromes, than when the belief occurred in the context of primary psychiatric disorders. The spousal association may be a product of the delusion occurring in older patients with neurodegenerative conditions as they will likely have a stronger affinity to a partner than a parent, if there is even one still living. Not unexpectedly, visual hallucinations were reported to be more common in those with co-morbid neurological disease, again as exemplified by our case. Despite believing her husband to have been replaced she did not become aggressive. Indeed, this is usually the case in misidentification syndromes and has been called 'double bookkeeping' (Bortolotti, 2010), where a delusional patient fails to act on their reported beliefs. Nevertheless, increased rates of homicide and violence in those with Capgras delusion have been reported so it is important to assess and manage risk proactively (Casu et al, 1994).

Our case demonstrated bilateral high signal on MRI with predominance in the right hemisphere. This issue of laterality is interesting and contended. Right hemispheric dysfunction has been suggested by several researchers

(Christodoulou, 1991; Dietl et al., 2003) and Cutting (1990) proposed that judging familiarity is a non-dominant hemisphere function. Bilateral or right dominant neuropathology was observed in 80% of Pandis et al.'s (2019) reported cases. However, in a large clinical sample of cases identified from electronic medical records, Bell et al. (2017) found no evidence for predominant right sided neuroimaging abnormalities, then went on to replicate this in another smaller although still sizable clinical population identified through similar methods (Currell et al., 2019). The numbers with reported neuroimaging (7) were insufficient for definitive conclusions to be drawn, however, and the question of laterality remains unresolved.

In a functional imaging study of Capgras syndrome, Thiel et al. (2014) found reduced activation in the left hemisphere extended face processing system, and noted that this dysfunction, together with a right frontal lesion, may be critical for the development of the syndrome. Our own case would broadly support this view, given the combination of visuoperceptual and executive dysfunction, perhaps in the context of a high level of anxiety. Again, this conforms to the findings in Pandis et al. (2019) who found memory, visuoperceptual, and executive impairments were frequently identified in many Capgras patients who underwent neuropsychological evaluation, especially those in whom it was associated with neurological disease. This would be in keeping with two-stage theories of delusion formation, which require first an abnormal experience and then faulty evaluation of that experience (Young, 2000; Coltheart et al., 2010). In the two-stage account, delusional content is attributed directly to the abnormal experience. In the case of Capgras' delusion, the absence of visuo-affective familiarity – involved in the dual recognition route (Ellis & Lewis, 2001) – for a close associate imbues the experience with an oddity and estrangement in want of explanation. The imposter idea immediately presents itself via unconscious Bayesian inference (Coltheart et al., 2010), although the prior probabilities assumed in this account have been challenged (McKay, 2012), implicating pathological bias in the process of inferencing itself. The second stage, involving executive dysfunction, is said to explain why the belief is not dismissed out of hand.

In some respects, this first stage accords well with the case presented above. The replicated subjects were those to whom Mrs X was closest – her husband and children. But there are inconsistencies too. The husband oscillated between being an imposter and himself. There may be dynamical fluctuations in the networks subserving affective familiarity that are beyond our current knowledge so this inconsistency is not ruinous for the model. Additionally, she mistook one son for another and her daughter for her sister. Surely an absence of affective familiarity would not cause the replacement of one offspring with another. One might suggest here that not all children are equal in the eyes of their parents and a diminished or altered affective response might be sufficient to modify recognition. Bell et al. (2017) have used such inconsistencies to argue that a significant minority (approx. 25%) of those with the Capgras delusion do not conform to the dual route model, so when the content involves strangers or inanimate objects a different first stage must account for this. Once formed, however, why is the thought that one's spouse is an imposter not rejected as implausible? Why indeed do those with Capgras delusion sometimes accept seemingly bizarre and outlandish notions such as the impersonator is really a robot (De Pauw & Szulecka, 1988)? The details of the second stage in two-stage accounts remains underspecified (Davies & Egan, 2013) but implicates executive dysfunction in the faulty evaluation of the belief to explain its persistence in the face of counter-evidence and contradictory knowledge.

In summary, we have described what to our knowledge is the first reported case of CJD presenting as Capgras syndrome. Perceptual and memory deficits were particularly prominent in the neuropsychological profile, and these probably played a key role in the formation of the delusions experienced by the patient.

References

Baiardi, S., Capellari, S., Stella, A., & Parchi, P. (2018). Unusual clinical presentations challenging the early clinical diagnosis of Creutzfeldt-Jakob disease. *Journal of Alzheimer's Disease, 64*, 1051–1065.

Bell, V., Marshall, C., Kanji, Z., Wilkinson, S., Halligan, P., & Deeley, Q. (2017). Uncovering Capgras delusion using a large-scale medical records database. *British Journal of Psychiatry Open, 3*(4), 179–185. https://doi.org/10.1192/bjpo. bp.117.005041

Bortolotti, L. (2010). *Delusions and other irrational beliefs.* Oxford University Press.

Caine, D., Tinelli, R. J., Hyare, H., De Vita, E., Lowe, J., Lukic, A., Thompson, A., Porter, M. C., Cipolotti, L., Rudge, P., Collinge, J., & Mead, S. (2015). The cognitive profile of prion disease: a prospective clinical and imaging study. *Annals of Clinical and Translational Neurology, 2*(5), 548–558. https://doi.org/10.1002/ acn3.195

Cannas, A., Meloni, M., Maschia, M. M. et al. (2016). Capgras syndrome in Parkinson's disease: Two new cases and literature review. *Neurological sciences, 38*(2), 225–231.

Capgras, J., & Carette, J. (1924). Illusion des sosies et complexe d'Oedipe. *Annales Médico-Psychologiques, 2*, 48.

Capgras, J., & Reboul-Lachaux, J. (1923[1994]). L'illusion des 'sosies' dans un délire systématisé chronique. *History of Psychiatry, 5*, 119–133.

Casu, G., Cascella, N., & Maggini, C. (1994). Homicide in Capgras' syndrome. *Psychopathology, 27*, 281–284.

Christodoulou, G. N. (1991). The delusional misidentification syndromes. *British Journal of Psychiatry, 159*(1), 65–69.

Coltheart, M., Menzies, P., & Sutton, J. (2010). Abductive inference and delusional belief. *Cognitive Neuropsychiatry, 15*(1), 261–287.

Cooper, S. A., Murray, K. L., Heath, C. A., Will, R. G., & Knight, R. S. (2005). Isolated visual symptoms at onset in sporadic Creutzfeldt-Jakob disease: The clinical phenotype of the 'Heidenhain variant'. *The British Journal of Ophthalmology, 89*(10), 1341–1342. https://doi.org/10.1136/bjo.2005.074856

Currell, E. A., Werbeloff, N., Hayes, J. F., & Bell, V. (2019). Cognitive neuropsychiatric analysis of an additional large Capgras delusion case series. *Cognitive Neuropsychiatry*, *24*(2), 123–134.

Cutting, J. (1990). *The right cerebral hemisphere and psychiatric disorders*. Oxford University Press, 1990.

Davies, M., & Egan, A. (2013). Delusion: Cognitive approaches – Bayesian inference and compartmentalization. In K. W. M. Fulford, M. Davies, R. G. T. Gipps, G. Graham, J. Z. Sadler, G. Stanghellini, & T. Thornton (Eds.), *The Oxford handbook of philosophy and psychiatry* (pp. 689–727). Oxford University Press.

De Pauw, K. W., & Szulecka, T. K. (1988). Dangerous delusions: Violence and the misidentification syndromes. *British Journal of Psychiatry*, *152*(1), 91–96.

Dietl, T., Herr, A., Brunner, H., & Friess, E. (2003). Capgras syndrome: Out of sight, out of mind? *Acta Psychiatrica Scandinavica*, *108*(6), 460–462.

Ellis, H. D., & Lewis, M. B. (2001). Capgras delusion: A window on face recognition. *Trends in Cognitive Sciences*, *5*(4), 149–156.

Ellis, H. D., & Young, A. W. (1990). Accounting for delusional misidentifications. *British Journal of Psychiatry*, *157*, 239–248.

Gluckman, L. K. (1968). A case of Capgras syndrome. *Australian & New Zealand Journal of Psychiatry*, *2*, 39–43.

Harciarek, M., & Kertesz, A. (2008). The prevalence of misidentification syndromes in neurodegenerative diseases. *Alzheimer Disorder & Associated Disorders*, *22*, 163–169.

Hillis, A. E. (1999). Selnes O: Cases of aphasia or neglect due to Creutzfeldt-Jakob disease. *Aphasiology*, *13*, 743–754.

Javed, Q., Alam, F., Krishna, S., & Jaganathan, G. (2010). An unusual case of sporadic Creutzfeldt-Jakob disease (CJD). *British Medical Journal case reports*, *2010*, bcr12.2009.2576. https://doi.org/10.1136/bcr.12.2009.2576

Kapur, N., Abbott, P., Lowman, A., Will, R. G. (2003). The neuropsychological profile associated with variant Creutzfeldt-Jakob disease. *Brain*, *126*, 2693–2702.

Kaufman, K. R., Newman, N. B., & Dawood, A. (2014). Capgras delusion with violent behaviour in Alzheimer dementia: Case analysis with literature review. *Annals of Clinical Psychiatry*, *26*(3), 187–191.

Kropp, S., Schulz-Schaeffer, W. J., Finkenstaedt, M., Riedemann, C., Windl, O., Steinhoff, B. J., Zerr, I., Kretzschmar, H. A., & Poser, S. (1999). The Heidenhain variant of Creutzfeldt-Jakob disease. *Archives of Neurology*, *56*(1), 55–61. https://doi.org/10.1001/archneur.56.1.55

Lovestone S. (2009). Alzheimer's disease and other dementias (including pseudodementias). In A. S. David, S. Fleminger, M. D. Kopelman, S. Lovestone & J. D. C. Mellers (Eds.), *Lishman's Organic Psychiatry* (pp. 543–615). Wiley-Blackwell.

Mandell, A. M., Alexander, M. P., Carpenter, S. (1989). Creutzfeldt- Jakob disease presenting as isolated aphasia. *Neurology*, *39*: 55–58.

McKay, R. (2012). Delusional inference. *Mind & Language*, *27*, 330–355.

Pandis, C., Agrawal, N., & Poole, N. A. (2019). Capgras' delusion: A systematic review of 255 published cases. *Psychopathology*, *52*(3), 161 –173.

Qi, C., Zhang, J. T., Zhao, W., Xing, X. W., & Yu, S. Y. (2020). Sporadic Creutzfeldt-Jakob disease: A retrospective analysis of 104 cases. *European Neurology*, *83*(1), 65–72. https://doi.org/10.1159/000507189

Reimers, K., Emmert, N., Shah, H., Benedict, R. H., & Szigeti, K. (2014). Capgras-like visual decomposition in Lewy body dementia with therapeutic response to donepezil. *Neurology. Clinical Practice*, *4*(6), 467–469. https://doi.org/10.1212/CPJ.0000000000000068

Snowden, J. S., Mann, D. M., & Neary, D. (2002). Distinct neuropsychological characteristics in Creutzfeldt-Jakob disease. *Journal of Neurology, Neurosurgery & Psychiatry*, *73*, 686–694.

Thiel, C. M., Studte, S., Hildebrandt, H., Huster, R., & Weerda, R. (2014). When a loved one feels unfamiliar: A case study on the neural basis of Capgras delusion. *Cortex: A Journal Devoted to the Study of the Nervous System and Behavior*, *52*, 75–85. https://doi.org/10.1016/j.cortex.2013.11.011

Wall, C. A., Rummans, T. A., Aksamit, A. J., Krahn, L. E., & Pankratz, V. S. (2005). Psychiatric manifestations of Creutzfeldt-Jakob disease: A 25-year analysis. *The Journal of Neuropsychiatry and Clinical Neurosciences*, *17*(4), 489–495. https://doi.org/10.1176/jnp.17.4.489

Young, A. W. (2000). Wondrous strange: The neuropsychology of abnormal beliefs. In M. Coltheart & M. Davies (Eds.), *Pathologies of belief* (pp. 47–74). Blackwell.

5 A rare and challenging differential diagnosis

Prosopagnosia and reduced empathy in right-variant semantic dementia – where *'understanding does not map onto reality'*

Julia Cook

Introduction

Dementia (otherwise known as Major Neurocognitive Disorder; APA, 2013) is an umbrella term for syndromes involving progressive cognitive impairment relative to previous ability in at least one cognitive domain that affects daily functioning, over and above that seen in normal ageing. Cortical dementias (e.g., Alzheimer's disease (AD) and fronto-temporal dementia (FTD)) directly affect specialised cortical areas (Shaik & Varna, 2012). Dementia subtypes are identified by triangulating clinical symptoms, course, neuropathological indicators, and selective impairment profiles (Burrell & Piguet, 2015). An illustrative case is provided to demonstrate the process and value of triangulation between these factors in rare dementias. The case, Victor, presented with progressive cognitive difficulties in semantic understanding, object agnosia, prosopagnosia and reduced empathy.

The imperative challenge of differential dementia diagnosis

Disease modifying treatments for dementia remain in their infancy and are not currently licensed for use in clinical practice. Nevertheless, identification of dementia subtype is important in predicting clinical course, informing early post-diagnostic education, intervention, and symptomatic treatment (Kumfor et al., 2018; Livingston et al., 2020). Crucially, acetylcholinesterase inhibitors used in AD treatment may exacerbate behavioural change in FTDs (Mendez et al., 2007). Caregiver stress can also be greater in FTDs than AD due to earlier loss of insight (Kamminga et al., 2015; Koyama et al., 2018).

Initial symptoms of dementia can be misattributed to aging, personal experiences, or personality and this can significantly delay help-seeking (Iliffe & Wilcock, 2017). Delays to diagnosis are particularly common in rarer dementias and those with young-onset dementia, and impact significantly upon the support and interventions available to the individual and their family.

DOI: 10.4324/9781003228226-6

Approximately 40% of those with FTD are misdiagnosed; common misdiagnoses involve attribution of symptoms including apathy, personality, and behaviour changes to psychiatric conditions, or attribution of cognitive symptoms to AD (Wylie et al., 2013; Mendez et al., 2020). Reaching a diagnosis of FTD often takes longer than for other types of dementia, both due to longer referral delays and delay to diagnosis (Leroy et al., 2021). As a subtype of FTD, Snowden et al. (2018) noted that 'a striking feature of semantic dementia patients is that they come to medical attention relatively late in the course of their disease' (pp. 200). This creates further challenges to differential diagnosis in these patients, because with progression, cognitive profiles become more homogenous across dementia syndromes.

To highlight the diagnostic complexity inherent in dementia diagnosis, the following literature review addresses the overlapping nature of neuropsychological deficits across the core neurodegenerative conditions considered relevant in Victor's case.

FTD

FTD is an umbrella term. Behavioural variant FTD (bvFTD) accounts for 70% of FTD cases (Snowden et al., 2002) and is associated with pathology in orbitofrontal (OFC), anterior insular cortices, and the amygdala (Kumfor et al., 2013). Social disinhibition, personality/behavioural change, loss of empathy, and executive dysfunction are characteristic (bvFTD diagnostic criteria: Rascovsky et al., 2011).

Semantic dementia (SD)

Patients with SD typically present with verbally mediated semantic memory deficits and fluent speech that lacks content (Kashibayashi et al., 2010). Neuroimaging shows bilateral, anteromedial temporal lobe (ATL) atrophy (Mion et al., 2010) with left-sided predominance. Atypical presentations associated with right ATL predominance occur in approximately 25% of cases (right-semantic dementia (r-SD); Hodges et al., 2010).

Patients with r-SD present with early deterioration in perceptual understanding, including familiar face recognition and visual associative object agnosia, outweighing lexical-semantic difficulties (Thompson et al., 2003). Episodic memory impairments have also been identified in r-SD (Chan et al., 2009). Together with visuospatial impairments, this leads to challenges in differentiating between this condition, Alzheimer's disease (AD) and its 'visuospatial' variant, posterior cortical atrophy (PCA), particularly given that people with SD tend to present to diagnostic services relatively late in the neurodegenerative course.

AD

AD is the most common form of dementia in older people, with well-defined neuropathological changes. Accumulation of beta-amyloid (Aβ) and hyper-phosphorylated tau proteins lead to senile plaques and neurofibrillary tangles (Gendron & Petrucelli, 2009). Pathology progressively extends from the medial temporal lobes through temporal, parietal, and frontal association areas (Braak & Braak, 1998). Loss of memory for recent episodes characterises typical AD, followed by deficits in word-finding, visuospatial skills, and executive functioning (McKhann et al., 2011).

Posterior cortical atrophy

Posterior cortical atrophy (PCA) is generally classed as a rare, atypical subtype of dementia, predominantly associated with AD pathology, affecting the parietal, occipito-temporal, and occipital lobes initially (Crutch et al., 2012). PCA presents with early and predominant visuospatial and visuoperceptual impairments; object agnosia tends to be apperceptive or pre-semantic and prosopagnosia can also feature (Humphreys & Riddoch, 2006; Lehmann et al., 2011).

Differential diagnosis: cognitive profiles in r-SD, SD, bvFTD, AD, and PCA

Due to overlapping neuropsychological profiles, dementia types are best discriminated by early cognitive symptoms in core domains.

Language, perception, and social cognition

The right ATL is instrumental in construction of representations based on perceptual information, whereas the left-ATL is specialised for language-mediated representations (Gainotti, 2015). Differential ATL involvement in perceptual vs language-mediated information is supported by evidence that, in early SD presentations, language-mediated semantic associative errors are found in typical SD (deficits on word-based semantic memory tasks), and perceptually mediated associative errors in r-SD (deficits on picture-based semantic memory tasks; Snowden et al., 2018; 2019; Pozueta et al., 2019). Accordingly, deficits in letter fluency are anticipated in typical SD due to lexical-semantic difficulties. They are also anticipated in bvFTD due to executive difficulties, but less so in early r-SD (Snowden et al., 2018; Johnen & Bertoux, 2019).

In r-SD, loss of person-specific semantic information (e.g., voice/face recognition) is greater than in typical SD (Gainotti, 2007). This has been attributed to a 'multi-modal person recognition' disorder, primarily driven by loss of perceptual understanding (e.g., affecting recognition of faces/voices; Snowden et al., 2004; Gainotti & Marra, 2011; Ding et al., 2020). Initially, person-recognition may be facilitated by verbal cues (e.g., names, Evans et al., 1995). With progression, atrophy spreads contralaterally and ipsilaterally from the ATL and connectional pathways become disrupted (Rohrer et al., 2008; Mann & Snowden, 2017); degraded conceptualisation ultimately spans all sensory modalities (Goll et al., 2012).

Whilst semantic/associative errors underlie visual difficulties in r–SD, in PCA and AD pre-semantic apperceptive errors underlie agnosia (Humphreys & Riddoch, 2006; Crutch et al., 2012). However, more generalised visuospatial impairments are not uncommon in both r–SD and bvFTD with progression to advanced dementia, as right-parietal connectivity degrades (Geser et al., 2009; Morbelli et al., 2016; Ulugut-Erkoyun et al., 2020).

Due to r–ATL involvement in basic behavioural and emotional functions including familiarity judgements through connectivity with OFC and limbic areas, r–SD leads to earlier, more pronounced change in social cognition/interpersonal behaviour than typical SD (and AD/PCA), bearing resemblance to bvFTD (Kumfor et al., 2016; Binney et al., 2016).

Memory

Encoding, consolidation, and storage deficits are well-documented in AD and occur with progression in PCA (Lowndes et al., 2008; Crutch et al., 2017). In SD and r–SD memory deficits appear to depend on task conceptualisation requirements, and in FTDs generally, relate to organisational strategies during encoding and retrieval (Chan et al., 2009; Hornberger & Piguet, 2012).

Executive functioning

In addition to social cognition impairments previously noted in r–SD and bvFTD, people with early r–SD, SD, and AD may show less executive dysfunction compared to those with bvFTD. PCA generally does not present with early executive dysfunction (Josephs et al., 2009; Bertoux et al., 2016).

Given overlapping profiles, quantitative and qualitative examination of performance is vital within the triangulation between formal test results, neuroimaging, and information provided by the patient and family (Thompson et al. 2005; Woollams et al. 2008). The nature of preliminary cognitive deficits in each condition is outlined in Table 5.1.

Table 5.1 Patterns of impairment across suspected conditions in early stages

	Executive function	Social cognition	Semantic knowledge Visual (inc. faces)	Verbal	Episodic memory	Language	Working memory/attention	Information processing speed	Verbal fluency	Visuo-construction/spatial
r-SD	+	++	++ (associative)	+		+(associative)				
SD	+/-	+	-	+	+	++	-	-	++	-/+(associative)
Bv	++	++	-		+/-	-	+	+	+	-
FTD	+	+		-	+/-					
AD	+	-	+(apperceptive)	+	++	+	-(verbal)	+	+	+(apperceptive)
PCA	-	-	+(apperceptive)	-	+/-	+	+	+	+	++(apperceptive)

++ significant impairment
+ impairment
– no impairment

Source: This table draws on data from the following papers: Crutch et al. (2013), Bertoux et al. (2016), Busigny et al. (2009), Ding et al. (2020), Firth et al. (2019), Gainotti (2007), Gorno-Tempini et al. (2011), Hornberger and Piguet (2012), Josephs et al. (2009), Kamath et al. (2019), Kamminga et al. (2015), Lowndes et al. (2008), Neitzel et al. (2016), Piguet et al. (2011), Pozueta et al. (2019), Snowden et al. (2019), Stopford et al. (2012), Thompson et al. (2003), Thompson et al. (2005), Woollams et al. (2008).

Case presentation

Reason for referral

Victor was a right-handed British gentleman in his mid-seventies. His wife, Pam raised concerns regarding cognitive changes to his GP who referred him to the dementia assessment service multidisciplinary team (MDT). Neuropsychological assessment was requested by the team to support differential diagnosis of dementia.

Background information

Victor was born in India to English parents, speaking English as his first and only fluent language. He met all developmental milestones and attained five O-Level equivalents at an English-speaking school, before returning to England aged 17 years.

Victor worked in sales, retiring aged 65. He and Pam had one daughter and three grandchildren.

Victor had diet-controlled hypertension. He was an ex-smoker, did not drink alcohol, and had no reported mental health history. There was no family history of neurological or degenerative conditions.

Victor was involved in a car accident two months prior to referral and was subsequently banned from driving. There was no loss of consciousness or post-traumatic amnesia, or any other injuries recorded. A computerised tomography (CT) brain scan was unremarkable.

Initial MDT investigations

Dementia blood screens were normal. During MDT review of the CT, possible right-anterior temporal atrophy was identified.

Cognitive screening gave a score of 78/100 (Addenbrooke's Cognitive Examination-III; cut-off 82/100). Victor lost points on free recall, semantic fluency, and serial 7s. He incorrectly identified two incomplete letters and two confrontation naming items.

Occupational therapy (OT) assessments revealed difficulties in kitchen tasks (e.g., mistaking a prune for a teabag). Conversation was described as simultaneously circumscribed and tangential, with occasional fluent anomia and absent turn-taking.

Presenting concerns

Victor acknowledged occasional word-finding problems but otherwise considered himself to function well. Scores on the Hospital Anxiety and Depression Scale (HADS) fell within the moderate range for depression and in the sub-clinical range for anxiety. Victor attributed all mood and cognitive difficulties to frustration about his driving ban.

Separate clinical interviews were conducted with Pam and their daughter, with Victor's agreement. Five years previously, Victor became uncharacteristically short-tempered and argumentative, and easily overwhelmed by the noise of his grandchildren crying. He also experienced 'memory difficulties' (e.g., not understanding that a friend had died after a long illness). His family noted that his report of events in these recent years was inaccurate (e.g., his account of his travels around the world). A two-year history of egocentricity/reduced empathy was reported, including out-of-character, disinhibited comments about Pam in public; for example, Victor would tell Pam that she had become shorter and/or fatter, and said he needed to measure her. When Pam broke her ankle during a shopping trip, Victor was uncharacteristically unsympathetic, would not let the supermarket staff telephone an ambulance, and became lost whilst trying to find their parked car.

Eighteen months prior to assessment, Victor struggled to recognise distant family members and experienced severe topographical disorientation at an airport which was previously highly familiar to him. He became preoccupied with Indian history and compulsively tidied his clothes.

Three months prior to assessment, Victor developed difficulties recognising close family members. He occasionally misidentified Pam and prevented her from using their shower. Victor 'appeared lost' in highly familiar locations, and had difficulties understanding finances and road signs. Most recently, changes in verbal understanding and expression had developed, together with difficulties using familiar objects (e.g., trolley coin-release mechanisms).

Victor did not demonstrate awareness of his cognitive difficulties, or the support Pam provided. Pam reported 'Victor's understanding does not map on to reality'.

Pam was experiencing significant carer strain. She frequently became tearful in conversation, and believed she needed to 'tread carefully'.

Initial formulation and hypotheses

Victor presented with cognitive changes progressing over a five-year period, into which he had limited insight. Family reported personality and behavioural changes, difficulties with social and visual understanding, changes in visual and verbal memory, and recent word-finding difficulties affecting functioning and associated with carer strain.

Considering Victor's symptoms and investigations to date, it was hypothesised that Victor was presenting with a dementia; likely r-SD. However, due to the rarity of this condition and overlapping neuropsychological profiles, the following possibilities were considered:

1. AD (primarily impaired learning and recall)
2. PCA (primarily visuospatial impairments)

3. bvFTD (primarily executive functioning and social cognition deficits)
4. SD/r-SD (primarily semantic deficits which may be person-specific, cross-modal, and/or more pronounced in visual or verbal tasks).

Neuropsychological assessment

Given post-diagnostic support implications, testing focused primarily on differentiation between FTDs and AD, and secondarily on subtypes. A process approach was taken, assessing across core domains whilst robustly testing the identified hypotheses (Milberg et al., 2009). Emphasis was given to visuospatial, semantic, memory, and executive functions, given their relevance to differential diagnosis.

Behaviour during assessment

Following pre-assessment counselling, Victor consented to proceed (LaFontaine et al., 2014). At each appointment, Victor did not recognise the assessor but showed awareness that he was being assessed. Speech was fluent and verbose with occasional anomia.

Performance validity

Victor passed embedded and standalone performance validity assessments (Rey-15 Item Test; Reliable Digit Span).

Premorbid functioning

The Test of Premorbid Functioning (TOPF) estimated premorbid intellectual functioning fell within the 'average' range (approximately 68th percentile), consistent with educational and occupational attainment, and current best performance.

Speed of processing, attention, and working memory

Processing speed performance was slow (Repeatable Battery for the Assessment of Neurological Status, RBANS-Coding, Wechsler Adult Intelligence Scale (WAIS-IV) WAIS-Symbol Search: both 0.1st percentile), with errors that reflected difficulties with visual understanding.

Victor's WAIS-IV Working Memory Index (WMI) fell within the 'borderline' range (6th percentile), significantly lower than estimated premorbid ability (base rate: 0.18%).

Auditory-verbal attention and working memory fell within the 'average' range (WAIS-IV Digit Span Forwards & Digit Span Backwards: 25th percentile). Auditory-verbal sequencing performance was 'borderline' (WAIS-IV Digit Span Sequencing: 5th percentile). These differences were not statistically or clinically significant (base rates: 21–40%). Mental arithmetic performance fell within the 'low average' range (WAIS-IV Arithmetic; 9th percentile).

Visuospatial/constructional skills

Victor passed the Visual Object and Space Perception (VOSP) battery shape-detection screening task but failed all other measures of object perception (VOSP Object Decision, Incomplete Letters, Silhouettes). Performance was error-free on a simple measure of space perception and simultaneous processing (VOSP Dot Counting). Outwith *identifying* famous people by their faces, he was able to provide qualitatively accurate descriptions of people on a bespoke famous faces test (FFT; e.g., 'an old man with crazy hair' for Einstein).

Victor's RBANS visuospatial index fell in the 'extremely low' range (0.3rd percentile). Spatial perception was impaired (RBANS Line Orientation; <2nd percentile). Victor passed the practice task with support but found it difficult to adhere to instructions (e.g., stating that he would 'add them up'). Organisational difficulties were observed on constructional tasks (e.g., starting with internal 'objects') resulting in spatial errors (RBANS Figure Copy: 0.1st percentile). Victor used verbal descriptions (e.g., describing three circles as 'baubles') to aid performance.

Perceptual reasoning skills were impaired (WAIS-IV Picture Completion; 5th percentile; VOSP Cube Analysis: below cut-off).

Language and semantic knowledge

Confrontation naming fell within the 'borderline-low average' range (RBANS Picture Naming; 3–9th percentile). Errors either described object function (circumlocutory error) or reflected semantic deficits (e.g., giraffe: 'tall, could be a horse'). Victor did not benefit from semantic cues.

Retrieval of factual information was intact (WAIS-IV Information; 75th percentile) but qualitatively, Victor struggled when asked about people's identities; for example, he was unable to provide information about a famous Indian civil rights leader. Performance was impaired on semantic knowledge tasks; Victor failed the Pyramids and Palm Trees (PPT) pictures practice task. For PPT-words performance was 'Extremely Low' (<0.01st percentile). Semantic word-retrieval was also 'Extremely Low' (DKEFS Category Fluency; 0.1st percentile).

Victor obtained a familiarity score of 5/10 on an FFT, correctly naming only the Queen (1/10) and incorrectly identifying two ordinary people as famous. When given the *names* of the famous people depicted, he could provide identifying semantic information for 4/9 people.

A bespoke task revealed that Victor was unable to identify two famous landmarks from pictures without verbal cues (including the Taj Mahal). On non-famous scenes, Victor could describe people depicted (e.g., young woman/boy/man-eyes closed) but could not visually infer behaviour (praying) or probable relationships (mother and son).

Memory

Victor's immediate verbal memory performance fell in the 'borderline' range (RBANS Immediate Memory Index: 5th percentile). List Learning ability was in the 'low average' range (9th percentile), demonstrating some learning across trials (i.e., learning curve: 2, 5, 6, 6 of a possible 10 per trial) with non-word intrusions (e.g., saddage; hador) and repetitions. RBANS Story Memory was 'borderline' (5th percentile) with considerable improvement on second repetition. On a more complex story learning task, Victor's response lacked semantic detail (WMS-IV Logical Memory, LM-I: 0.4th percentile; 'extremely low'). Paired word list learning performance was 'borderline' (WMS-IV Verbal Paired Associates I, VPA-I: 2nd percentile). Overall, learning performance suggested inconsistent encoding abilities affected by executive encoding strategies and processing speed.

Free recall of the word list was adequate (RBANS List Recall: 17–25th cumulative percentile, 'low average–average') but cueing had limited benefit (List Recognition: 16/20;<2nd percentile; 'extremely low') and story recall was poor (RBANS Story Recall; 1st percentile; 'extremely low').

Delayed recall of a more complex story was 'extremely low' (WMS-IV LM-II: 1st percentile; LM-I = LM-II; Contrast Scaled Score [CSS] = 10); with minimal semantic detail. Cueing benefited performance (10–16th cumulative percentile; LM Recognition>Recall; CSS = 3). On cued paired associate recall, Victor performed in the 'average' range (VPA-II: 25th percentile) representing a strength within his profile (VPA-II>VPA-I; CSS = 17). Pairs recalled after a delay had been recalled on at least one learning trial and were meaningfully associated. VPA-II Recognition performance was 'low average–average' ($17-25^{th}$ cumulative percentile), whereas VPA-II Word Recall was 'borderline' (5th percentile).

Recall of a complex figure also fell within the 'extremely low' range (RBANS-Figure Recall: 1st percentile).

Overall, Victor's delayed memory profile was characterised by benefits from initial encoding accuracy and cueing paradigms.

Executive functioning

Phonemic fluency (Delis-Kaplan Executive Function System (DKEFS) Letter Fluency; 50th percentile) was considerably stronger than semantic fluency (DKEFS-Category Fluency; 0.1st percentile); this discrepancy was highly unusual (CSS = 19). Poor performance was observed on both switching and accuracy of responses (DKEFS Category Switching: 1st percentile), constrained by reduced overall semantic fluency (Category Switching>Category Fluency-CSS = 12; percent switching accuracy: 25th percentile). Victor perseverated across trials, making many repetition and set-loss errors (0.1st percentile), and displaying no use of strategy. Repetition errors were most evident for letter fluency and set-loss errors were most evident on semantic fluency.

Inhibitory control was impaired (Hayling Errors; 0.8th percentile) with adequate initiation response times (Hayling 1 and 2 timing scores: 40th and 23rd percentiles). Planning was inefficient, slow and likely ineffective (Behavioural Assessment of the Dysexecutive Syndrome (BADS) Key Search).

Informant-reported measures of executive function (BADS-Dysexecutive Questionnaire; Frontotemporal Dementia Rating Scale) revealed difficulties with self-monitoring, social behaviour, memory (confabulation), and insight, with 'severe decline' over time. A 29-point discrepancy was seen between Victor and Pam's DEX ratings potentially reflecting reduced insight.

Social cognition

Performance on the Reading the Mind in the Eyes Task (RMET) was weak (approx. 2nd percentile) with poor discrimination of anger and fear.

Summary

Neuropsychological testing suggested performance on episodic memory and visuospatial–constructional tasks were reflective of executive difficulties. Impairments in visuospatial object perception were primarily seen when required to identify items or where tasks were somewhat abstract, indicating associative and executive (reasoning) errors respectively, whilst basic visual processing (including face processing) appeared relatively intact. On memory tasks, improved performance was observed with cues and on recognition trials, suggesting preserved consolidation and that deficits in encoding and free recall were likely to be mediated executively. Victor experienced particular difficulties with visual semantic information, in addition to difficulties on verbal semantic tasks, despite preserved verbal 'general knowledge'.

Results were evaluated against initial hypotheses and triangulated with collateral information to form an opinion on diagnosis and consider interventions (Wilson & Betteridge, 2019).

Hypotheses

In keeping with a dementia diagnosis, Victor experienced objective impairment in multiple cognitive domains, impact on activities of daily living, and Pam reported progression over time.

Evaluating whether Victor was experiencing AD, Victor's memory profile was consistent with executively-mediated difficulties, rather than encoding, consolidation and storage deficits. Together with evidence of early change in behaviour/personality, this hypothesis was rejected.

There was some evidence of visuospatial impairments, consistent with PCA. However, errors were executive and associative in nature rather than apperceptive/spatial (e.g., correct perception of giraffe as an animal, but inability to name due to partial semantic access). Dot counting, which does not require associative/abstract reasoning, was preserved, as was basic face processing. Together with evidence of executive dysfunction, lexical-semantic errors and behaviour/personality change, this hypothesis was rejected.

In relation to the possibility of bvFTD, Victor's social cognition was impaired and test performance was consistent with descriptions from daily life. Deficits on verbal mental flexibility tasks appeared mediated by semantic task requirements. Initiation of verbal responses and phonemic fluency were preserved, but there were difficulties with inhibition, planning, self-monitoring and organisation, in addition to qualitative evidence of executive dysfunction on memory and visuospatial tasks. Difficulties with elements of executive function, taken together with early change in personality, behaviour and empathy partially supported this hypothesis.

In evaluating whether Victor experienced SD or r-SD, this was supported by Victor's deficits on visual tasks tapping object identification and/or semantics (e.g., PPT, face, and landmark recognition). Verbal cues aided identification, consistent with r-SD (e.g., Evans et al., 1995). This semantic deficit was weighted toward visual-perceptual tasks, appeared to affect person recognition, and had cross-modal elements (e.g., impaired semantic fluency; in line with Snowden et al., 2018). Verbal comprehension (i.e. 'general knowledge') and phonemic fluency were preserved. This was likely to be inconsistent with a typical SD diagnosis: verbal comprehension is associated with left posterior temporal lobe lesions (Snowden et al., 2018), and single-word comprehension and lexical access are affected in typical SD (e.g., Grossman & Moore, 2005).

Considering the evidence evaluated, and collateral reports of symptom development over time, Victor's symptoms were considered consistent with probable FTD, with r-SD the most likely subtype. Table 5.2 provides an overview.

Formulation

Alongside cognitive difficulties affecting semantic knowledge, memory, executive functioning, and social cognition in keeping with FTD-rSD, Victor's identity had been affected by loss of valued roles (e.g., driving; Hennelly et al., 2021), contributing to low mood. Reduced insight negated Victor's opportunities to build his understanding of his difficulties and develop compensatory strategies (see Figure 5.1) which placed Pam under considerable carer strain.

Given the rarity of this dementia subtype, Victor was offered magnetic resonance imaging (MRI). This showed 'moderate asymmetrical atrophy, most marked in the right anteromedial temporal lobe', providing further support for the FTD-rSD diagnosis.

Table 5.2 Victor's neuropsychological profile and differentials

	Executive function	Social cognition	Semantic knowledge Visual (inc. faces)	Semantic knowledge Verbal	Episodic memory	Language	Working memory/ attention	Information processing speed	Verbal fluency	Visuo-construction/ spatial
r-SD	+	++	++ (associative)	+	+/-	+	-	+	+	+(associative)
Profiles in dementia syndromes under consideration										
SD	+	+	+ (associative)	++	+/-	++	-	-	++	-/+(associative)
Bv	++	++	-		+/-	-	+	+	+	-
FTD										
AD	+	-	+(apperceptive)	+	++	+	+	+	+	+(apperceptive)
PCA	-	-	+(apperceptive)	-	+/-	+	-(verbal)	+	+	++(apperceptive)
Victor's profile										
	+	+	++	+	+/-	+	-/+ (executive)	+	+	+(associative)

++ significant impairment
+ impairment
- no impairment

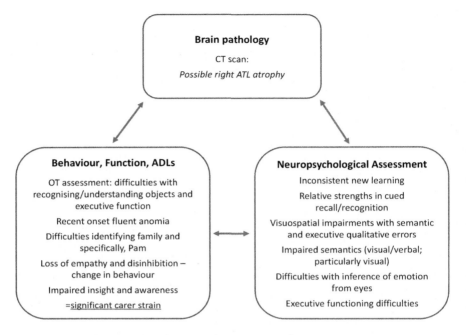

Figure 5.1 Triangulation formulation (Wilson & Betteridge, 2019)

Treatment and Outcome

The diagnosis was shared with Victor and Pam in a joint session with Psychology and Psychiatry. Victor did not express concern about the diagnosis but was frustrated about loss of role and identity following his driving licence being revoked. He was offered post-diagnostic support focused on self-identity, including life story work (Parker et al., 2020). Victor engaged well with the support worker and they co-created a 'This Is Me' booklet based on Victor's life story (cultural and family background, things that were important to him) and choices about future care (e.g., communication, personal care routines, and preferences).

Caregiver stress can be comparatively high in r-SD due to apathy, disinhibition, and difficulties with person recognition (Thompson et al., 2003; Koyama et al., 2018), which dovetailed with Pam's experience. Based on the neuropsychological formulation, Pam was offered personalised psycho-education and carer support, focused on external compensatory strategies for Victor's loss of visual semantic knowledge (e.g., using her name in conversations with Victor; Kumfor et al., 2018) and coping with changes in Victor's cognition and behaviour (NICE, 2018), including compassion-focused self-care (Collins et al., 2018). Pam responded well to these interventions, which were provided by OT, noting that they bolstered her ability to cope with the challenges that she and Victor were experiencing. Pam was also referred to the local Admiral Nurse service for ongoing carer support.

Victor later developed a combination of 'delusional misidentification syndromes'. In particular, Victor experienced reduplicative paramnesia for people and places (believing there were two showers and many versions of the same woman in the house (Pam)). The emotional salience that Victor had associated with 'Pam' progressively reduced, despite her verbal cues (i.e., in addition to not recognising Pam by face, Victor believed Pam to be an imposter; akin to Capgras syndrome). Meaningful speech content declined (despite preservation of motor speech, phonology, and syntax), and Victor developed swallowing difficulties. It was no longer possible for Pam to maintain Victor's safety at home. When Victor's condition progressed requiring admission to respite care and later, a care home, the 'This Is Me' document enabled formal caregivers to support Victor more effectively and. over time, Victor settled well into this environment.

Conclusions

Right-variant semantic dementia is a complex condition to diagnose, with unique implications for support and intervention. Neuropsychology has a pivotal role in the assessment, formulation, diagnosis, and treatment of rare forms of dementia. Despite Victor's late presentation to services, neuropsychological assessment supported identification of this particular form of dementia through using both standardised and non-standardised assessment, grounded in neuropsychological models, together with a process-based approach to assessment. In particular, given the known challenges of formally assessing executive and social cognitive functioning (Mesulam, 1986), careful triangulation between observations, collateral information, and clinical investigations was essential to formulation (Wilson & Betteridge, 2019). This also avoided identification of impairments solely on test scores and introduction of type-I errors ('false positives'; Binder et al., 2009).

Neuropsychological formulation contributed to this case in numerous ways. Diagnostic accuracy was enhanced through formulation clarifying the nature of the difficulties (e.g., visuospatial problems of an associative nature; memory problems driven by executive and semantic difficulties). Use of bespoke measures enabled neuropsychological formulation of informant-reported facial and topographical recognition difficulties. This also supported the MDT's understanding of Victor's rarer form of dementia. Using 'real world' tasks such as these also facilitated family understanding of post-diagnostic recommendations (e.g., Pam identifying herself verbally in conversation to support person recognition). Victor did not experience potential iatrogenic harm through anticholinergic medications, which could inadvertently increase agitation. Finally, formulation indicated that Victor experienced numerous psychological threats to his sense of personhood, including loss of role and identity, which indicated a particular role for life story work in this case.

Acknowledgements

I would like to express my sincere gratitude to Victor and Pam, who gave me the opportunity to apply neuropsychological principles to supporting them. I would also like to thank Dr Gaby Parker for developing my understanding of the Boston process approach and for supporting me to write Victor's case into a book chapter.

Note

1 All identifying details were changed to protect anonymity and confidentiality. 'Victor' and 'Pam' provided informed consent for their anonymised details to be used in this case study.

References

American Psychiatric Association (2013). *Diagnostic and statistical manual of mental disorders* (5th ed.). American Psychiatric Association.

Bertoux, M., O'Callaghan, C., Dubois, B., & Hornberger, M. (2016). In two minds: executive functioning versus theory of mind in behavioural variant frontotemporal dementia. *Journal of Neurology, Neurosurgery & Psychiatry, 87*, 231–234. https://doi.org/10.1136/jnnp-2015-311643

Binder, L. M, Iverson, G. L., & Brooks, B. L. (2009). To err is human: 'abnormal' neuropsychological scores and variability are common in healthy adults. *Archives of Clinical Neuropsychology, 24*(1), 31–46. https://doi.org/10.1093/arclin/acn001

Binney, R. J., Henry, M. L., Babiak, M., Pressman, P. S., Santos-Santos, M, A., Narvid, J., Mandelli, M. L., Strain, P. J., Miller, B. L., Rankin, K. P., Rosen, H. J. & Gorno-Tempini, M. L. (2016). Reading words and other people: A comparison of exception word, familiar face and affect processing in the left and right temporal variants of primary progressive aphasia. *Cortex, 82*, 147–163. https://doi.org/10.1016/j.cortex.2016.05.014

Braak, H., & Braak, E. (1998). Evolution of neuronal changes in the course of Alzheimer's disease. *Journal of Neural Transmission Supplement, 53*, 127–140. https://doi.org/10.1007/978-3-7091-6467-9_11

Burrell, J. R., & Piguet, O. (2015). Lifting the veil: How to use clinical neuropsychology to assess dementia. *Journal of Neurology, Neurosurgery & Psychiatry, 86*(11), 1216–1224. https://doi.org/10.1136/jnnp-2013-307483

Busigny, T., Robaye, L., Dricot, L., & Rossion, B. (2009). Right anterior temporal lobe atrophy and person-based semantic defect: a detailed case study. *Neurocase, 15*(6), 485–508. https://doi.org/10.1080/13554790902971141

Chan, D., Anderson, V., Pijnenburg, Y., Whitwell, J., Barnes, J., Scahill, R., Stevens, J. M., Barkhof, F., Scheltens, P., Rossor, M.N. & Fox, N.C. (2009). The clinical profile of right temporal lobe atrophy. *Brain, 132*(5), 1287–1298. https://doi.org/10.1093/brain/awp037

Collins, R. N., Gilligan, L. J., & Poz, R. (2018). The evaluation of a compassion-focused therapy group for couples experiencing a dementia diagnosis. *Clinical Gerontologist, 41*(5), 474–486. https://doi.org/10.1080/07317115.2017.1397830

Crutch, S. J., Lehmann, M., Schott, J. M., Rabinovici, G. D., Rossor, M. N., & Fox, N. C. (2012). Posterior cortical atrophy. *The Lancet. Neurology, 11*(2), 170–178. https://doi.org/10.1016/S1474-4422(11)70289-7

Crutch, S. J., Lehmann, M., Warren, J. D., & Rohrer, J. D. (2013). The language profile of posterior cortical atrophy. *Journal of Neurology, Neurosurgery & Psychiatry, 84*(4), 460–466. https://doi.org/10.1136/jnnp-2012-303309

Crutch, S. J., Schott, J. M., Rabinovici, G. D., Murray, M., Snowden, J. S., van der Flier, W. M., Dickerson, B. C., Vandenberghe, R., Ahmed, S., Bak, T. H., Boeve, B. F., Butler, C., Cappa, S. F., Ceccaldi, M., de Souza, L. C., Dubois, B., Felician, O., Galasko, D., Graff-Radford, J., Graff-Radford, N. R., … Alzheimer's Association ISTAART Atypical Alzheimer's disease and Associated Syndromes Professional Interest Area. (2017). Consensus classification of posterior cortical atrophy. *Alzheimer's & Dementia: Journal of the Alzheimer's Association, 13*(8), 870–884. https://doi.org/10.1016/j.jalz.2017.01.014

Ding, J., Chen, K., Liu, H., Huang, L., Chen, Y., Lv, Y., Yang, Q., Guo, Q., Han, Z., & Lambon Ralph, M. A. (2020). A unified neurocognitive model of semantics, language, social behaviour and face recognition in semantic dementia. *Nature Communications, 11*(1), 2595. https://doi.org/10.1038/s41467-020-16089-9

Evans, J. J., Heggs, A. J., Antoun, N. & Hodges, J. R. (1995). Progressive prosopagnosia with selective right-temporal lobe atrophy: a new syndrome? *Brain, 118,* 1–13. https://doi.org/10.1093/brain/118.1.1

Firth, N. C., Primativo, S., Marinescu, R. V., Shakespeare, T. J., Suarez-Gonzalez, A., Lehmann, M., Carton, A., Ocal, D., Pavisic, I., Paterson, R. W., Slattery, C. F., Foulkes, A., Ridha, B. H., Gil-Néciga, E., Oxtoby, N. P., Young, A. L., Modat, M., Cardoso, M. J., Ourselin, S., Ryan, N. S., … Crutch, S. J. (2019). Longitudinal neuroanatomical and cognitive progression of posterior cortical atrophy. *Brain, 142*(7), 2082–2095. https://doi.org/10.1093/brain/awz136

Gainotti, G. (2007). Different patterns of famous people recognition disorders in patients with right and left anterior temporal lesions: A systematic review. *Neuropsychologia, 45,* 1591–1607. https://doi.org/10.1016/j.neuropsychologia.2006.12.013

Gainotti, G., & Marra, C. (2011). Differential contribution of right and left temporo-occipital and anterior temporal lesions to face recognition disorders. *Frontiers in Human Neuroscience, 5,* 55. https://doi.org/10.3389/fnhum.2011.00055

Gainotti G. (2015). Is the difference between right and left ATLs due to the distinction between general and social cognition or between verbal and non-verbal representations?. *Neuroscience and Biobehavioral Reviews, 51,* 296–312. https://doi.org/10.1016/j.neubiorev.2015.02.004

Gendron, T. F. & Petrucelli, L. (2009). The role of tau in neurodegeneration. *Molecular Neurodegeneration, 4*:13. https://doi.org/10.1186/1750-1326-4-13

Geser, F., Martinez-Lage, M., Robinson, J., Uryu, K., Neumann, M., Brandmeir, N. J., Xie, S. X., Kwong, L. K., Elman, L., McCluskey, L., Clark, C. M., Malunda, J., Miller, B. L., Zimmerman, E. A., Qian, J., Van Deerlin, V., Grossman, M., Lee, V. M., & Trojanowski, J. Q. (2009). Clinical and pathological continuum of multisystem TDP-43 proteinopathies. *Archives of Neurology, 66*(2), 180–189. https://doi.org/10.1001/archneurol.2008.558

Goll, J. C., Ridgway, G. R., Crutch, S. J., Theunissen, F. E., & Warren, J. D. (2012). Nonverbal sound processing in semantic dementia: A functional MRI study. *Neuroimage, 61*(1), 170–180. https://doi.org/10.1016/j.neuroimage.2012.02.045

Gorno-Tempini, M. L., Hillis, A. E., Weintraub, S., Kertesz, A., Mendez, M., Cappa, S. F., Ogar, J. M., Rohrer, J. D., Black, S., Boeve, B. F., Manes, F., Dronkers, N. F., Vandenberghe, R., Rascovsky, K., Patterson, K., Miller, B. L., Knopman, D. S., Hodges, J. R., Mesulam, M. M., & Grossman, M. (2011). Classification of primary progressive aphasia and its variants. *Neurology, 76*(11), 1006–1014. https://doi.org/10.1212/WNL.0b013e31821103e6

Grossman, M., & Moore, P. (2005). A longitudinal study of sentence comprehension difficulty in primary progressive aphasia. *Journal of Neurology, Neurosurgery & Psychiatry, 76*(5), 644–649. https://doi.org/10.1136/jnnp.2004.039966

Hennelly, N., Cooney, A., Houghton, C., & O'Shea, E. (2021). Personhood and dementia care: A qualitative evidence synthesis of the perspectives of people with dementia. *The Gerontologist, 61*(3), e85–e100. https://doi.org/10.1093/geront/gnz159

Hodges, J. R., Mitchell, J., Dawson, K., Spillantini, M. G., Xuereb, J. H., McMonagle, P., Nestor, P. J., & Patterson, K. (2010). Semantic dementia: Demography, familial factors and survival in a consecutive series of 100 cases. *Brain, 133*(Pt 1), 300–306. https://doi.org/10.1093/brain/awp248

Hornberger, M., & Piguet, O. (2012). Episodic memory in frontotemporal dementia: A critical review, *Brain, 135*(3), 678–692, https://doi.org/10.1093/brain/aws011

Humphreys, G. W., & Riddoch, M. J. (2006). Features, objects, action: The cognitive neuropsychology of visual object processing, 1984–2004. *Cognitive Neuropsychology, 23*(1), 156–183. https://doi.org/10.1080/02643290542000030

Iliffe, S., & Wilcock, J. (2017). The UK experience of promoting dementia recognition and management in primary care. *Zeitschrift fur Gerontologie und Geriatrie, 50*(Suppl 2), 63–67. https://doi.org/10.1007/s00391-016-1175-1

Johnen, A., & Bertoux, M. (2019). Psychological and cognitive markers of behavioral variant frontotemporal dementia: A clinical neuropsychologist's view on diagnostic criteria and beyond. *Frontiers in Neurology, 10*, 594. https://doi.org/10.3389/fneur.2019.00594

Josephs, K. A., Whitwell, J. L., Knopman, D. S., Boeve, B. F., Vemuri, P., Senjem, M. L., Parisi, J. E., Ivnik, R. J., Dickson, D. W., Petersen, R. C., & Jack, C. R., Jr (2009). Two distinct subtypes of right temporal variant frontotemporal dementia. *Neurology, 73*(18), 1443–1450. https://doi.org/10.1212/WNL.0b013e3181bf9945

Kamath, V., Chaney, G. S., DeRight, J., & Onyike, C. U. (2019). A meta-analysis of neuropsychological, social cognitive, and olfactory functioning in the behavioral and language variants of frontotemporal dementia. *Psychological Medicine, 49*(16), 2669–2680. https://doi.org/10.1017/S0033291718003604

Kamminga, J., Kumfor, F., Burrell, J. R., Piguet, O., Hodges, J. R., & Irish, M. (2015). Differentiating between right-lateralised semantic dementia and behavioural-variant frontotemporal dementia: An examination of clinical characteristics and emotion processing. *Journal of Neurology, Neurosurgery and Psychiatry, 86*(10), 1082–1088. https://doi.org/10.1136/jnnp-2014-309120

Kashibayashi, T., Ikeda, M., Komori, K., Shinagawa, S., Shimizu, H., Toyota, Y., Mori, T., Ishikawa, T., Fukuhara, R., Ueno, S., & Tanimukai, S. (2010). Transition of distinctive symptoms of semantic dementia during longitudinal clinical observation. *Dementia and Geriatric Cognitive Disorders, 29*(3), 224–232. https://doi.org/10.1159/000269972

Koyama, A., Hashimoto, M., Fukuhara, R., Ichimi, N., Takasaki, A., Matsushita, M., Ishikawa, T., Tanaka, H., Miyagawa, Y., & Ikeda, M. (2018). Caregiver burden in semantic dementia with right- and left-sided predominant cerebral atrophy and in behavioral-variant frontotemporal dementia. *Dementia and Geriatric Cognitive Disorders Extra, 8*(1), 128–137. https://doi.org/10.1159/000487851

Kumfor, F., Ibanez, A., Hutchings, R., Hazelton, J. L., Hodges, J. R., & Piguet, O. (2018). Beyond the face: How context modulates emotion processing in frontotemporal dementia subtypes. *Brain, 141*(4), 1172–1185. https://doi.org/10.1093/brain/awy002

Kumfor, F., Irish, M., Hodges, J. R., & Piguet, O. (2013). Discrete neural correlates for the recognition of negative emotions: Insights from frontotemporal dementia. *Plos One, 8*(6), e67457. https://doi.org/10.1371/journal.pone.0067457

Kumfor, F., Landin-Romero, R., Devenney, E., Hutchings, R., Grasso, R., Hodges, J. R., & Piguet, O. (2016). On the right side? A longitudinal study of left- versus right-lateralized semantic dementia. *Brain, 139*(Pt 3), 986–998. https://doi.org/10.1093/brain/awv387

LaFontaine, J., Buckell, A., Knibbs, T., & Palfrey, M. (2014). Early and timely intervention in dementia: Pre-assessment counselling. *Clinical psychology in the early stage dementia pathway* (pp. 6–30). British Psychological Society.

Leroy, M., Bertoux, M., Skrobala, E., Mode, E., Adnet-Bonte, C., Le Ber, I., Bombois, S., Cassagnaud, P., Chen, Y., Deramecourt, V., Lebert, F., Mackowiak, M. A., Sillaire, A. R., Wathelet, M., Pasquier, F., Lebouvier, T., & Méotis network (2021). Characteristics and progression of patients with frontotemporal dementia in a regional memory clinic network. *Alzheimer's Research & Therapy, 13*(1), 19. https://doi.org/10.1186/s13195-020-00753-9

Lehmann, M., Barnes, J., Ridgway, G. R., Wattam-Bell, J., Warrington, E. K., Fox, N. C., & Crutch, S. J. (2011). Basic visual function and cortical thickness patterns in posterior cortical atrophy. *Cerebral Cortex, 21*(9), 2122–2132. https://doi.org/10.1093/cercor/bhq287

Livingston, G., Huntley, J., Sommerlad, A., Ames, D., Ballard, C., Banerjee, S., Brayne, C., Burns, A., Cohen-Mansfield, J., Cooper, C., Costafreda, S. G., Dias, A., Fox, N., Gitlin, L. N., Howard, R., Kales, H. C., Kivimäki, M., Larson, E. B., Ogunniyi, A., Orgeta, V., … Mukadam, N. (2020). Dementia prevention, intervention, and care: 2020 report of the Lancet Commission. *Lancet (London, England), 396*(10248), 413–446. https://doi.org/10.1016/S0140-6736(20)30367-6

Lowndes, G. J., Saling, M. M., Ames, D., Chiu, E., Gonzalez, L. M., & Savage, G. R. (2008). Recall and recognition of verbal paired associates in early Alzheimer's disease. *Journal of the International Neuropsychological Society, 14*(4), 591–600. https://doi.org/10.1017/S1355617708080806

Mann, D., & Snowden, J. S. (2017). Frontotemporal lobar degeneration: Pathogenesis, pathology and pathways to phenotype. *Brain pathology (Zurich, Switzerland), 27*(6), 723–736. https://doi.org/10.1111/bpa.12486

McKhann, G. M., Knopman, D. S., Chertkow, H., Hyman, B. T., Jack, C. R., Jr, Kawas, C. H., Klunk, W. E., Koroshetz, W. J., Manly, J. J., Mayeux, R., Mohs, R. C., Morris, J. C., Rossor, M. N., Scheltens, P., Carrillo, M. C., Thies, B., Weintraub, S., & Phelps, C. H. (2011). The diagnosis of dementia due to Alzheimer's disease: Recommendations from the National Institute on Aging – Alzheimer's Association workgroups on diagnostic guidelines for Alzheimer's disease. *Alzheimer's & Dementia, 7*(3), 263–269. https://doi.org/10.1016/j.jalz.2011.03.005

Mendez, M. F., Chavez, D., Desarzant, R. E., & Yerstein, O. (2020). Clinical features of late-onset semantic dementia. *Cognitive and Behavioral Neurology, 33*(2), 122–128. https://doi.org/10.1097/WNN.0000000000000229

Mendez, M. F, Shapira, J. S, McMurtray, A., & Licht, E. (2007). Preliminary findings: behavioral worsening on donepezil in patients with frontotemporal dementia. *American Journal of Geriatric Psychiatry, 15,* 84–87. https://doi.org/10.1097/01. JGP.0000231744.69631.33

Mesulam M. M. (1986). Frontal cortex and behavior. *Annals of Neurology, 19*(4), 320–325. https://doi.org/10.1002/ana.410190403

Milberg, W. P., Hebben, N., & Kaplan, E. (2009). The Boston process approach to neuropsychological assessment. In K. Adams (Ed.), *Neuropsychological assessment of neuropsychiatric and neuromedical disorders* (pp. 42–65). Oxford University Press.

Mion, M., Patterson, K., Acosta-Cabronero, J., Pengas, G., Izquierdo-Garcia, D., Hong, Y. T., Fryer, T. D., Williams, G. B., Hodges, J. R., & Nestor, P. J. (2010). What the left and right anterior fusiform gyri tell us about semantic memory. *Brain, 133*(11), 3256–3268. https://doi.org/10.1093/brain/awq272

Morbelli, S., Ferrara, M., Fiz, F., Dessi, B., Arnaldi, D., Picco, A., Bossert, I., Buschiazzo, A., Accardo, J., Picori, L., Girtler, N., Mandich, P., Pagani, M., Sambuceti, G. & Nobili, F. (2016). Mapping brain morphological and functional conversion patterns in predementia late-onset bvFTD. *European Journal of Nuclear Medicine and Molecular Imaging, 43*(7):1337–1347. https://doi.org/10.1007/s00259-016-3335-3

National Institute for Health and Care Excellence. (2018). *Dementia: Assessment, management and support for people living with dementia and their carers.* NICE Guideline 97. NICE.

Neary, D., Snowden, J. S., Gustafson, L., Passant, U., Stuss, D., Black, S., Freedman, M., Kertesz, A., Robert, P. H., Albert, M., Boone, K., Miller, B. L., Cummings, J., & Benson, D. F. (1998). Frontotemporal lobar degeneration: a consensus on clinical diagnostic criteria. *Neurology, 51*(6), 1546–1554. https://doi.org/10.1212/wnl.51.6.1546

Neitzel, J., Ortner, M., Haupt, M., Redel, P., Grimmer, T., Yakushev, I., Drzezga, A., Bublak, P., Preul, C., Sorg, C., & Finke, K. (2016). Neuro-cognitive mechanisms of simultanagnosia in patients with posterior cortical atrophy. *Brain, 139*(Pt 12), 3267–3280. https://doi.org/10.1093/brain/aww235

Parker, G., Gridley, K., Birks, Y., & Glanville, J. (2020). Using a systematic review to uncover theory and outcomes for a complex intervention in health and social care: A worked example using life story work for people with dementia. *Journal of Health Services Research & Policy, 25*(4): 265–277. https://doi.org/10.1177/1355819619897091

Piguet, O., Hornberger, M., Mioshi, E., & Hodges, J. R. (2011). Behavioural variant frontotemporal dementia: Diagnosis, clinical staging and management. *Lancet Neurology, 10,* 162–172. https://doi.org/10.1016/S1474-4422(10)70299-4

Pozueta, A., Lage, C., García-Martínez, M., Kazimierczak, M., Bravo, M., López-García, S., Riancho, J., González-Suarez, A., Vázquez-Higuera, J. L., de Arcocha-Torres, M., Banzo, I., Jiménez-Bonilla, J., Berciano, J., Rodríguez-Rodríguez, E., & Sánchez-Juan, P. (2019). Cognitive and behavioral profiles of left and right semantic dementia: Differential diagnosis with behavioral variant frontotemporal dementia and Alzheimer's disease. *Journal of Alzheimer's Disease, 72*(4), 1129–1144. https://doi.org/10.3233/JAD-190877

Rascovsky, K., Hodges, J. R., Knopman, D., Mendez, M. F., Kramer, J. H., Neuhaus, J., van Swieten, J. C., Seelaar, H., Dopper, E. G., Onyike, C. U., Hillis, A. E., Josephs, K. A., Boeve, B. F., Kertesz, A., Seeley, W. W., Rankin, K. P., Johnson, J. K., Gorno-Tempini, M. L., Rosen, H., Prioleau-Latham, C. E., … Miller,

B. L. (2011). Sensitivity of revised diagnostic criteria for the behavioural variant of frontotemporal dementia. *Brain*, *134:* 2456–2477. https://doi.org/10.1093/brain/awr179

Rohrer, J. D., McNaught, E., Foster, J., Clegg, S. L., Barnes, J., Omar, R., Warrington, E. K., Rossor, M. N., Warren, J. D., & Fox, N. C. (2008). Tracking progression in frontotemporal lobar degeneration: Serial MRI in semantic dementia. *Neurology*, *71*(18), 1445–1451. https://doi.org/10.1212/01.wnl.0000327889.13734.cd

Shaik, S. S., & Varna, A. R. (2012). Differentiating the dementias: A neurological approach. *Progress in Neurology and Psychiatry*, *16*(1), 11–18. https://doi.org/10.1002/pnp.224

Snowden, J. S., Harris, J. M., Saxon, J. A., Thompson, J. C., Richardson, A. M., Jones, M., & Kobylecki, C. (2019). Naming and conceptual understanding in frontotemporal dementia. *Cortex*, *120*, 22–35. https://doi.org/10.1016/j.cortex.2019.04.027

Snowden, J. S., Harris, J. M., Thompson, J. C., Kobylecki, C., Jones, M., Richardson, A. M., & Neary, D. (2018). Semantic dementia and the left and right temporal lobes. *Cortex*, *107*, 188–203. https://doi.org/10.1016/j.cortex.2017.08.024

Snowden, J. S., Neary, D., & Mann, D. M. (2002). Frontotemporal dementia. *British Journal of Psychiatry*, *180*, 140–143. https://doi.org/10.1192/bjp.180.2.140

Snowden, J. S., Thompson, J. C. & Neary, D. (2004). Knowledge of famous faces and names in semantic dementia. *Brain*, *127*(4), 860–872. https://doi.org/10.1093/brain/awh099

Snowden, J. S., Thompson, J. C., Stopford, C. L., Richardson, A. M., Gerhard, A., Neary, D. & Mann, D. M. (2011). The clinical diagnosis of early-onset dementias: Diagnostic accuracy and clinicopathological relationships. *Brain*, *134*(9), 2478–2492. https://doi.org/10.1093/brain/awr189

Stopford, C. L., Thompson, J. C., Neary, D., Richardson, A. M., & Snowden, J. S. (2012). Working memory, attention, and executive function in Alzheimer's disease and frontotemporal dementia. *Cortex*, *48*(4), 429–446. https://doi.org/10.1016/j.cortex.2010.12.002

Thompson, S. A., Patterson, K., & Hodges, J. R. (2003). Left/right asymmetry of atrophy in semantic dementia: Behavioral-cognitive implications. *Neurology*, *61*, 1196–1203. https://doi.org/10.1212/01.wnl.0000091868.28557.b8

Thompson, J. C., Stopford, C. L., Snowden, J. S., & Neary, D. (2005). Qualitative neuropsychological performance characteristics in frontotemporal dementia and Alzheimer's disease. *Journal of Neurology, Neurosurgery & Psychiatry*, *76*(7), 920–927. https://doi.org/10.1136/jnnp.2003.033779

Ulugut-Erkoyun, H., Groot, C., Heilbron, R., Nelissen, A., van Rossum, J., Jutten, R., Koene, T., van der Flier, W. M., Wattjes, M. P., Scheltens, P., Ossenkoppele, R., Barkhof, F., & Pijnenburg, Y. (2020). A clinical–radiological framework of the right temporal variant of frontotemporal dementia. *Brain*, *143*(9), 2831–2843. https://doi.org/10.1093/brain/awaa225

Wilson, B., & Betteridge, S. (2019). *Essentials of neuropsychological rehabilitation*. Guilford Press.

Woollams, A. M., Cooper-Pye, E., Hodges, J. R., & Patterson, K. (2008). Anomia: A doubly typical signature of semantic dementia. *Neuropsychologia*, *46*(10), 2503–2514. https://doi.org/10.1016/j.neuropsychologia.2008.04.005

Wylie, M. A., Shnall, A., Onyike, C. U., & Huey, E. D. (2013). Management of frontotemporal dementia in mental health and multidisciplinary settings. *International Review of Psychiatry*, *25*(2), 230–236. https://doi.org/10.3109/09540261.2013.776949

References: tests and analyses

Baron-Cohen, S., Wheelwright, S., Hill, J., Raste, Y., & Plumb, I. (2001). The 'Reading the Mind in the Eyes' Test revised version: A study with normal adults and adults with Asperger syndrome or high-functioning autism. *Journal of Child Psychology & Psychiatry, 42*(2), 241–251.

Burgess, P. W., & Shallice, T. (1997). *The Hayling and Brixton tests.* Thames Valley Test Company.

Delis, D. C., Kaplan, E., & Kramer, J. H. (2001). *The Delis–Kaplan executive function system: Examiner's manual.* The Psychological Corporation.

Howard, D., & Patterson, K. (1992). *The Pyramids and Palm Trees Test: A test for semantic access from words and pictures.* Thames Valley Test Company.

James, M., Plant, G. T., & Warrington, E. K. (2001). *CORVIST: Cortical vision screening test.* Thames Valley Test Company.

Randolph, C. (2012). *Repeatable battery for the assessment of neuropsychological status update (RBANS Update).* The Psychological Corporation.

Warrington, E. K., & James, M. (1991). *The visual object and space perception battery.* Thames Valley Test Company.

Wechsler, D. (2010). *Test of pre-morbid functioning UK version (ToPF-UK).* Pearson.

Wechsler, D. (2010). *Wechsler Adult Intelligence Scale UK* (4th ed.) *(WAIS-IV-UK).* Pearson.

Wechsler, D. (2010). *Wechsler Memory Scale UK* (4th ed.) *(WMS-IV-UK).* Pearson Ltd.

Wilson, B., Alderman, N., Burgess, P., Emslie, H., & Evans, J. (1996). *Behavioural assessment of the dysexecutive syndrome (BADS).* Thames Valley Test Company

Zigmond, A. S., & Snaith, R. P. (1983). The Hospital Anxiety and Depression scale. *Acta Psychiatrica Scandinavica, 67*(6), 361–370. https://doi.org/10.1111/j.1600-0447.1983.tb09716.x

6 A life in *Portrait* mode

Living with Balint's syndrome

Jwala Narayanan

Introduction

Balint's syndrome is a rare neuropsychological syndrome, first described by Reszo Bálint, a Hungarian psychiatrist and neurologist (Bálint, 1909). The syndrome is characterised by a triad of features: impaired visually guided reaching (optic ataxia), impaired voluntary eye movements (optic apraxia), and impaired processing of more than one stimulus in a scene (simultanagnosia). The common pathology in Balint's syndrome consists of bilateral infarcts in the watershed area between the territory of the middle and posterior communicating arteries (Rafal, 2003). The reported aetiologies have been diverse and interesting. Between 1900 and the 1950s vascular lesions and trauma (gunshot injuries) were the common causes. From the 1950s to 2021 there have been reports of vascular lesions, trauma, tumours, demyelinating disorders, epilepsy, Creutzfeldt-Jacob disease, cardiac arrest, anoxia, systemic hypotension, and more recently, COVID-related stroke leading to Balint's syndrome (Jacob et al., 2002 Bhattacharya, 2015; Parvathaneni & Das, 2022; Narayanan et al., 2020). Ghoneim et al. (2018) also reported an idiopathic case, wherein the patient reported no preceding brain insult before developing Balint's syndrome. Typically, Balint's syndrome follows damage to bilateral parietal lobes and parieto-occipital regions (Bálint, 1909; Hecaen & De Ajuriaguerra, 1954; Rafal, 2003; Rizzo & Vecera, 2002; Chechlacz et al., 2012.)

Rizzo and Vecera (2002), in their detailed account of the psychological and anatomical substrates of Balint's syndrome, conclude as follows:

> Visual cues convey a wealth of information on physical objects and their relations. We construct our reality from serial glimpses, and our impression of a seamless and richly detailed visual world is an illusion. Damage to visual cortex and white matter in Bálint's syndrome can destroy this illusion, resulting in a piecemeal experience of the visual world (simultanagnosia/visual disorientation) and impaired visual control of eye movements (ocular apraxia) and hand movements (optic ataxia).
>
> (p. 175)

DOI: 10.4324/9781003228226-7

The impact of Balint's syndrome is often so serious that patients appear to behave as if they are blind (Kerkhoff & Heldmann, 1999). They may walk with their hands outstretched to feel their way around, they may bump into things and may need assistance for vision-related tasks. While some patients have no awareness of their visual deficits, others may feel they are blind, despite being partly able to see. The syndrome can be extremely disabling even when other cognitive domains are well functioning. People can have difficulty with basic abilities including walking, judging bumps on the road, finding things around the house, pouring water for themselves, and more complex tasks like cooking, using a phone, and reading.

The other cognitive deficits often reported with the classic triad of Balint's syndrome are of working memory, apraxia, hemispatial neglect, prosopagnosia, anosognosia, and in a few patients apperceptive agnosia (Rose et al., 2016; Wilson et al., 1997; Jacob et al., 2002; Narayanan et al., 2020).

The Balint's syndrome literature is dominated by case reports, hence there are no clear data on its prevalence. Only a few studies give a detailed description of the condition, its impact on everyday life and rehabilitation (Bálint, 1909; Rose et al., 2016; Wilson, 2009). Although the syndrome is rare, it can be diverse in its presentation, aetiologies, neural substrates, and recovery. Chechlacz and Humphreys (2014) and Rizzo and Vecera (2002), in their examinations of Balint's syndrome, evaluated underlying mechanisms to the functional deficits and emphasised the need for better understanding of the condition. Rizzo and Vecera (2002) described each of the symptoms seen in Balint's syndrome and proposed the possible interactions of visuoperceptual deficits with other cognitive deficits, including attention and working memory impairments that contribute to the experience of this syndrome. They suggest that the experience of vision is a result of complex interactions across brain networks and hence Balint's syndrome cannot be simply explained by damage to one area.

There are few cases that have reported full recovery from Balint's syndrome, and such cases usually occur following a temporary ischaemia. In most cases, the prognosis is poor. Patients usually have to compensate for their deficits, live in altered environments, and need some assistance (Parvanthaneni & Das, 2022).

Some retraining exercises include visual scanning and frequent practice in reading. Task-specific retraining (e.g. route finding, dressing, or using public transport) have been shown to improve independent functioning (AL-Khawaja & Haboubi, 2001). However, most rehabilitation interventions include compensatory strategies, the use of assistive technology, and altering the environment so that patients can be more independent (Heutink et al., 2019).

The case of QB is unique because she is the only reported case of Balint's syndrome that we are aware of following Dengue encephalitis. She is one of the younger cases to have been diagnosed with Balint's syndrome, and is also struggling with apperceptive agnosia. KV was one of the first cases of Balint's syndrome to have been reported following COVID-related stroke

(Narayanan et al., 2020), and there have been a few more COVID-related cases reported subsequently (Panico et al., 2020; Storti et al., 2021.

Clinical presentation

QB was 18 years of age when she presented with a diagnosis of Dengue encephalitis, and an incidental diagnosis of diabetic ketoacidosis in the July of 2019. She was hospitalised for over a month, requiring intensive care for a large proportion of her admission. She experienced seizures and was not completely alert or oriented; she had to be intubated and was put on mechanical ventilation. Her MRI was reported as showing *diffuse neuroparenchymal atrophy*. She was medically stable by the end of August 2019 and was discharged from the hospital. Another MRI at discharge indicated *bilateral symmetrical cortical hyperintensities* involving predominantly the parieto-occipital lobes and a few gyri in the right fronto-temporal region. At discharge she was alert, ambulant, and oriented. She was diagnosed with cortical blindness by her neurologist and referred to neuropsychology for rehabilitation.

KV tested COVID-19 positive in April 2020, aged 62. She developed acute respiratory distress syndrome and was on ventilator support for 45 days. She then developed sepsis with multi-organ dysfunction and acute kidney failure. She subsequently suffered a haemorrhagic stroke affecting bilateral parieto-occipital regions. Her MRI indicated *hyperintense signals corresponding to bilateral watershed pattern of infarcts*, especially involving parieto-occipital regions. She required medical intervention to manage bilateral internal jugular vein thrombus, adrenal insufficiency, sleep disturbance, agitation, and restlessness. She further received physiotherapy and occupational therapy to improve her range of movement, sitting balance, and strengthening of all four limbs. When admitted to the neurorehabilitation unit, it was noted that her vision was poor and that she could only identify red light at 3 inches from her face. At discharge from the neurorehabilitation unit, her vision was improving, although blurred, and she was diagnosed with cortical blindness. KV presented to us in a wheelchair. She complained of poor vision and feeling 'blind'. She also reported being in pain and discomfort. She was unable to carry out chores independently and required assistance for self-care. She has been on medication (duloxetine) for a depressive disorder for ten years. She was diagnosed with hypothyroidism about two years ago and has been managed well with medication (thyronorm 25mg). She has also been on medication for vertigo for about a year prior to her admission in 2020.

Background

QB grew up in a small town in the state of Karnataka, India. She came to Bangalore aged 18 to start a Bachelor's degree in Architecture. She was admitted in hospital on what should have been her first day at university. Her parents described her as a very active and social person. She loved to dance and enjoyed engaging in creative activities, including sketching and painting. She was a diligent student, meticulous, and a *perfectionist*. Her mother described her as mature and responsible; she often oversaw household chores as her mother was a busy doctor. Just like any teenager she liked shopping, spending time with friends, and dressing up.

KV grew up in the Eastern part of India but later moved to Bangalore. She completed a Master's degree in history and certificate courses in teaching. She had a difficult childhood and a troubled marriage. However, she was strong willed and raised her children as a single parent. She also had a successful career as an educationist, including teaching children with special needs, developing and designing curricula, and teacher training. At the time of her illness, aged 62, she was living with her son, daughter-in-law, and granddaughter. Her family described her as being an active, independent, and social person.

QB's and KV's visual deficits and their impact on daily life

QB's and KV's visual abilities at discharge were very limited. For the initial few days at home, they could only differentiate light from dark. When they came to the neuropsychology service, they were able to see form and some shapes; however, they could not always identify the edges of forms. They found locating items in space quite difficult. They had difficulty identifying shapes and colours.

Their lives had been completely turned upside down. From being very independent people, a young lady who was used to running the house for her mother, and a mother who raised her children and looked after her granddaughter, they had now both become extremely dependent on their families. They had to be accompanied everywhere they went. They could not take a walk without holding on to someone. They were unable to find their things around the house, and they needed help for self-care activities, including bathing, putting toothpaste on the toothbrush, and dressing. They also needed help eating and serving themselves food. QB was unable to return to college, she wanted to pursue studies in Architecture but her family deferred her admission. QB's biggest disappointment was her inability to connect with her friends and her loss of privacy, as all her calls and messages had to be coordinated by her parents. KV was unable to return to work, or engage in zentangling (a form of meditative art using structured drawing patterns), a hobby she had taken up recently.

Over two years, both have shown some recovery, have adapted well to their condition, and are working hard to lead independent lives as far as possible. KV and QB describe their vision as being blurred and some aspects that come into focus to be clearer. QB described this as seeing things in a *portrait* camera mode, wherein you can focus on a particular object by blurring the background.

Balint's syndrome and the impact it has had on their families

Balint's syndrome has impacted both QB's and KV's families. QB's family initially travelled to various doctors seeking advice and therapies. It was particularly difficult for the parents to see QB so incapacitated. They had expected QB to recover completely in a few months and didn't think her difficulties would continue to considerably change her life. QB's mother was particularly affected as she was very proud of her independent and capable daughter. She took a break from work and tried transfer location to be closer to QB.

For KV, who had always been a fighter and had always found ways to sail through difficult times on her own, being faced with a condition that made her highly dependent on others, even for seemingly minor self-care activities, was a major challenge. This impacted her identity to a large extent, and to that of her family, who needed to engage full-time care for KV. All are still adapting to this change.

Neuropsychological assessment

A summary of the neuropsychological assessment for QB and KV can be found in Table 6.1. Their performance on neuropsychological tests differed, possibly due to the extent of pathology. KV's stroke seemed to involve a larger area of the brain, likely affecting a number of cognitive functions, while QB's impairment was more specific to tests related to vision and working memory.

KV and QB presented approximately a month after their brain injuries. They were both oriented to person and place. KV was not oriented to time, while QB was. They were cooperative with testing and responded to questions appropriately, though KV's speech was tangential. They both had difficulty organising their thoughts and expressing themselves coherently. KV was confused about the sequence of events in her life; when asked about her current job, she described a job she had been doing about five years ago, although she acknowledged the work she was doing prior to her stroke when specifically asked about it. QB seemed better oriented to the series of events in her life prior to the injury.

Their speech was generally fluent, although both displayed word-finding difficulty at the time of presentation. Their comprehension seemed relatively preserved. They both seemed to have awareness about their difficulties, but their account of the experience of their vision was impoverished. During conversations, they would both look in the general direction of people speaking to them but struggled to make eye contact. KV often indicated she was blind and hoped her vision would return. KV was able to recognise familiar faces and objects displayed to her. QB reported she could see, although she indicated that her difficulty was more apparent to her when she was carrying out an activity or was being tested. QB found it difficult to recognise faces and objects when presented to her; she initially denied having these difficulties, and it was only known to her when we tested her.

Table 6.1 QB's and KV's neuropsychological test findings

Test	QB'S raw score	QB's statistic scores & comments	KV'S raw score	Statistic scores & comments
Memory				
AVLT learning trails	4,8,12,14,15,15/15		1,4,3,3,5/15	
AVLT total learning	68/75	75th %ile	16/75	<5th %ile
AVLT trial delayed recall	15/15	>95th %ile	0/15	<5th %ile
Recognition	15/15	>95th %ile	6/15	<5th %ile
Famous faces	0/33	<5th %ile	12/30	5th %ile
Modified naming test★	4/30	<5th %ile	17/30	5th %ile
Visuospatial ability				
Motor free visual perception test – picture matching	discontinued		discontinued	
Corsi blocks (WMS III)	0	<5th %ile	0	<5th %ile
VOSP	**score**	**cutoff**	**score**	**cutoff**
Screening	18	15	6	15
Incomplete letters	1	17	1	17
Silhouettes	0	16	1	16
Object decision	0	15	0	15
Progressive silhouettes	0	14	0	14
Dot counting	0	8	1	8
Position discrimination	13	15	9	15
Number location	0	7	0	7
Cube analysis	1	6	0	6
Executive functions and intellectual functioning				
Digit span forward	6 (span – 4)		10 (span – 6)	
Digit span backward	4 (span – 3)		2 (span – 2)	
Digit span total	10	Scaled score 5	12	Scaled score 7
Vocabulary	37	Scaled score 10	20	Scaled score 6
Arithmetic	6	Scaled score 4	6	Scaled score 4
Similarities	26	Scaled score 12	20	Scaled score 10

KV and QB were severely impaired on tests of visual perception including the visual object and space perception (VOSP) battery (Warrington & James, 1991), the Corsi block tapping test from the Wechsler Memory Scale (WMS III), and the motor free visual perception test (MVPT-3; Colarusso & Hammill, 2003). The MVPT-3 had to be discontinued as they were unable to see pictures in order to match similar-looking designs. On the Corsi block tapping test, they were unable to reach out and tap even one block accurately. On the VOSP, KV was below cut-off values on all subtests. KV also failed the screening test of the VOSP, where she was required to detect a fragmented 'X' amongst a noisy background. Passing this test is an indication that there is no gross deficit of visual acuity (Warrington & James, 1991). KV was unable to recognise any of the items from the silhouettes subtest except the camel; she identified all the animals as 'animals', and the others as not being animals. In the progressive silhouettes subtest, she was only able to identify the object (a gun) on the final, complete, representation. QB did a little better than KV on the screening test of the VOSP; however, all her other scores fell under cut-off values and her performance was at floor. Unlike KV, QB was unable to identify any silhouettes. Their poor performance on the visual perception tests seemed in part secondary to a difficulty in visually fixating on an object and finding it in space. QB seemed to also have difficulty in perceiving the gestalt, indicative of apperceptive agnosia.

Owing to her apperceptive agnosia, QB was unable to read words or identify single letters. She was able to write, but unable to see or read what she was writing. KV denied being able to read; however, when she was presented with words she would read them or call them out without realising she had read the word accurately. However, KV was unable to read sentences, secondary to her simultanagnosia.

QB and KV displayed simultanagnosia when asked to identify an array of objects presented in front of them. They were only able to *see* one or two objects at a time. They would need prompting to scan the table to try and identify other objects. Simultanagnosia was also evident on the dot counting test from the VOSP, and when asked to describe the Cookie Theft Picture, KV reported seeing a *chef* in the picture and nothing further. QB indicated not being able to identify anything and seeing *dots* and *blotches* on the Cookie Theft Picture. They also showed great difficulty while reaching for things on a table; they would reach out in the direction of the object, but miss it by a few inches.

An object-naming test and a test of famous faces were administered to both KV and QB. KV identified 12/30 of the faces and QB was unable to identify any face. The famous faces test consists of 30 people rated as being famous amongst adults in urban Bangalore. The test stimuli include politicians, actors, freedom fighters, sports personalities, industrial entrepreneurs, and spiritual leaders. The object-naming test consists of 30 pictures of objects culturally appropriate for urban Bangalore with varying word frequency. KV identified 17/30 objects accurately, while QB was able to identify only four objects. She was only able to name pictures that were visually unique and had colour cues to help identify the image (e.g. the tricolours of the Indian national flag, the head of a pineapple, grapes, and a star). When these objects/famous people were presented to her via verbal description, she was able to identify and name them without much difficulty indicating no general semantic memory deficits. Unlike QB, KV did not seem to have apperceptive agnosia based on her ability to perceive a person in the cookie theft picture, and her ability to identify famous faces (12/30) and name objects (17/30). Her inability to name all of the faces/objects appeared secondary to being unable to focus on the cards, naming difficulty and fatigue.

On other tests of cognitive function, KV and QB showed mild deficits on tests of working memory including Digit Span backward and the Arithmetic subtest of the Wechsler Abbreviated Intelligence Scale (WAIS) III. KV had a span of six digits forwards, but only two backwards. QB had a span of four forward and three backwards. They both had a scaled score of four for Arithmetic. QB also struggled with spelling.

QB's performance on a verbal learning and memory task (WHO–UCLA Auditory Verbal Learning Test) was above average. Her performance was at ceiling for short–term and delayed recall. Her excellent memory ability was also reflected in her learning of new tasks. However, KV displayed impairment in verbal learning and memory on the same task. QB and KV both showed relatively spared performance on the WAIS III Vocabulary and Similarities subtests.

Rehabilitation

The process of rehabilitation began with psychoeducation – providing information about the brain injury and the process of rehabilitation. QB, KV, and their families were introduced to the diagnosis of Balint's syndrome and explained the difficulties they were having. They were also given information about the condition and resources for their own reading. The initial few sessions involved goal setting, which was discussed with QB, KV, and their families. Making adjustments to the home environment, including de-cluttering spaces and maintaining safety, was emphasised. The weekly sessions included setting goals for the week and assigning exercises that they carried out with assistant psychologists or family on a daily basis.

One of the earliest exercises we gave them was colour and form recognition. Their cortical blindness seemed to be improving and they were soon able to identify colour with minimal error. Their ability to recognise form improved in the first few weeks. QB still struggles with irregular shapes or objects out of context. QB tends to use her general intelligence and memory well to identify things around her. One of her early goals was to read and hence she worked on exercises to read numbers and alphabets. She learnt numbers 0 to 9 within a few days, but when presented in different fonts, she was unable to recognise them. She was trained on numbers across fonts and she seemed to be able to recognise numbers in different fonts and handwriting within an average of about five seconds for a number. The same process was carried out with the alphabet. However, she found this much more challenging.

Both patients were given exercises to locate things in space and try to differentiate one from the other. The therapist would keep objects in different parts of the room and they would have to scan and locate the objects. Another scanning exercise included different coloured panels in a row and they would have to name each colour from left to right. This task helped them focus (increase awareness) on object boundaries, moving their gaze from one object to another. This exercise was found to generalise to other activities in everyday life. QB also enjoyed playing some card games including *UNO* and *Fletter* that reinforced her exercises in therapy, improving her ability to recognise numbers and word building.

About eight months following QB's rehabilitation, it was time for her to think about going back to college. We had sessions to discuss various career options and courses and she decided she wanted to do a course that interested her rather than thinking of a career. She was interested in journalism and public affairs and hence chose to study International Relations.

KV's goals concerned activities of daily living (ADLs), including walking without support, jogging, serving herself food, being independent using the toilet, and pouring herself a glass of water. Each of these activities was broken into steps and carried out in a sequential manner to facilitate independent performance. She also wanted to engage in activities related to her work. She discussed the possibilities of running workshops on life skills for children. Training for these workshops was also part of the rehabilitation programme with psychology assistants.

Assistive technology

QB was resistant to any type of assistive technology early in her rehabilitation. She was very keen on exercising and retraining her vision. She wanted to be able to see everything on her own. The idea of using technology or any assistive aids upset her greatly. Nevertheless, she became more flexible in her views over time and the first assistive technology she agreed to use was voice-to-text and text-to-voice on her phone – this gave her the freedom to communicate with her friends directly without a mediator! The software was hard to use initially, but she soon got used to it. As she was unable to read the names of her friends in the contact list, she saved their names with an emoticon that helped her identify who she wanted to call; e.g., her mother was represented by a red heart alongside the name, and my own name had a green heart next to it.

We looked at various technology options for QB's studies. The family did some research and we also liaised with people with low vision on the best technology for QB. She finally settled on an iPad, since it seemed to be the most user friendly and with superior voice command technology compared to other similar devices.

By the time QB applied for her course, the COVID-19 pandemic had begun. This worked to her advantage in some respect – she had time to get into the college routine and had the time and space to make new friends virtually.

The Amazon *Echo Dot* also proved to be very helpful to KV. She uses it to keep reminders, make lists, and obtain information. She listens to podcasts and audiobooks as a substitute to reading, which she still misses. As she found using the phone extremely confusing and effortful, she is still not independent in using it. However, she keeps in touch with friends and family by sending/receiving voice messages, which she treasures.

Other assistive technology resources

There is a wide range of assistive technology devices and apps available for people with low vision and the blind. As noted, the iPad came highly recommended and was found to be useful. The OrCam also seemed like a promising product – however, was not pursued as QB was not ready to use an external aid and we thought it may have been a little complex for KV given her other cognitive deficits. The OrCam is also an expensive investment, as patient families would have to pay for it themselves. OrCam is a wearable device with a camera attached that can be fitted onto a pair of glasses (see www.orcam.com/en/myeye2/). It recognises objects, people, and things around you and it can also read and feedback to the individual through voice output. Another helpful device is the Amazon *Echo Show*, an interactive device like the *Echo Dot* that has a show-and-tell feature. An individual can show an item to the device and it would recognise the object and name it; it even reads labels. Both devices seemed ideal for QB, particularly given her apperceptive agnosia, which makes it difficult for her to recognise objects; however, QB still wanted to use her own skills rather than relying on technology. KV is using the *Echo Dot* and she finds it very useful for accessing information and keeping reminders. She described it as her *bodyguard* and reported that she felt more independent using it. There are a few apps that are potentially more accessible than stand-alone devices in low-cost settings. *Aipoly*, an app using the camera feature of smartphones, is helpful to point and capture something to get more information about it. Another *heart-warming* app is *Be My Eyes*. Here the individual points and takes a picture of something and volunteers from around the world identify it or read it out to the individual. These are just a few examples of some of the technologies out there and it is certainly not an exhaustive list. Another helpful source is Professor Gordon Dutton's website on cerebral visual impairment, https://cvi.aphtech.org/. It is an excellent resource to share with patients and their family to understand visual impairments better and to find resources that may be relevant to them.

Other therapies and activities

QB joined a gym and a contemporary dance class that she really enjoyed. In both, she had teachers who were very supportive and understanding. QB found they helped elevate her mood. She has also been working with a visual therapist, who has been working more specifically on reading. She can now read three letter words, although it is still time consuming and effortful.

KV had regular physiotherapy and occupational therapy for her physical difficulties. She made good progress and is now able to jog and use her right lower limb more effectively, although she still struggles with fine motor skills. She also underwent Ayurvedic treatment and consulted alternate healing therapists, who contributed to her improvement as reported by her and the family. In addition, KV is also part of regular meditation and spiritual practices that she attends via Zoom calls.

At the time of writing

QB is pursuing a graduation degree in International Relations. She requires a scribe for exams but is able to attend classes and complete assignments with little assistance. She is able to find things around the house, is fairly independent with most ADLs, including applying make-up. She takes the dog for a walk and is able to walk independently and carefully. She remains unable to read signs or recognise people. She can identify most numbers and letters if given some time. Her optic ataxia seems to have improved, although it is still present and her oculomotor apraxia also seems to have improved. She continues to have simultanagnosia. She remains unable to type on her mobile phone. QB is intelligent and tries to compensate for her deficits using cues; she works hard, but is easily discouraged if she makes errors.

KV is able to do most self-care activities on her own, with supervision from a carer. She is able to find most of her things on her own, but may require some assistance at times. She uses the *Echo Dot* for reminders and information, and this gives her a great sense of independence. With the help of the assistant psychologists, KV has been working on curating and delivering life skills workshops for children via Zoom. She has conducted three such workshops successfully. She is also working on narrating her story for a book.

Conclusion

Balint's syndrome is a rare condition that can be easily missed or misdiagnosed. It can present following various aetiologies and can present along with other visuoperceptual disorders (e.g. apperceptive agnosia/neglect) and other cognitive deficits (e.g. working memory impairment). The approach to rehabilitation is a combination of compensatory strategies, changes in environment, using assistive technology, and retraining exercises (e.g. scanning). Rehabilitation needs to be tailored to the needs of the individual, bearing in mind their socio-cultural background, interests, and aspirations. Psycho-education about Balint's syndrome to the patient and family is an important aspect of the process of rehabilitation. Conveying the prognosis of Balint's syndrome can be challenging. Although complete recovery has been observed in some, in many cases full recovery may not be possible and patients may have to adjust to living with Balint's syndrome. Even though much of the evidence points in the direction of compensatory strategies, education, and altering the environment, QB, KV, and their families were not ready to accept such suggestions in the early stages of rehabilitation. For QB and her mother, accepting assistive technology meant accepting defeat. QB was highly motivated to engage in retraining exercises, even though they were effortful and tiring. The retraining sessions gave them hope in some sense. KV indicates that her vision is much better when she reminds herself to 'focus' or 'sharp focus'. QB says that she has adapted well, and feels her vision is better, but still sees things in 'portrait mode', hence the title to this chapter.

Acknowledgements

I would like to thank QB and KV and their families for consenting to the reporting of their cases. I am grateful to Prof. Narinder Kapur for his comments on the first draft of this chapter. I would like to acknowledge all the hard work by the assistant psychologists, Vyushti Johari, Priyanka Kuppuswamy, Vandhana Easwaran, and Divya Pawar who have worked closely with QB and KV through their rehabilitation.

References

AL-Khawaja, I., & Haboubi, N. H. J. (2001). Neurovisual rehabilitation in Balint's syndrome. *Journal of Neurology, Neurosurgery & Psychiatry, 70*, 416.

Bálint, R. (1909). Seelenlähmung des 'Schauens', optische Ataxie, räumliche Störung der Aufmerksamkeit. *Monatschrift für Psychiatrie und Neurologie, 25*, 51–181.

Bhattacharya, A., Rao, B. B., & Fasanella, K. E. (2015). Balint's syndrome with metastatic pancreatic cancer: A case report. *American Journal of Gastroenterology, 110*, S74–S75.

Chechlacz, M., Rotshtein, P., Hansen, P. C., Riddoch, J. M., Deb, S., & Humphreys, G. W. (2012). The neural underpinnings of simultanagnosia: Disconnecting the visuospatial attention network. *Journal of Cognitive Neuroscience, 24*, 718–735. https://doi.org/10.1162/jocn_a_00159

Chechlacz, M., & Humphreys, G. W. (2014). The enigma of Balint's syndrome: Neural substrates and cognitive deficits. *Frontiers in Human Neuroscience, 8*, 123.

Colarusso, R.P., & Hammill, D. D. (2003). *Motor-free visual perception test. 3*. Academic Therapy Publications.

Ghoneim, A., Pollard, C., Greene, J., & Jampana, R. (2018). Balint syndrome (chronic visual–spatial disorder) presenting without known cause. *Radiology Case Reports Journal, 13*, 1242–1245.

Hécaen, H., & de Ajuriaguerra, J. (1954). Bálint's syndrome (psychic paralysis of visual fixation) and its minor forms. *Brain*, *77*, 373–400.

Heutink, J., Indorf, D. L., & Cordes, C. (2019). The neuropsychological rehabilitation of visual agnosia and Balint's syndrome. *Neuropsychological Rehabilitation*, *29*(10), 1489–1508. https://doi.org/10.1080/09602011.2017.1422272

Jacob, S. S., Jacob, S., Albornoz, A. M., & Biswas, D. (2002). Bálint's syndrome – missed or mistaken?, Letter to the Editor. *American Journal of Medicine*, *112*, 509–510.

Kerkhoff, G., & Heldmann, B. (1999). Balint-Syndrom und assoziierte Störungen. Anamnese–Diagnostik–Behandlungsansätze [Balint syndrome and associated disorders. Anamnesis–diagnosis–approaches to treatment]. Nervenarz, *70*(10), 859–69. [German]

Narayanan, J., Wilson, B. A., & Evans, J. J. (2020). A case of Balint's syndrome after Covid-19. *Newsletter of the International Neuropsychological Society*, *3*, 27–31.

Parvathaneni, A. M., & Das, J. (2022). *Balint syndrome.* [Updated 2021, June 30]. StatPearls [Online]. StatPearls Publishing. www.ncbi.nlm.nih.gov/books/NBK544347/#_NBK544347_pubdet_

Panico, F., Arini, A., Cantone, P. Crisci, C., & Trojano, L. (2020). Balint-Holmes syndrome due to stroke following SARS-CoV-2 infection: A single-case report. *Neurological Sciences*, *41*(12), 3487–3489. https://doi.org/10.1007/s10072-020-04860-1

Rafal, R. (2003). Balint's syndrome: A disorder of visual cognition. In M. D'Esposito (Ed.), *Neurological foundations of cognitive neuroscience* (27–40). MIT Press.

Rizzo, M., & Vecera, S. P. (2002). Psychoanatomical substrates of Balint's syndrome. *Journal of Neurology, Neurosurgery and Psychiatry*, *72*, 162–178.

Rose, A., Wilson, B. A., Manolov, R., & Florschutz, G. (2016). Seeing red: Relearning to read in a case of Balint's syndrome. *NeuroRehabilitation*, *39*(1), 111–117.

Storti, B., Cereda, D., Balducci, C. Santangelo, F., Ferrarese, C., & Appollonio, I. (2021). Who is really blind in the time of coronavirus: The patient or the doctor? A rare case of Balint's syndrome. *Neurological Sciences*, *42*, 2079–2080. doi.org/10.1007/s10072-020-04934-0

Warrington, E. K., & James, M. (1988). Visual apperceptive agnosia: A clinico-anatomical study of three cases. *Cortex*, *24*, 13–32.

Wilson, B. A., Clare, L., Young, A. W., & Hodges, J. R. (1997). Knowing where and knowing what: A double dissociation. *Cortex*, *33* (3), 529–541.

Wilson, B. (2009). Malcolm: Coping with the effects of Balint's syndrome and topographical disorientation. In B. Wilson, F. Gracey, J. Evans, & A. Bateman (Eds), *Neuropsychological rehabilitation: Theory, models, therapy and outcome* (pp. 304–316). Cambridge University Press. https://doi.org/10.1017/CBO9780511581083.022

7 Exploring the unknown

Shared discovery in rare mitochondrial disease

Ben Marram

Introduction

Human genetics and mitochondria

An organism's complete set of deoxyribonucleic acid (DNA) is referred to as a genome, or all of the genetic material of an organism. A chromosome is a long DNA molecule of which there are 23 pairs (the twenty-third of which determines sex, e.g. XX and XY). When thinking about the contribution of a segment of DNA to our functioning, we refer to this as a gene. These are important terms in how we begin to understand the nature of mitochondrial disease. Genes are composed of DNA and each rung or ladder consists of two paired chemicals called 'bases'. Each individual has thousands of genes and billions of base pairs of DNA and these determine individual characteristics which we refer to as genetic traits (Lewis, 2016).

Mitochondria and mitochondrial disease

Mitochondrial diseases are chronic, genetic, often inherited disorders that occur when mitochondria fail to produce enough energy for the body to function properly. They create energy from fuel (i.e. food) and oxygen for virtually every human cell. Although most of the cell's DNA is contained in the cell nucleus (or what is referred to as nuclear DNA), the mitochondrion has its own independent genome (mtDNA). Mitochondrial diseases are highly heterogeneous conditions as a consequence of significant variability in mtDNA gene mutation. As a result, the symptoms of the condition can affect any major organ in the human body that uses a lot of energy, such as the brain. Symptoms of impaired brain function include seizures, myoclonus, stroke, dementia, and migraine (McFarland et al., 2010). Vast efforts are taking place to catalogue the significant number of potential mitochondrial mutations and estimates suggest that mitochondrial mutations affect a minimum of 1 in 10,000 adults in the UK (Schaefer et al., 2008), although other reports suggest the burden of disease may be much more common (Abramov et al., 2010).

DOI: 10.4324/9781003228226-8

What causes mitochondrial disease?

Under normal circumstances, a child inherits genes in pairs; one each from the mother and father. A child with a mitochondrial disease does not receive a normal pair of genes from the parents (Rötig & Poulton, 2009). Learning the way in which a mitochondrial disease has been inherited helps predict the chance of passing on the disease(s) to future children (Rötig & Poulton, 2009). In autosomal recessive inheritance, the child receives one mutated copy of a gene from each parent. In autosomal dominant inheritance, the child receives one mutated copy of a gene from either parent. Sometimes genes develop a mutation of their own that is not inherited from a parent. Mitochondrial inheritance is more unique; the mitochondria contain their own DNA (mtDNA). Only mitochondrial disorders caused by mutations in the mitochondrial DNA are exclusively inherited from mothers. If this is the way a mitochondrial disease was inherited, there is a 100% chance that each child in the family will inherit a mitochondrial disease.

Grier et al. (2018) found that patients saw on average eight clinicians before receiving a diagnosis of mitochondrial disease. The first clinician consulted was typically a primary care physician (56.7%), although 35.2% initially sought a specialist. A neurologist delivered the diagnosis in 55.2% of cases, a clinical geneticist in 18.2%, and a metabolic disease specialist in 11.8%. A majority (54.6%) received 1 or more non-mitochondrial diagnoses before their final mitochondrial diagnosis. In their pursuit of a diagnosis, 84.8% of participants received blood tests, 71% a muscle biopsy, 60.5% MRI, and 38.6% urine organic acids. In addition, 39.5% underwent mitochondrial DNA sequencing, 19% sequencing of nuclear gene(s), and 11.4% whole-exome sequencing. This demonstrates the diagnostic odyssey of patients with mitochondrial disease is complex and burdensome. It features multiple consultations and tests, and, often, conflicting diagnoses. These reflect disease variety, diagnostic uncertainty, and clinician unfamiliarity. With the introduction of specialist centres and increased knowledge of mitochondrial-related conditions this is improving.

Mitochondrial myopathy, encephalopathy, lactic acidosis, and stroke-like episodes (MELAS)

MELAS syndrome is a mitochondrial multisystem disorder caused by the A3243G mutation (Karkare et al., 2009). It is associated with stroke-like episodes before the age of 40, encephalopathy with epileptic seizures, dementia, or both (Kraya et al., 2019). These episodes occur in 84–99% of affected individuals and present clinically with partially reversible aphasia, cortical vision loss, motor weakness, headaches, altered mental status, and seizures (El-Hattab et al., 2015). The affected areas in neuroimaging do not correspond to classic vascular distribution, are asymmetric, involve predominantly the temporal, parietal, and occipital lobes and can be restricted to cortical areas or involve subcortical white matter (El-Hattab et al., 2015).

In cerebral Magnetic Resonance Imaging (MRI) stroke-like lesions, hyperintensities in T2-weighted sequences are typical. Dementia is frequently described in patients with MELAS (Hirano & Pavlakis, 1994; Sproule & Kaufmann, 2008), but the criteria for dementia have not yet been clearly defined (Kraya et al., 2019. Structural changes commonly include basal ganglia calcification, ventricular enlargement, and cortico-subcortical infarctions (Sartor et al., 2002).

Neuropsychological performance in the context of MELAS

The profile and trajectory of cognitive impairment in MELAS is poorly defined. Moore et al. (2020) completed a systematic review of cognitive deficits in adult mitochondrial disease. The study, which adhered to the Preferred Reporting Items for Systematic Reviews and Meta-Analyses guidelines (Page et al., 2021), included 168 articles. The review found that conventions for reporting cognitive impairment varied, with studies using (a) the number of cognitive domains impaired e.g. >5 of the seven assessed (Majamaa-Voltii et al., 2006), (b) scores below a cut-off (e.g. Z-score below −1.65, standard score below six or percentile below five (Fromont et al., 2009), score below the tenth percentile (Bosbach et al., 2003) or (c) difference from the normative mean (Turconi et al., 1999; Moore et al., 2019). Global impairments were found across studies, with specific deficits found in verbal and non-verbal memory, attention, language, comprehension, processing speed and executive function, as well as deficits in arithmetic, motor co-ordination and personality. Moore et al., (2019) found that compared to matched controls, patients performed worse on all domains, except memory and executive function.

Studies that have reported the results of neuropsychological testing are much less indicative of general cognitive impairment and dementia than is suggested by the findings of case reports and review articles. These results provide strong support for a profile of focal cognitive deficits, rather than global difficulties, in areas such as visuospatial functioning, memory, attention, processing speed, and executive functions (Moore et al., 2020).

Focal pathology or functional impairment in the context of a global pathological process

It is unclear if neuropsychological impairment in MELAS is caused by stroke-like episodes alone or by an additional neurodegenerative process caused by mitochondrial disease (Kraya et al., 2019). One of the challenges of examining neuropsychological difficulties in MELAS is the complex interplay between focal pathology caused by metabolic stroke-like episodes in the context of global mitochondrial disturbance. Whilst literature on this issue is limited, it can be closely related to vascular dementia (VaD). Mendez and

Cummings (2003) include MELAS mitochondrial encephalopathies in their list of vascular aetiologies capable of producing vascular cognitive disorder.

Case presentation

Reason for referral

Rebecca[1] was referred by her neurologist for neuropsychological assessment to examine her cognitive functioning. She was diagnosed with the pathogenic m.3243A>G mitochondrial DNA mutation. Following her diagnosis, she noticed deterioration in her cognition, affecting her work performance. This deterioration coincided with a number of stroke-like episodes, consistent with m.3243A>G mitochondrial encephalomyopathy, lactic acidosis, and stroke-like episodes (MELAS).

Social history

Rebecca was a 22-year-old, Caucasian British, right-handed woman. She was premature at birth weighing 1 pound 15 ounces. Whilst she met all developmental milestones, she reported significant exercise intolerance and had a small stature. She attended mainstream school until the age of 16 before completing NVQs in beauty and hairdressing. Rebecca reported 'school was difficult'. She could not recall her grades, but said she 'hadn't done very well'. She subsequently started a full-time role at McDonald's restaurant. At the time of assessment, Rebecca was part of the domestic services team.

Diagnosis

Rebecca first attended the NHS service for rare mitochondrial disease in September 2018. Her initial symptoms included exercise intolerance and temporomandibular joint disorder. She was diagnosed with the pathogenic m.3243A>G mtDNA mutation in January 2019. Heteroplasmy is the presence of more than one mtDNA type (Melton, 2004), with the greater percentage representing more pathogenesis. For Rebecca, it had been detected at high levels (suggesting a greater burden of disease), with 63% in blood-derived DNA samples, 74% in urine-derived DNA and 77% in buccal epithelial-derived DNA samples.

Stroke-like episodes

Rebecca experienced her first suspected stroke-like episode in November 2019. She described a 'confused period' at work. This was accompanied by 'a circle of white noise' in her visual field that disappeared after 'an hour'. A few weeks later, she experienced a migrainous attack which resulted in her attending Accident and Emergency. She complained of occipital headaches without photophobia and described 'flaky bits' affecting both right and left hemifields simultaneously. Computerised Tomography (CT) scan was reported as 'normal'. Rebecca slept 'the entire next day', but otherwise made a full recovery.

In January 2020, Rebecca had a further stroke-like episode. She reported anxiety and blurred vision. She called out to her father that she could not see then repeated 'bird, bird', and then a little later 'line, line'. She later developed an occipital headache.

Medical investigations

Following this second stroke-like episode she underwent MRI, showing generalised volume loss and signal change to the left inferior posterior temporal lobe.

Rebecca also underwent electroencephalogram (EEG) study. The study concluded that the general background appearances were acceptable but there were a number of transient anterior predominant bursts; however, these were not significant enough for a diagnosis of an epilepsy.

Rebecca's view of her presenting difficulties

Rebecca reported new difficulties with vision, processing speed, memory, and topographical orientation. She reported 'getting lost on the bus', and 'can't seem to figure out where I am once I get lost'. Rebecca also reported feeling guilty after losing her iPhone, a device she used to help her memory.

Rebecca recognised deterioration to cognitive function and vision following her stroke-like episodes. She described worry and low mood both in response to this deterioration, as well as her awareness of disease progression after losing her mother to mitochondrial disease.

Views of family

Rebecca's father, Ron recognised a number of changes. He thought Rebecca had 'lost her edge'. He spent more time explaining simple concepts to Rebecca, and noted that she required more prompts and reminders. Of most concern to Ron were Rebecca's difficulties with topographical orientation. He reported that she needed simple directions to travel along familiar routes. He had also noticed change in her behaviour, with Rebecca frequently misinterpreting visual information in her environment (e.g. thinking specks of dirt were bugs).

Ron thought Rebecca was becoming increasingly more vulnerable due to her cognitive difficulties. Having lost his wife to mitochondrial disease, Ron was concerned about the early onset of these difficulties as well as the increasing frequency of stroke-like episodes and what this might mean for Rebecca's prognosis.

Neuropsychological assessment

The service provides specialist neuropsychological assessment and where possible brief intervention for patients living with mitochondrial disease. Typically, this will involve liaising with local neuropsychology and neurore-habilitation services to support intervention in the person's locality.

Rationale for assessment

Considering the literature and evidence in this area (Kraya et al., 2019; Moore et al., 2019; Neargarder et al., 2007), a flexible hypothesis-driven battery was selected to assess global cognitive functioning including verbal and visual memory, attention, verbal comprehension, perceptual reasoning, executive function, and information processing with consideration of motor speed. It was also important to include functional assessment to assess topographical orientation and other functional abilities (i.e. managing money) to better understand these abilities in everyday tasks. Finally, a shorter battery was selected to account for fatigue, given the potential impact of metabolic changes on performance.

The following a priori hypotheses were generated, which, if supported, would mean Rebecca would meet DSM-V criteria for major neurocognitive disorder:

- There will be evidence of significant changes (>1.5 standard deviation difference relative to pre-morbid estimates) to memory, processing speed, attention, language, visuospatial/visuo-perceptual abilities, and executive function.
- Given changes to the inferior posterior temporal lobe, there will be evidence of difficulties with visual object agnosia (e.g. naming difficulties without preserved semantic knowledge of the object such as ability to gesture use).

Presentation during assessment

Rebecca was independently mobile, but required distant support from her father to navigate to the clinic room, e.g. 'this way'. There was no evidence of expressive aphasia or speech apraxia, though Rebecca presented with word finding difficulty. She gave little eye contact yet was motivated and keen to 'understand what is going on', particularly her difficulties with getting lost, losing belongings and 'seeing funny things'.

Assessment results

Performance validity

Performance validity testing is contraindicated where moderate or severe dementia is a consideration (Walter et al., 2014) and, in this case, embedded measures of effort together with Rebecca's presentation gave no indication of sub-optimal effort.

Estimating pre-morbid functioning

The test of premorbid functioning (TOPF-UK) and Crawford and Allan (1997) regression equation was used to estimate pre-morbid abilities, given the potential confounding visuo-perceptual and reading difficulties. On both measures her abilities were estimated to lie within the 'low average' range (FSIQ = 84.1 and 84.6 respectively, 14th percentile) reflecting a consistent and accurate estimate of pre-morbid ability.

Memory and Learning

Rebecca's performance was impaired across all verbal memory measures including list learning (List Learning; RBANS (Repeatable Battery for the Assessment of Neurological Status)), story recall (Story Memory; RBANS), and figure recall, at immediate and delayed test, and in recognition as well as recall format.

Visuoconstructional abilities

Rebecca's performance on a measure of visuoconstructional abilities (Figure Copy; RBANS) fell within the 'Impaired' range (0.1st percentile). Despite scoring within the impaired range, Rebecca was able to perceive aspects of the drawing but demonstrated difficulty with the spatial element of the task.

Visuospatial abilities

Rebecca's performance on a simple visuospatial task (Line Orientation; RBANS) fell within the 'Impaired' range (<2nd percentile). Qualitative analysis of her performance showed mild errors (i.e. answers either side of the correct answer), but overall performance was poor (e.g. 9/20).

Rebecca's visuo-spatial, sequencing, and planning abilities were assessed using the Clock Drawing (ACE-III) task. Her approach was as follows (Figure 7.1):

1. Rebecca used the clock in the room as a reference point.
2. She wrote out all numbers first.
3. She then added in the hands when instructed to put them at 'ten past five'.
4. She completed the circle.

Processing speed

Rebecca's performance on a measure of information processing speed (Speed of Information Processing; BMIPB) was below expectations and fell within the 'Borderline' range (6th percentile). When accounting for motor speed,

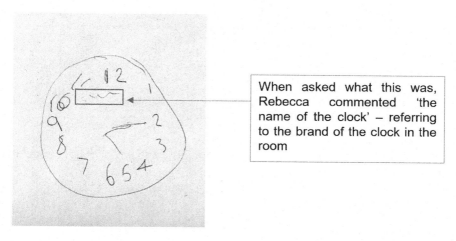

> When asked what this was, Rebecca commented 'the name of the clock' – referring to the brand of the clock in the room

Figure 7.1 Rebecca's clock drawing

there was no significant improvement (6th percentile). Errors were common (15% errors; <0.1st percentile).

Language

Rebecca's performance on a measure of confrontation naming (Picture Naming; RBANS) was significantly below expectations ('Impaired' range, <2nd percentile). Rebecca retained semantic knowledge of the item and how it would be used. She referred to items as 'thingy-mabobby's' whilst pantomiming their functional use.

Working memory

Rebecca's auditory verbal attention span (Digit Span; WAIS–IV) was significantly below expectations ('Borderline' range, 2nd percentile). There was a significant discrepancy between performance on Digit Span Backward and Digit Span Sequencing, only seen in 12.5% of age-related peers. In Rebecca's case, this may be accounted for by the additional working memory demands of the Digit Span Sequencing task.

Perceptual Reasoning

Rebecca's nonverbal reasoning abilities (Block Design; WAIS–IV) fell significantly below expectations ('Borderline' range, 2nd percentile), with evidence of reduced problem-solving speed (e.g. correctly completing item 7 outside the time limit). Her ability to analyse and synthesise abstract visual stimuli (Visual Puzzles; WAIS–IV) was also significantly below expectations ('Borderline' range, 2nd percentile).

Table 7.1. Evaluation of functional task using Knight, Alderman and Burgess (2002) Multiple Errands Test (hospital version)

Error type	Description of error
Inefficiencies	• Slow to take environmental cues, despite familiarity • Fixed on the type of Ribena, i.e. not clearly specified – diet or not
Rule breaks	• None specified in this example • Didn't check change
Interpretation failure	• None noted
Task failure	• N/A – task completed

Executive function

Rebecca's ability to retrieve phonemically linked information from memory (Semantic Fluency; RBANS*)* was significantly lower than expected ('Impaired' range, 0.1st percentile) and showed evidence of reduced cognitive flexibility, focusing entirely on Fruits.

Functional assessment

A procedure akin to the Knight, Alderman and Burgess (2002) multiple errands test for hospital settings was developed. Rebecca, who was familiar with the hospital environment, was asked to:

1. Leave the clinic room and find the nearest shop.
2. Purchase a bottle of Ribena using a five-pound note provided by the assessor.
3. Check change is correct and return this to the assessor.

Rebecca was informed that this task would form part of our assessment. She understood, though lacked confidence (e.g. she asked 'will you be right next to me?'). She was provided with a handout with instructions. Using the 'errors' template (Knight, Alderman & Burgess, 2002), the observations in Table 7.1 were made:

Psychological Factors

Mood and anxiety

On the Beck Depression Inventory (BDI-II), Rebecca's score fell within the 'minimal' range. On the Beck Anxiety Inventory (BAI), Rebecca's score fell within the 'moderate' range.

Self-esteem

Using the Rosenberg Self-Esteem Scale (RSES), Rebecca's score was suggestive of low self-esteem. She subjectively reported increasing awareness of her deteriorating health which made her feel negatively about herself.

Neuropsychological formulation

To understand Rebecca's difficulties with topographical orientation, evaluation was made of the data against the Riddoch and Humphries (1993) model of object perception (see Table 7.2). This highlighted specific difficulties with naming and allocentric orientation across both standardised and non-standardised measures.

Rebecca was a young woman with a pathogenic variant of the m.3243A>G gene. This inherited neurodegenerative condition had resulted in functional changes to her performance at work and at home. Rebecca had marked cognitive impairment in areas of verbal and visual memory, attention, processing speed, language, attention, and executive function. As a result of these significant changes, as well as a metacognitive awareness of her worsening health, she could feel overwhelmed by sensory information in her environment that left her unable to independently problem solve. As such, she became lost in both familiar and unfamiliar situations. Whilst an early hypothesis was of a focal visual agnosia, analysis of the standardised and non-standardised data, informant reporting, and clinical history suggested that her difficulties more likely represented distinct difficulties in key cognitive domains that, as a whole, produce functional impairment, e.g. problem solving, attention, and memory. Her low-level seizure activity, ongoing disease burden and risk of additional metabolic stroke-like episodes increased her risk of further deterioration. Rebecca's reduced cognitive reserve increased her risk in the short term, and she was aware of her risk. Given the severity of her difficulties coupled with wider confusion about the meaning of dementia or neurodegeneration in a person of her age, it was hard for Rebecca and those around her to make sense of her place in the world. This resulted in fear and anxiety which, coupled with fluctuating energy levels, compounded her cognitive symptoms.

Treatment

Rebecca and Ron attended a feedback appointment. We focused on discussing external strategies to maintain her well-being and independence in the community (e.g. using her iPhone to set reminders and prompts) and family support (e.g. providing clear, unambiguous directions or feedback). We also talked about her experience of confusing visual stimuli, validating and normalising her experience by sharing our biopsychosocial formulation. This

Table 7.2 Functional assessment against Riddoch and Humphries (1993) model of object perception

Component in hierarchy	Evidence gathered during assessment	
	Standardised	Non-standardised
Size/Length/ Orientation/Location	• Line orientation performance (<2nd percentile) • Speed of information processing performance (6th percentile) • Picture naming performance – adequately experiencing percept (demonstrated by mime use)	• Use of iPhone • Ability to navigate space, e.g. walking into room • Ability to judge space, e.g. sitting on chair • Ability to read/see stimuli in test situation • Ability to visit shop to buy fizzy drink etc.
Figure/ground	• Block design performance (2nd percentile) • Focusing on RBANS stimulus book to complete visuoperceptual tasks	• Use of iPhone • Ability to navigate space, e.g. walking into room • Ability to judge space, e.g. sitting on chair • Ability to read/see stimuli in test situation • Ability to visit shop to buy fizzy drink etc. • Ability to orientate self to shop
Viewpoint invariant processing	• Block design performance • Line orientation performance (<2nd percentile) • Visual puzzles performance (2nd percentile – *allocentric orientation changes*)	
Stored knowledge of shape	• Picture naming performance ('It's one of them thingy mabobbies')	• Purchasing drink • Ability to describe elements of journey to appointment • Subtle evidence – 'please take a seat'?
Stored knowledge of function and between-object **Name**	• Picture naming performance (<2nd percentile) • Block design performance (2nd percentile) • Visual puzzles performance (2nd percentile) • Picture naming performance – *evidence of difficulties with naming*	• Opening door to clinic room • Use of iPhone/headphones • Money/bottles/shop • iPhone • Pen • Clock • Other generic items in clinic room

was coupled with some basic brain injury awareness using materials from the Brain Injury Workbook (Powell, 2017).

Rebecca was referred to a local authority social worker with recommendations based on her needs and provided information about mitochondrial disease. This contained information specifically about changes to her cognitive function, decision making, and considerations around future care planning. Following this, Rebecca's local care team were provided with extensive information about mitochondrial disease. As well as a comprehensive assessment of her social care needs, Rebecca was also referred for tertiary care neurorehabilitation for adapted psychotherapeutic intervention. This was completed in parallel with emotional support for Rebecca's father as he adjusted to further experience of loss and change in the context of mitochondrial disease. This collaborative work allowed for early discussions around advance care planning and thoughts around capacity to consent to the appointment of a Lasting Power of Attorney. However, it was agreed that there was a trade-off between prioritising this discussion due to the neurodegenerative nature of MELAS, whilst also allowing time for Rebecca to process the emotional and psychological impact of her diagnosis and changing health.

In our shared work, Ron and I focused on establishing relevant coping resources early on. His profound experience of loss and the uncertainty surrounding mitochondrial prognosis resulted in feelings of guilt and shame, compounded by the genetic nature of the condition, e.g. 'I am responsible'. As such, we used a compassion-focused approach with education about mitochondrial disease, as well as an emphasis on maintaining behaviours associated with his role as a proud and supportive father (consistent with his values). In doing this, we highlighted the importance of Ron maintaining his role as 'dad', a role no-one else could fulfil with Rebecca. This emphasis on 'just being dad' allowed Ron to engage in a more compassionate response to challenge (e.g. 'we would usually have a laugh about this') and maintain a more 'typical' relationship with Rebecca. His increased knowledge of mitochondrial disease, as well as his bravery in discussing difficult topics such as advanced care planning, reduced some of the uncertainty he experienced. Ron established the mantra of 'focus on what I can control' as another way of managing uncertainty, supported by his emphasis on being the 'best dad' he could be.

Conclusion

In this case example, Rebecca was 22 years old when she started to experience her first stroke-like episodes characteristic of MELAS. The trajectory of the disease process is dependent on both the location and severity of metabolic stroke-like episodes as well as the underlying burden of disease. Neuropsychology has an important role in the assessment and treatment of mitochondrial conditions as demonstrated in this chapter. The specialist skill of using standardised and non-standardised assessment, triangulation of relevant biological, psychological, and social factors and expert knowledge of brain/behaviour link supports the understanding and therefore application of individualised treatment plans and guidance for non-experts, including families (who are experts in their own right). Where standardised assessment may be more challenging, e.g. where fatigue or sensory difficulties are present (as they often are in MELAS), neuropsychologists can explore models of cognitive neuropsychology and human cognition to better formulate neuropsychological strengths and weaknesses, improving the quality, appropriateness, and timeliness of intervention, and educate other health professionals on what is and isn't relevant. This may be particularly helpful in making important decisions around issues of mental capacity and best interests, clearly identifying factors such as the causative nexus, i.e. the link between difficulties associated with the neurological condition and the diagnostic test of mental capacity. In MELAS, formulation should pay particular attention to family experience of the disease and illness process, use of standardised and non-standardised assessment methods to understand individual strengths and weaknesses, and informant reporting where possible. Developmental factors may be particularly important, as well as the person's previous experience of health services due to the diagnostic uncertainty.

Note

1 All identifying details were changed to protect anonymity and confidentiality. 'Rebecca' provided informed consent for her anonymised details to be used in this case study.

References

Abramov, A. Y., Smulders-Srinivasan, T. K., Kirby, D. M., Acin-Perez, R., Enriquez, J. A., Lightowlers, R. N., & Turnbull, D. M. (2010). Mechanism of neurodegeneration of neurons with mitochondrial DNA mutations. *Brain*, *133*(3), 797–807. https://doi.org/10.1093/brain/awq015

Bosbach, S., Kornblum, C., Schroder, R., & Wagner, M. (2003). Executive and visuospatial deficits in patients with chronic progressive external ophthalmoplegia and Kearns-Sayre Syndrome. *Brain*, *126*, 1231–1240. https://doi.org/ 10.1093/brain/awg101

Crawford, J. R., & Allan, K. M. (1997). Estimating premorbid WAIS-R IQ with demographic variables: Regression equations derived from a UK sample. *The Clinical Neuropsychologist*, *11*(2), 192–197.

El-Hattab, A. W., Adesina, A. M., Jones, J., & Scaglia, F. (2015). MELAS syndrome: Clinical manifestations, pathogenesis, and treatment options. *Molecular Genetics and Metabolism*, *116*(1–2), 4–12. https://doi.org/10.1016/j.ymgme.2015.06.004

Fromont, I., Nicoli, F., Valero, R., Felician, O., Lebail, B., Lefur, Y., & Vialettes, B. (2009). Brain anomalies in maternally inherited diabetes and deafness syndrome. *Journal of Neurology*, *256*(10), 1696–1704. https://doi.org/10.1007/s00415-009-5185-4

Grier, J., Hirano, M., Karaa, A., Shepard, E., & Thompson, J. L. (2018). Diagnostic odyssey of patients with mitochondrial disease: Results of a survey. *Neurology Genetics*, *4*(2), 1– 7. https://doi.org/10.1212/NXG.0000000000000230

Hirano, M., & Pavlakis, S. G. (1994). Topical review: mitochondrial myopathy, encephalopathy, lactic acidosis, and stroke-like episodes (MELAS): Current concepts. *Journal of Child Neurology, 9*(1), 4–13. https://doi.org/10.1177/088307389400900102

Humphreys, G. W., & Riddoch, M. J. (1993). Interactions between object and space systems revealed through neuropsychology. In D. E. Meyer & S. Kornblum (Eds.), *Attention and performance XIV: Synergies in experimental psychology, artificial intelligence, and cognitive neuroscience* (pp. 143–162). MIT Press.

Karkare, S., Merchant, S., Solomon, G., Engel, M., & Kosofsky, B. (2009). MELAS with A3243G mutation presenting with occipital status epilepticus. *Journal of Child Neurology, 24*(12), 1564–1567. https://doi.org/10.1177/0883073809334386

Knight, C., Alderman, N., & Burgess, P. W. (2002). Development of a simplified version of the multiple errands test for use in hospital settings. *Neuropsychological Rehabilitation, 12*(3), 231–255. https://doi.org/10.1080/09602010244000039

Kraya, T., Neumann, L., Paelecke-Habermann, Y., Deschauer, M., Stoevesandt, D., Zierz, S., & Watzke, S. (2019). Cognitive impairment, clinical severity and MRI changes in MELAS syndrome. *Mitochondrion, 44*, 53–57. https://doi.org/10.1016/j.mito.2017.12.012

Lewis, R. (2016). *Human genetics: The basics.* Garland Science. https://doi.org/10.4324/9781315406985

Majamaa, K., Turkka, J., Kärppä, M., Winqvist, S., & Hassinen, I. E. (1999). The common MELAS mutation A3243G in mitochondrial DNA among young patients with an occipital brain infarct. *Neurology, 49*, 1331–1334. https://doi.org/10.1212/wnl.49.5.1331

McFarland, R., Taylor, R. W., & Turnbull, D. M. (2010). A neurological perspective on mitochondrial disease. *The Lancet Neurology, 9*(8), 829–840. https://doi.org/10.1016/S1474-4422(10)70116-2

Melton, T. (2004). Mitochondrial DNA heteroplasmy. *Forensic Science Review, 16*(1), 1–20.

Mendez, M. F., & Cummings, J. L. (2003). *Dementia: A clinical approach.* Butterworth-Heinemann.

Moher, D., Altman, D. G., Liberati, A., & Tetzlaff, J. (2011). PRISMA statement. *Epidemiology, 22*(1), 128. https://doi.org/10.1097/EDE.0b013e3181fe7825

Moore, H. L., Kelly, T., Bright, A., Field, R. H., Schaefer, A. M., Blain, A. P., & Gorman, G. S. (2019). Cognitive deficits in adult m. 3243A> G-and m. 8344A> G-related mitochondrial disease: Importance of correcting for baseline intellectual ability. *Annals of Clinical and Translational Neurology, 6*(5), 826–836. https://doi.org/10.1002/13.736

Moore, H. L., Blain, A. P., Turnbull, D. M., & Gorman, G. S. (2020). Systematic review of cognitive deficits in adult mitochondrial disease. *European Journal of Neurology, 27*(1), 3–17. https://doi.org/10.1111/ene.14068

Neargarder, S. A., Murtagh, M. P., Wong, B., & Hill, E. K. (2007). The neuropsychological deficits of MELAS: evidence of global impairment. *Cognitive and Behavioral Neurology, 20*(2), 83–92. https://doi.org/10.1097/WNN.0b013e3180335faf

Page, M. J., McKenzie, J. E., Bossuyt, P. M., Boutron, I., Hoffmann, T. C., Mulrow, C. D., & Moher, D. (2021). The PRISMA 2020 statement: An updated guideline for reporting systematic reviews. *British Medical Journal, 372.* www.bmj.com/content/bmj/372/bmj.n71.full.pdf

Powell, T. (2017). *The brain injury workbook: Exercises for cognitive rehabilitation.* Routledge.

Riddoch, M. J., & Humphreys, G. W. (1993). *BORB: Birmingham Object Recognition Battery.* Lawrence Erlbaum.

Rötig, A., & Poulton, J. (2009). Genetic causes of mitochondrial DNA depletion in humans. *Biochimica et Biophysica Acta (BBA)-Molecular Basis of Disease, 1792*(12), 1103–1108. https://doi.org/10.1016/j.bbadis.2009.06.009

Sartor, H., Loose, R., Tucha, O., Klein, H.E., Lange, K.W., (2002). MELAS: A neuropsychological and radiological follow-up study. Mitochondrial encephalomyopathy, lactic acidosis and stroke. *Acta Neurologica Scandinavica, 106*, 309–313. https://doi.org/10.1034/j.1600-0404.2002.01089.x

Schaefer, A. M., McFarland, R., Blakely, E. L., He, L., Whittaker, R. G., Taylor, R. W., & Turnbull, D. M. (2008). Prevalence of mitochondrial DNA disease in adults. *Annals of Neurology: Official Journal of the American Neurological Association and the Child Neurology Society, 63*(1), 35–39. https://doi.org/10.1002/ana.21217

Sproule, D. M., & Kaufmann, P. (2008). Mitochondrial encephalopathy, lactic acidosis, and stroke-like episodes: Basic concepts, clinical phenotype, and therapeutic management of MELAS syndrome. *Annals of the New York Academy of Sciences, 1142*(1), 133–158. https://doi.org/10.1196/annals.1444.011

Turconi, A. C., Benti, R., Castelli, E., Pochintesta, S., Felisari, G., Comi, G., & Bresolin, N. (1999). Focal cognitive impairment in mitochondrial encephalomyopathies: A neuropsychological and neuroimaging study. *Journal of the Neurological Sciences, 170*(1), 57–63. https://doi.org/10.1016/s0022-510x(99)00199-9

Walter, J., Morris, J., Swier-Vosnos, A., & Pliskin, N. (2014). Effects of severity of dementia on a symptom validity measure. *The Clinical Neuropsychologist, 28*(7), 1197–1208. https://doi.org/10.1080/13854046.2014.960454

Wilson, B. A., & Betteridge, S. (2019). *Essentials of neuropsychological rehabilitation.* Guilford Publications.

Test references

Beck, A. T., Steer, R. A., & Brown, G. (1996). Beck depression inventory–II. *Psychological Assessment.* Psychological Cororation.

Hsieh, S., Schubert, S., Hoon, C., Mioshi, E., & Hodges, J. R. (2013). 'Validation of the Addenbrooke's Cognitive Examination III in frontotemporal dementia and Alzheimer's disease'. *Dementia and Geriatric Cognitive Disorders, 36* (3–4), 242–250.

Peak, C., & Teager, A. (2020). *Estimated premorbid intelligence calculator based on demographic variables.* www.researchgate.net/publication/338865079_Estimated_Premorbid_Intelligence_Calculator_based_on_Demographic_Variables

Randolph, C. (2012). *Repeatable Battery for the Assessment of Neuropsychological Status (RBANS) UK-Update.* The Psychological Corporation.

Riddoch, M. J., & Humphreys, G. W. (1993). *Birmingham object recognition battery.* Lawrence Erlbaum.

Rosenberg, M. (1965). Rosenberg self-esteem scale (RSE). *Acceptance and commitment therapy. Measures package, 61*(52), 18.

Steer, R. A., & Beck, A. T. (1997). *Beck Anxiety Inventory.* Springer.

Warrington, E. & Merle, J. (1991). *Visual Object and Space Perception battery (VOSP).* Pearson.

Wechsler, D. (2010). *Test of Pre-morbid Functioning – UK version (ToPF-UK).* Pearson.

Wechsler, D. (2010). *Wechsler Adult Intelligence Scale – UK* (4th ed.). *(WAIS-IV-UK).* Pearson.

8 Galactosaemia

A rare metabolic disorder associated with 'hidden' deficits and social vulnerability

Stephanie Satariano, Louise Edwards, and Roshni Vara

Introduction

Galactosaemia (CG; OMIM: 230400) is a rare autosomal recessive metabolic disorder with an incidence between 1:16.000 and 1:60.000 in Europe and the USA (Hermans et al., 2019).

Galactosaemia affects the body's ability to convert galactose (ingested in the form of lactose, a sugar found in milk) to glucose. These are a group of disorders due to enzyme deficiencies in the galactose metabolism pathway. Classical galactosaemia (CG) results from a severe deficiency of the enzyme galactose-1-phosphate uridyl transferase (GALIPUT) due to mutations in the *GALT* gene. Clinical presentation is usually in the first few days or weeks of life with poor feeding, failure to thrive jaundice, liver dysfunction, and cataracts. The Duarte variant galactosaemia is a more common type in which children usually show about 25% the normal level of GALIPUT activity in red blood cells, in contrast to CG where activity is usually less than 1%. Treatment for CG is a strict lactose-free diet. Dietary intervention for the Duarte variant is unclear; however, more recent evidence shows that lactose restriction is not required (Carlock et al., 2019). There can also be deficiency of other enzymes in the pathway, galactokinase and galactose epimerase, which are rarer forms; dietary intervention is not required for these forms.

Despite early intervention and adherence to dietary treatment, the long-term outcomes of CG are suboptimal with complications such as learning difficulties, speech and language disorders, including motor speech disorders, primary ovarian failure, and osteoporosis (Lewis et al., 2013; Romani, 2018; Timmers et al., 2012). The incidence of cognitive impairment in patients with CG is not yet clear; therefore, both clinicians and researchers encountering patients with CG need to be aware of possible cognitive impairments. Although there is some evidence that indicates that very early restriction of lactose can have favourable results on health-related outcomes (Kotb et al., 2018), it does not show favourable cognitive outcomes (Bosch, 2011; Hughes et al., 2009; Welsink-Karssies et al., 2020). Furthermore, highly compliant dietary restrictions also did not show an improvement in long-term outcomes (Hughes et al., 2009; Kotb et al., 2018; Kotb et al., 2019).

DOI: 10.4324/9781003228226-9

Welling et al. (2019) found that there are groups of children who show no cognitive impairment but display a 'social vulnerability', particularly due to a breakdown in gaining and maintaining friendships. Some research is lending itself to the notion of language impairments; however, to date these have not been well evidenced in the research (Welsink-Karssies et al., 2020). According to Potter et al. (2008), those with typical cognitive development showed a greater likelihood of having expressive language disorder. Whereas a systematic review by Hermans et al. (2019) found mixed findings regarding expressive language outcomes.

We do not yet have a clear understanding of why the deficits exist, particularly given good dietary adherence. There is some evidence to suggest reduced white matter in patients with CG (Hughes et al., 2009), will lend itself to the reduction in IQ, however this does not provide an explanatory framework for the language difficulties. Moreover, some deficits may be better understood in CG as being social skills deficits as these skills derive from across the brain, for example frontal and temporal lobe interaction along with involvement of the subcortical structures such as the amygdala (Elleseff, 2015).

Case presentation

H was a 14-year-old diagnosed with galactosaemia at seven days old, following abnormal liver function and jaundice. She has shown good dietary adherence since this date. Overall, she remains in good health. Her early developmental milestones were noted to be within expected norms. The first difficulties noted in the nursery were around expressive language skills. She received speech and language therapy (SLT) input between two and five years of age. H's parents could not recall the nature of the intervention but it more likely represented traditional, developmental rather than bespoke SLT intervention.

Throughout her education H was reported to have low academic attainment. She was reported to be a hard-working girl, who showed excellent behaviour in school. School reports noted difficulties with expressing herself, for example, putting her thoughts onto paper, and rarely contributing to classroom discussions or debates.

H was in a small mainstream school, which had 14 girls in each class. Socially, she tended to be quite isolated. She had friends over the years but was unable to sustain any friendships. Now in her teenage years, she has struggled to keep up with her friends. Interestingly, this appears to be in keeping with emerging literature around the 'social vulnerability' of children with galactosaemia (Welling et al. 2019). Her parents noted that she liked to please those around her, and therefore was very compliant.

Of note, H loved drama and found it easy to learn her lines when on stage. However, she reportedly found all other subjects very difficult. She noted that, whilst she was able to understand what the teacher was saying, she struggled to execute the work assigned.

Neuropsychological assessment

During assessment H was very well-mannered and compliant. She put in good effort through the assessment, which was noticeable through the level of fatigue observed at the end of the assessment. A formal assessment of effort was carried out that showed adequate effort.

Intellectual ability

H's intellectual ability was assessed using the Wechsler Intelligence Scale Children's – 5th Version (WISC®-V, Q interactive version: Wechsler, 2014). This was a follow-up assessment with an initial assessment carried out using the WISC®-IV (Wechsler, 2003) eight years prior.

H's verbal intellectual ability as measured by the Verbal Comprehension Index was found to be in the 'average' range (standard score = 92). Her visual and auditory working memory and processing speed were found to be in line with this (standard scores 97, 89, and 108 respectively). On the Visual Spatial Index (VSI), she performed significantly lower with a standard score of 69.

H was found to have significant strength in her non-verbal intellectual ability as measured by the Fluid Reasoning Index (FRI), where she scored a standard score of 121.

H's verbal intellectual ability, visual spatial ability, and working memory were broadly in keeping with the previous assessment. However, her performance on the FRI subtests was significantly higher than previously assessed. H noted that she felt more comfortable and relaxed in this assessment than the previous one. Furthermore, without breaking standardisation, the examiner presented instructions in a clear and structured manner, using short sentences. It is acknowledged this may have supported H's ability to respond to the instructions, enabling her improved accessibility and to feel more comfortable with the tasks.

Language

Throughout the assessment, it was highly noticeable that H struggled to express herself as she tended to speak in short sentences; as short as possible to get her message across. When longer sentences or responses were required she would say 'I don't know' and laugh or giggle. Functionally, this presents as a limitation of her expressive language skills and use of giggling diverts the attention of the listener and offers a release for the speaker. According to Aragón et al. (2015), these 'dimorphous expressions' of positive emotion (in this case laughing or giggling) may serve to regulate the individual.

On formal assessments of expressive language, the Formulated Sentences and Sentence Assembly (from the Clinical Evaluation of Language Fundamentals (CELF-5)), H scored in the borderline range. She performed somewhat better on another task of expressive language, the Word Classes subtest (9), however, this only requires single word responses. H's understanding of language on the Receptive Language Index from CELF-5 was found to be at the top of the low average range; this is noticeably weaker than her 'superior' nonverbal intellectual ability. H's verbal fluency was also assessed on the Verbal Fluency subtest from the Delis-Kaplan Executive Function System (D-KEFS) where she performed in the borderline range (for letter and category), and further emphasises difficulties with expressive language.

Table 8.1 (CELF-5) and Table 8.2 (D-KEFS) provide summaries of H's language scores.

As the results of the assessments demonstrate, H presents with significant expressive language difficulties. These needs are particularly prominent where a profile of strong non-verbal reasoning skills exists. For H the ability to

Table 8.1 Clinical Evaluation of Language Fundamentals – fifth edition (CELF-5) assessment results

Language		
Assessment Battery	*Subtest*	*Score*
CELF-5	Recalling sentences	9^1
	Understanding spoken paragraphs	7^1
	Semantic relationship	8^1
	Word classes	9^1
	Sentence assembly	6^1
	Formulated sentences	5^1
	Core Language Index Score	82^2
	Receptive Language Index	88
	Expressive Language Index	80

[1]Scaled Score [2]Standard Score

Table 8.2 Delis-Kaplan Executive Function System (D-KEFS) assessment results.

Language			
Assessment battery	*Test*	*Subtest*	*Scaled score*
D-KEFS	Verbal fluency	Letter fluency	6
		Category fluency	6
		Switching accuracy	9
		Switching total	10

understand and 'work out' the world but without being able to adequately contribute verbally may be frustrating and debilitating.

Without formal assessments on social cognition, understanding the real-life impact of social skills impairment on well-being and participation are little understood (Hermans et al., 2019). From the clinical observations and assessment, it is not possible to clarify whether H's social issues and difficulty with peer relationships are a direct result of her limited expressive language skills or whether there is a specific social cognitive deficit, or indeed both.

Further assessment of language needs

Whilst the CELF-5 offers the possibility of completing the 'pragmatic profile', inferring standard scores should be cautiously interpreted. H would have benefited from functional clinical, observational assessment that included observations of her skills in difficult social situations. Indeed, Elleseff (2015) notes that standardised assessments can 'compensate' for social communication deficits.

Considering social and expressive language skills in functional tasks, for example, explaining the plot of a familiar movie to peers or describing the consequences of a particular action or emotion may offer important observations of the successes and limitations of language.

Whilst being concerned with academic achievement is important for a young person of H's age, the impact of limited expressive language and social skills on peer relationships, and therefore identity and self-esteem is compelling. As noted, H was demonstrating evidence of social isolation, difficulties forming and maintaining peer relationships, and an overall reduction in well-being and participation.

Treatment

Established medical treatment to limit the progression of mortality and morbidity of galactosaemia exists. However, there is a significant knowledge gap with little to no literature available on the recommended therapeutic support, so as to aid the cognitive and language difficulties noted in such patients.

Welling et al. (2019) note in the 'International clinical guideline for the management of classical galactosemia', detailed recommendations on the assessment of children and young people (CYP) with CG; however, recommendation 17 refers to the 'standard' or traditional speech and language therapy approach for communication support. Whilst it could be argued that traditional speech and language therapy through a developmental model may have been supportive for H, she may have required more dynamic, focused intervention that addressed specific needs and skills.

Unfortunately, given the nature of the service H was seen in, her support ceased at a neuropsychological assessment, with onward referrals to community services. However, upon reflection, there are a number of important considerations and strategies that would have helped H in both academic and social scenarios:

Providing accurate and appropriate education and strategies for the school setting are vital in optimising H's contribution to the academic setting as well as her peers. Developing specific, targeted and meaningful communication strategies are important to give H opportunities to succeed in communication exchanges across environments and scenarios.

Ensuring H has access to additional support in a classroom setting is an important consideration. As noted, H has excellent nonverbal reasoning skills and therefore has a lot to contribute to academic discussion. Someone available to shape and expand H's expressive language skills will ensure she is able to actively participate in such discussions and make meaningful contributions.

Although often seen within primarily adult aphasia therapy, implementing a social approach to H's needs such as Communication Partner Training (CPT) may further support H and help others in their understanding and interaction with H. A CPT-type approach moves the focus of intervention to the communication partner to improve the 'language, communication, participation, and/or well being' of the affected individual (Simmons-Mackie, 2010).

Implementing this social approach may also reduce social vulnerability, for example where a trusted peer may be able to support H's access to a range of communication environments. However, caution is emphasised to ensure any supporting peers or CPTs themselves have support to minimise communication partner burden. Furthermore, this needs to be done sensitively, given the social dynamics that present themselves, particularly in the teenage years and with development of identity and peer relationships.

H may benefit from a Social Use of Language Programme (SULP, Rinaldi, 1992) type approach. This approach enables people with communication needs across the age spectrum to explore social rules and expectations. Whilst H has some understanding of social norms, having a safe space outside of education and peer relationships to practice interactions and expressive language may build confidence and skills.

As discussed, H has excellent nonverbal reasoning ability and better comprehension than expressive language skills. In order to succeed in academic and social environments she must find strategies that support access and success within communication opportunities. Whilst H is already showing successful use of 'fillers' such as 'I don't know', these phrases have limited use, particularly in rapid, emotive, or dynamic peer conversations. Therefore, H's enjoyment of drama offers an opportunity to utilise skills from drama to support her expressive language. Use of social scripts and predefined narratives are techniques utilised in speech and language therapy clinical practice to support expressive language skills, particularly in social situations. Whilst most notably used with autistic individuals, where understanding, expressive language, and social communication may be impaired, the use of narrative can support more challenging but frequently occurring social circumstances that require active and immediate interactions, for example responding to peer pressure.

Reducing the cognitive and linguistic load in communication environments and exchanges may provide an opportunity to explore the skills and needs of CYP with CG. Where verbal communication is particularly challenging, the use of augmentative communication methods, such as Talking Mats® may support the exploration of feelings or needs. Additionally, augmentative tools may help expansion of utterances, for example with visual reminders and prompts.

Conclusion

In summary, assessment over time found no change in H's cognitive functioning. She presents with a strong nonverbal intellectual ability with particular difficulties in her expressive language skills and visual-spatial construction skills. Interestingly, the expressive language difficulties were more apparent in her day-to-day life than on standardised assessments. Such a discrepancy in her cognitive abilities has resulted in those around her underestimating her ability. It has also impacted her ability to exhibit her knowledge and her self-confidence, and made the classroom environment and academic work overwhelming and challenging.

H does not present with low intellectual ability; however, she has specific areas of impairment. The expressive language difficulties and visual-spatial difficulties outlined above are likely an impact of her diagnosis of CG, and are in keeping with more recent research indicating a 'social vulnerability' (Welling et al., 2019). Her unique profile highlights the potential of hidden deficits amongst this group of patients, as the difficulties are difficult to pick up using standardised assessments, and therefore their identification relies on clinical experience and expertise. Additionally, presenting as a compliant, quiet individual means these deficits may be missed altogether.

Whilst CYP with CG presenting with cognitive and language deficits represent a low incidence caseload, they can have potentially significant high needs, particularly in school and social circumstances. Understanding the short- and long-term impacts of these deficits in a classroom setting and beyond is vital in understanding how these CYP can be supported in attaining not only academic achievements but also peer relationships and overall wellbeing. When there is a diagnosis of CG, educating the school on the risk factors and potential hidden deficits within this population will be essential in supporting them to optimally move along their developmental and academic trajectory.

It is also going to be critical to the rehabilitation of CYP with CG, that long-term studies looking at the trajectory within this population are carried out, to understand their unique vulnerability and optimise support. Identifying appropriate assessment methods including observations of functional communication across communication environments is important in recognising individual profiling. Furthermore, detailed analysis of clinical presentation will inform intervention.

Implementation of a developmental model of speech and language therapy input may not be appropriate for CYP with CG. Further understanding of bespoke, individualised approaches to communication needs of CYP with CG, considering the complex cognitive needs, is required to optimise outcomes and ensure success, participation, and well-being across communication environments.

References

Aragón, O. R., Clark, M. S., Dyer, R. L., & Bargh, J. A. (2015). Dimorphous expressions of positive emotion: Displays of both care and aggression in response to cute stimuli. *Psychological Science*, 26(3), 259–273. https://doi.org/10.1177/0956797614561044

Bosch, A. M. (2011). Classic galactosemia: Dietary dilemmas. *Journal of Inherited Metabolic Diseases*, 34, 257–260. https://doi.org/10.1007/s10545-010-9157-8

Carlock, G., Lynch, M. E., Potter, N., & Fisher, S. T. (2019). Developmental outcomes in Duarte galactosaemia. *Pediatrics*, 143(1). E20182516. https://doi.org/10.1542/peds.2018-2516

Delis, D. C., Kaplan, E., & Kramer, J. H. (2001). Delis-Kaplan Executive Function System: Technical Manual. San Antonio, TX: Harcourt Assessment Company. Delis-Kaplan Executive Function System™ (D-KEFS™).

Elleseff, T. (2015). Assessing social communication abilities of school-aged children. *Perspectives on School-Based Issues*, 16, 79. https://doi.org/10.1044/sbi16.3.79

Hermans, M. E., Welsink-Karssies, M. M., Bosch, A. M. Oostrom, K. J., & Geurtsen, G. J. (2019). Cognitive functioning in patients with classical galactosemia: A systematic review. *Orphanet Journal of Rare Diseases*, 14, 226. https://doi.org/10.1186/s13023-019-1215-1

Hughes, J., Ryan, S., Lambert, D., Geoghegan, O., Clark, A., Rogers, Y., Hendroff, U., Monavari, A., Twomey, E., & Treacy, E. P. (2009). Outcomes of siblings with classical galactosemia. *The Journal of Pediatrics*, 154 (5), 721–726. https://doi.org/10.1016/j.jpeds.2008.11.052

Kotb, M. A., Mansour, L., & Shamma, R. A. (2019). Screening for galactosemia: Is there a place for it? *International Journal of General Medicine*, 23(12), 193–205. https://doi.org/10.2147/IJGM.S180706

Kotb, M. A., Mansour, L., William Shaker Basanti, C., El Garf, W., Ali, G. I. Z., Mostafa El Sorogy, S. T., Kamel, I. E. M., & Kamal, N. M. (2018). Pilot study of classic galactosemia: Neurodevelopmental impact and other complications urge neonatal screening in Egypt. *Journal of Advanced Research*, 12, 39–45. https://doi.org/10.1016/j.jare.2018.02.001

Lewis, F. M., Coman, D. J., Syrmis, M., Kilcoyne, S., & Murdoch, B. E. (2013). Impaired language abilities and pre-linguistic communication skills in a child with a diagnosis of galactosaemia. *Early Child Development and Care*, 183(12), 1747–1757. https://doi.org/10.1080/03004430.2012.751101

Potter, N. L., Lazarus, J. A., Johnson, J. M., Steiner, R. D., & Shriberg, L. D. (2008). Correlates of language impairment in children with galactosaemia. *Journal of Inherited Metabolic Diseases*, 31(4), 524–532. https://doi.org/10.1007/s10545-008-0877-y

Rinaldi, W. (1992). *The social use of language programme.* NFER-Nelson.

Romani, C. (2018). Cognitive impairments in inherited metabolic diseases: Promises and challenges. *Cognitive Neuropsychology, 35* (3–4), 113–119. https://doi.org/10.10 80/02643294.2017.1417249

Simmons-Mackie, N., Raymer, A., Armstrong, E., Holland, A., & Cherney, L. R. (2010). Communication partner training in aphasia: A systematic review. *Archives of Physical Medicine and Rehabilitation, 91*(12), 1814–1837. https://doi.org/10.1016/j. apmr.2010.08.026

Talking Mats®. www.talkingmats.com/

Timmers, I., Jansma, B. M., & Rubio-Gozalbo, M. E. (2012). From mind to mouth: Event related potentials of sentence production in classic galactosemia. *PLoS ONE, 7*(12), e52826. https://doi.org/10.1371/journal.pone.0052826

Wechsler, D. (2014). *WISC-V: Technical and interpretive manual.* Pearson.

Wechsler, D. (2003). *Wechsler intelligence scale for children,* 4th ed. PsychCorp.

Welling, L., Meester-Delver, A., Derks, T. G., Janssen, M. C. H, Hollak, C. E. M., de Vries, M., & Bosch, A. M. (2019). The need for additional care in patients with classical galactosaemia. *Disability and Rehabilitation, 41*(22), 2663–2668. https://doi. org/10.1080/09638288.2018.1475514

Welsink-Karssies, M. M., Oostrom, K. J., Hermans, M. E., Hollak, C. E. M., Janssen, C. H., Langendonk, J. G., Oussoren, E., Rubio Gozalbo, M. E., de Vries, M., Geurtsen, G. J., & Bosch, A. M. (2020). Classical galactosemia: Neuropsychological and psychosocial functioning beyond intellectual abilities. *Orphanet Journal of Rare Diseases, 15,* 42. https://doi.org/10.1186/s13023-019-1277-0

9 Anti-N-methyl-D-aspartate receptor antibody encephalitis

Post-acute neuropsychological consequences and rehabilitation in adolescence

Catherine Harter and Fergus Gracey

Introduction

Rare inflammatory brain diseases have been increasingly identified in children (see Celluci et al., 2020 for review). Anti-N-methyl-D-aspartate receptor (anti-NMDAR) antibody encephalitis is a non-infectious, autoimmune encephalopathy that causes an acute inflammatory disorder of the brain in a small number of individuals, typically identified when they present to psychiatric services (Dalmau et al., 2011). This antibody mediated central nervous system (CNS) disorder has been characterised by a psychiatric onset followed by later movement disorder, with antibody levels correlated with illness severity (Irani & Vincent, 2011). Substantial gains have been made in the last decade in terms of identification, diagnosis, and treatment (see Graus et al., 2016 for a review), although the route to specialist neurological/neuropsychological services can often be protracted, particularly for those who do not have access to neuropsychological support.

Anti-NMDAR encephalitis is seen in individuals who present with atypical forms of psychiatric illnesses (e.g. Zandi et al., 2011), particularly acute first onset psychosis (Steiner et al, 2020). Recent UK population surveillance estimates an incidence of 0.85 per million children per year (Wright et al., 2015). Across population age ranges, 70–75% are females, with 58% of patients showing an underlying tumour (most commonly ovarian teratoma). However, in children, only 31% of those under 18 years old and 9% of children under 14 years old had evidence of a tumour (Remy et al., 2017). Diagnostic criteria include the rapid onset of abnormal psychiatric behaviour and cognitive symptoms, speech dysfunction, seizures, movement disorder, decreased levels of consciousness and autonomic dysfunction/hypoventilation, with laboratory test confirmation by either abnormal electroencephalogram (EEG) or cerebrospinal fluid with pleocytosis or oligoclonal bands (Graus et al., 2016). Review studies note that some children may develop anti-NMDAR antibodies as part of an immune response to other pathogens

DOI: 10.4324/9781003228226-10

(Remy et al., 2017). Symptom onset progresses from a viral-like prodrome to alterations in memory or other aspects of cognition, behaviour, psychosis, seizures, and dyskinesias (orofacial, limb, and trunk), and prognosis tends to follow a slow, relapsing recovery with eventual improvement in residual symptoms (Rosenfeld & Dalmau 2011; Irani & Vincent, 2011, Dalmau et al., 2011). Children and young adults are believed to represent about 40% of all anti-NMDAR encephalitis cases (Rosenfeld & Dalmau, 2011), with anti-NMDAR antibodies reported in children as young as three months of age (Remy et al., 2017). Three phases including a prodromal stage, early psychosis/seizure phase through to a later hyperkinetic phase have been described (Remy et al., 2017).

There are suggestions of persisting brain injury related effects. Whilst 80% of patients make a substantial recovery, and there are continued improvements up to two years after symptom presentation, some people experience persistent difficulties including with impulsivity, behaviour disinhibition, memory, planning, attention, and social interaction (Armangue et al., 2012; Finke et al., 2016).

Causal theories and pathology

Pathogenesis

There are varying causal explanations and, related to this, challenges in making a swift diagnosis. Irani and Vincent (2011) suggest that anti-NMDAR encephalitis is caused either by antibodies or B cells traversing the blood–brain barrier, which initiates or mediates the infection prodrome. At a molecular level, Irani and Vincent (2011) suggest that the NMDA receptor antibodies reduce the surface expression of the NMDA receptors on neurons. Most patients have abnormal cerebrospinal fluid (CSF) with abnormal MRI, when present, detailing increased T2 signal in cerebral or cerebellar cortex, medial temporal lobes, and also the corpus callosum or brainstem (Rosenfeld & Dalmau, 2011). Of note, typical brain MRI is reported in more than half of all paediatric patients, with imaging findings often nonspecific (e.g. Brenton & Goodkin, 2016). Multimodal imaging approaches examining hippocampal volumetric and microstructural integrity found that patients with anti-NMDAR encephalitis experience long-standing structural damage of the hippocampus consisting of reduced volumes of hippocampal input and output structures and impaired microstructural integrity related to disease severity and duration (Finke et al., 2016).

Treatments and their impact

Treatments that have been reported to have positive effects include tumour removal (where appropriate), and more widely the use of immunotherapies (including corticosteroids, intravenous immunoglobulins, plasma exchange), with the goal of reducing NMDA receptor antibody levels (Irani & Vincent, 2011). Response of children to immunotherapy is variable (Rosenfeld & Dalmau, 2011) with early and intensive immunotherapy often leading to better prognosis despite illness severity (Steiner et al., 2020). Of note, the neuropsychological consequences of anti-NMDAR encephalitis may be confounded by the impact of treatment. For example, long-standing studies document corticosteroid therapy can impact upon memory, frontal function, and mood (Naber et al., 1995; Lupien & McEwen, 1997; Belanoff et al., 2001; Sherwood Brown et al., 2004). The challenges of balancing the long-term implications of treatment on a developing neuroimmunological system, versus the risks of disease recurrence, have been noted (Brenton & Goodkin, 2016).

Neuropsychological features

In terms of neuropsychology, memory deficits are a key feature not included in diagnostic criteria due to assessment challenges in young children or those with psychosis or agitation (Graus et al., 2016). Early reviews have suggested that the NMDA subtype of glutamate receptor and long term potentiation (LTP) of synapse transmission may be essential mechanisms in learning and memory (Rison & Stanton, 1995). Other commonly documented characteristics that might endure after the acute phase include frontal lobe dysfunction incorporating poor attention, planning, impulsivity, behavioural disinhibition, and memory deficits (Rosenfeld & Dalmau, 2011).

In a key review, Barkus and colleagues (2010) reported that brain structures in the medial temporal lobes (hippocampus and amygdala) were likely candidates for where the NMDA receptors may exert their greatest effects, particularly the ventral part of the hippocampus. This notion is echoed by Heine et al. (2021) who postulated that memory problems and executive dysfunction seen in anti-NMDAR encephalitis are likely consequences of frontal and medial temporal NMDAR dysfunction, and that decoupling of the hippocampus and the medial prefrontal cortex detected via imaging has been found to be correlated with severity of memory deficits.

Neuropsychological case reports have detailed findings of impairments to verbal memory and working/short-term memory (Nicolle & Moses, 2018), attention, processing speed, oral language and executive functioning, visuospatial processing, and social cognition (e.g. Loughan et al., 2016, Nicolle & Moses, 2018; Gibson et al. 2020). Memory deficits tend to persist more chronically long-term, (McIvor & Moore, 2017, Nicolle & Moses, 2018) as do executive function difficulties (Nicolle & Moses, 2018).

Longitudinal studies are needed to map the recovery trajectory including how this affects an individual at different stages in their life. A recent study of 40 patients post anti-NMDAR encephalitis by Heine et al. (2021) found that all patients exhibited cognitive deficits after the acute stage, with 50% experiencing severe deficits in working memory, verbal episodic memory, and executive function at two years post onset. Similarly, long-term follow-up studies in paediatric population increasingly find that most children do not return to baseline levels of cognitive functioning. Persisting cognitive deficits include disruptions to short-term verbal memory, language, reduced sustained attention and speed, and executive dysfunction (e.g. Wilkinson-Smith et al., 2021; de Bruijn et al., 2018); or adaptive functioning skills (communication, social skills, independent living) and more rarely described impairments in fine motor speed, dexterity, and language (Wilkinson-Smith et al., 2021). A key finding was that fatigue was frequently reported as the most disabling persisting consequence, hampering normal participation, quality of life, and school attendance (de Bruijn et al., 2018).

Anti-NMDAR encephalitis in the developmental context

Given the potential for both primary and secondary disruption to brain function, the impact of anti-NMDAR encephalitis will be more complicated in the developmental context, with consequences causing downstream disruption of later development, as described by Gamino et al. (2009) in relation to brain injury in childhood.

Studies assessing neuropsychological functioning in children and young people with this condition are rare. Hinkle et al. (2017) followed up three teenagers, 12 months post onset of symptoms, and noted improved cognitive functioning during recovery, but persisting cognitive deficits in fine motor dexterity, language, and memory at long-term follow-up. Studies have documented minimal to intact cognitive recovery in two pediatric patients, believed to represent adequate functional recovery after illness, although persisting anxiety, reduced participation, and fatigue were noted (Moss et al., 2018). Given that disease severity and duration is associated with hippocampal damage (e.g. Finke et al., 2016), it is important that neuropsychologists are able to complete assessments in both the acute and chronic phase to track recovery or highlight risk of relapse.

Adolescence and interruptions to typical development

It is well established that brain development continues through to the third decade of life (Johnson et al., 2009), and the adolescent brain is considerably influenced by its environment, with hypersensitivity to encoding memories more deeply, and events triggering stronger emotions (Steinberg, 2014). Early stress and peer relationships can have a marked impact on the developing brain (Kolb & Gibb, 2011). Adolescence is a time of increased vulnerability to the onset of mental illness (Steinberg, 2014), disrupting independent skills, and the goals of adolescence being to move to attaining adult social roles, responsibilities, and status (Vijayakumar et al., 2018). Blakemore (2018) emphasises that adolescents are particularly sensitive to how they fit into their social environment, highlighting the importance of social inclusion by peers, with adverse effects or 'social stress' of being isolated. Finally, NMDAR encephalitis may present with particular challenges that are greater than those for other acquired brain injuries, through the protracted nature of symptom onset and progression, the typical delays in establishing the correct diagnosis and treatment, and the additional stress of coping with a condition that is not well understood. These cumulative stressors could limit recovery and adaptation. Social factors and understanding of illness and consequences perhaps represent non-injury factors that can be targeted by services to positively affect outcome and post-brain injury recovery.

Laura: neuropsychological assessment and rehabilitation for anti-NMDA receptor antibody encephalitis in adolescence

Laura was referred to our neuropsychological rehabilitation service aged 16 years and two months, after she had been discharged from hospital, five months after the onset of her first symptoms. The interdisciplinary assessment and formulation process undertaken in the service followed the World Health Organization–International Classification of Functioning (WHO–ICF, 2007) aiming to integrate social, family, and medical history, current neuropsychological, emotional, family, and social functioning in the context of everyday life and goals. A much-abbreviated summary of key information is provided here and in the case formulation diagram (Figure 9.2).

Clinical history

Laura's initial presentation was described by her parents as consisting of her acting strangely and out of character, arising in the context of a stressful build-up to school exams. She was referred to child and adolescent mental health services and diagnosed with an acute and transient psychotic episode. After several weeks of treatment with anti-psychotic medication, it emerged that this was an incorrect diagnosis, and she was transferred to hospital. NMDAR encephalitis was suspected, and Laura was treated with plasma exchange, steroids, and immunotherapies. After a further two episodes of relapse, where she was re-admitted into the Intensive Care Unit, following periods of being very unwell with reduced motor functioning, including drooling and being unable to walk, further treatment was delivered, including increased steroids, immunosuppressants, and an antibody infusion. Laura's condition finally stabilised, and she was discharged home exactly three months after her first presentation. Laura's mother reported that Laura had been conscious throughout her hospital stay, apart from when she was on her way to ICU during her first admission. Nonetheless, her memory of events was 'incomplete' and this period of acute illness traumatic to her parents. This included an attempt to end her life by medication overdose two weeks post discharge and she was hospitalised further for four days.

Developmental history

Laura's early developmental history was unremarkable. She reached all of her developmental milestones on time, although she had speech delay diagnosed and treated when she was aged three years and had been diagnosed with dyslexia aged eight years. Before her injury Laura was described as an outgoing person, who always organised her friends, was confident, independent, and involved at a high level in her active pastimes.

Information from school

Two months after discharge Laura returned to school part time, for one to two hours per week, although her adaptive functioning was limited by high levels of fatigue and the dissolution of formal teaching whilst her peers undertook statutory exams. A plan for a gradual return to education and a repeat of her current academic year had been put in place. Individual tuition for catching up in the summer holidays was scheduled.

Presenting problems at initial assessment

At initial referral, five months following onset of symptoms, Laura reported difficulties with memory, speech, and communication, confusion and, although fully mobile, was unsteady physically, including a hand tremor. She was unable to attend to her independent or self-care needs, and her parents felt that she could only be left independently for very brief periods. She had extreme fatigue and it was clear that she would be unable to cope with extensive neuropsychological testing.

Goals at initial assessment

Laura and her family set the following goals:

- To be less fatigued, because 'this affects everything'
- To be better at remembering things; 'things slip my mind'
- To do well in my GCSEs, A levels, and move on to university or an apprenticeship.

Initial neuropsychological assessment

In line with the literature and evidence that NMDA receptors are highly concentrated in the hippocampus and to a lesser extent the prefrontal cortex, memory and attention were targets for assessment. We had to ensure that our test selection allowed us to complete a fuller follow-up assessment following a period of further recovery, without contaminating measures or increasing practice effects. An alternative approach might have been to use statistical corrections, complete reliable change analyses, or multiple regression-based formulae predicting scores at different time points (e.g. McIvor & Moore, 2017). As this was an initial assessment, the NEPSY II (Korkman, Kirk & Kemp, 2007), was used in order to provide a baseline for how Laura was functioning at the early stage of her recovery and believed to be less demanding than other formal assessments.

Neuropsychological assessment results

Laura's focused and switching attention were within the extremely high to average range, respectively. Tests of sensorimotor functioning indicated that when repeating or copying sequences with both her dominant and non-dominant hand, she performed in the extremely low range. Her ability to recognise emotions in faces was within the average range. Laura's greatest difficulties were evidenced on tests of memory. Whilst narrative memory was relatively preserved, being within the low average range, she showed a rapid decay, with delayed narrative memory falling to within the extremely low range. Of note, Laura showed no advantage during cued recognition memory conditions, suggesting that she may not have been able to encode the information or use her implicit memory system. Her recognition memory for faces (at both short and long delay) was in the extremely low range, with recognition accuracy of just under 40%. Similarly, whilst she had a good ability to remember the spatial and content information of a series of designs, her long-term retention was low, with a significant drop of information retained, despite this being noted as a pre-illness strength. Whilst Laura's memory for names (matching names to a series of simplified line drawings), was intact on this measure, as with many areas, her delayed memory scores were weaker than her immediate recall. Working memory, as assessed by a word list interference task, was low for both the short-term (repetition) and working memory condition (ordered recall) of the task.

Table 9.1 Neuropsychological assessment data for Laura at Time 1 (initial assessment five months post symptom onset)

Cognitive domain	Test used	Test typical standard Score	Performance classification
Working memory: NEPSY-II	Word list interference repetition	3	Extremely low
	Word list interference recall	4	Low
Memory: NEPSY-II	Memory for faces immediate	2	Extremely low
	Memory for faces delayed	2	Extremely low
	Memory for names immediate	8	Average range

Cognitive domain	Test used	Test typical standard Score	Performance classification
	Memory for names delayed	6	Low average
	Narrative memory free recall	7	Low average
	Narrative memory free and cued recall	3	Extremely low
	Memory for designs immediate content	8	Average
	Memory for designs immediate spatial	4	Low
	Memory for designs delayed content	7	Low average
	Memory for designs delayed spatial	2	Extremely low
	Memory designs immediate combined	8	Average
	Memory designs delayed combined	6	Low average
Attention: NEPSY-II	Auditory attention	16	Extremely high
Sensorimotor: NEPSY-II	Auditory attention and response set	9	Average range
	Fingertip tapping repetitions	1	Extremely low
	Fingertip tapping sequences	2	Extremely low
	Fingertip tapping dominant hand	1	Extremely low
	Fingertip tapping nondominant hand	1	Extremely low
Social perception: NEPSY-II	Affect recognition	12	Average range
Emotion and behaviour: SDQ	Emotional symptoms	16	Slight concern
	Behavioural difficulties	10	Significant difficulties
	Attention/Hyperactivity	3	Slight concerns
	Peer problems	1	No concern
	Prosocial behaviour	2	No concern
	Total difficulties	15	No concern
Family impact: PEDS-QL	Total score	60	Average
	Parent HRQOL score	64	Average
	Family function summary score	78	Average
	Physical functioning	83	Above Average
	Emotional functioning	45	Below average
	Social functioning	63	Average
	Cognitive functioning	60	Average
	Communication	50	Below average
	Worry	25	Significantly below average
	Daily Activities	58	Average
	Family relationships	90	Above average
Emotional Functioning: BYI	Beck self concept Inventory	39	Much lower than average
	Beck anxiety inventory	57	Mildly elevated
	Beck depression inventory	53	Average
	Beck anger inventory	37	Average
	Beck disruptive behaviour inventory	41	Average
Resiliency scales	Sense of mastery	42	Below average
	Sense of relatedness	34	Low
	Emotional reactivity	42	Below average

Emotions and behaviour

Laura completed the Beck Youth Inventory (Beck et al., 2005), which examines levels of self-esteem, anxiety, depression, anger, and disruptive behaviour. Laura's scores indicated low levels of self-esteem, in addition to mildly elevated levels of anxiety.

The Child and Adolescent Resiliency Scale (Prince-Embury, 2007) measures factors that can predict positive coping. Laura rated her sense of mastery (in her achievements) and relatedness (relationships with her peers and feelings of available social support) as low. Laura rated her emotional reactivity as low, reflecting either good emotional self-regulation in the presence of adversity, possibly reduced insight, and ability to self-monitor her mood or neurologically reduced reactivity.

Laura reported some anxious and sad feelings, triggered especially in relation to worries about returning to school and about her friends moving on without her. Laura also expressed concerns about her ability to cope socially, how difficult things were for her, and people not realising her struggles.

Impact on the family

Laura's mother completed the Impact of Events Scale (Weiss, 2007). This questionnaire examines symptoms of stress and trauma following challenging life experiences. Her mother's scores were below the clinically elevated range, although the period when Laura was unwell was a considerable stressful life event for which there are continued intrusions and challenging emotions.

Second neuropsychological assessment

Eleven months after Laura's first onset of symptoms, she completed a more detailed neuropsychological assessment, close to six months after the baseline assessment. At this point, Laura's fatigue had recovered such that it was no longer a barrier to completion of a full neuropsychological assessment.

Laura's general ability (as measured on the Wechsler Intelligence Scale for Children, UK fifth edition, Wechsler, 2014) was within the average range for verbal comprehension, visual–spatial, and processing speed. She had strengths in fluid reasoning, which fell within the high average range. Her working memory continued to be low (low average picture span, low range digit span), for which the latter may have reflected *domain general* deficits associated with dyslexia in combination with some lingering effects of her illness. Academic attainment skills (Wechsler Individual Achievement Test, second edition, Wechsler, 2005) included average to high average maths skills, with reading falling into the low average range, perhaps reflecting her premorbid dyslexia rather than effects specific to anti-NMDAR encephalitis.

In terms of executive functioning, the trail-making test has been regularly used to track progress of people recovering from anti-NMDAR encephalitis,

Table 9.2 Neuropsychological assessment data for Laura at Time 2 (11 months after symptom onset)

Cognitive domain	Test used	Test standard /scaled score	Performance classification
Intellectual: WISC–IV	Verbal comprehension	106	Average
	Visual spatial	100	Average
	Fluid reasoning	118	High average
	Working memory	76	Very low
	Processing speed	92	Average
	Full scale	103	Average
	Cognitive proficiency Index	81	Low average
	General ability index	111	High average
Academics: WIAT–II	Word reading	89	Low average
	Pseudoword decoding	81	Low average
	Numerical operations	113	High average
	Mathematical reasoning	106	Average
DKEFS: Trail making	Visual scanning	8	Average range
	Number sequencing	4	Low range
	Letter sequencing	4	Low range
	Number–letter Sequencing	8	Average range
	Motor speed	6	Low average range
DKEFS: Colour word interference	Colour naming	4	Low
	Word reading	5	Low
	Inhibition	8	Average
	Inhibition/Switching	7	Low average
DKEFS: Verbal fluency	Letter fluency	6	Low average
	Category fluency	12	Average
	Category switching	11	Average
	Category switching accuracy	12	Average
Memory: CMS	Stories immediate	8	Average
	Stories total score	8	Average
	Stories long delay	12	Average
	Faces immediate	13	High average
	Faces delayed	11	Average
	Word pairs learning	6	Low average
	Word pairs total score	6	Low average
	Word pairs long delay	7	Low average
	Word pairs delayed recognition	11	Average
Emotion and Behaviour: SDQ	Emotional symptoms	8	No concern
	Behavioural difficulties	5	Significant concern
	Attention/Hyperactivity	0	No concern
	Peer problems	2	No concern

(Continued)

Table 9.2 Continued

Cognitive domain	Test used	Test standard /scaled score	Performance classification
	Prosocial behaviour	1	No concern
	Total difficulties	8	No concern
Family impact: PEDS-QL	Total score	51	Average
	Parent HRQOL score	55	Average
	family function summary score	50	Average
	Physical functioning	58	Average
	Emotional functioning	50	Average
	Social functioning	63	Average
	Cognitive functioning	50	Below average
	Communication	58	Average
	Worry	35	Average
	Daily activities	50	Average
	Family relationships	50	Below average

assessing flexibility of thinking and visual motor sequencing (Delis Kaplan Executive Functioning Scale, Delis, Kaplan, & Kramer, 2001). Laura's performance likely reflected good cognitive flexibility. She made no errors across the entire assessment but exhibited slower speed, particularly for the motor speed items, perhaps reflecting ongoing motor deficits which may also have artificially lowered her overall executive function performance score. Similar speed difficulties were perhaps detected on the colour word and verbal fluency subtests, where Laura had average levels of inhibition and cognitive flexibility as measured by the colour word tests, although slower naming and reading speed were detected. In terms of verbal fluency, Laura had average scores on category fluency and switching subtests, with weaker letter fluency, perhaps reflecting her premorbid dyslexia. Of greatest interest were the marked improvements to Laura's memory, particularly her long-term memory function. Laura displayed average performance on an episodic story recall measure, with her delayed recall in the high average range. Her visual memory for the location of dots on a grid fell within the average range, obtaining a perfect score by the third learning trial and her overall score moving to the high average range following a long delay. Her short-term recall for faces had moved into the high average range, with only a slightly lesser improvement into the average range on the long-term memory condition. Word pair learning was in the low average range; although, it is hypothesised that this reflects a specific phonological memory difficulty seen in individuals with dyslexia (Lit & Nation, 2014).

Figure 9.1 shows the changes to Laura's memory scores (different tests were used, but with a shared domain), with time and improved recovery, resumption of better long-term memory function, memory for faces, and short-term visual memory. Changes to verbal recall was more average. For

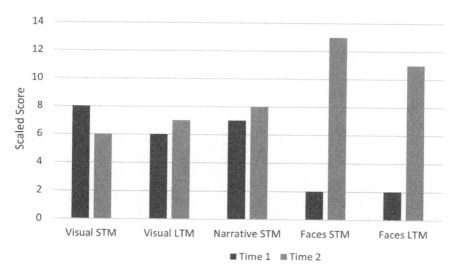

Figure 9.1 Laura's memory score changes time 1 (5 months after symptom onset) and
time 2 (11 months after illness onset). Please note, for ease of comparison
of functioning and change over time, at the two assessment time points,
scores are graphed by domain assessed, although different memory tests
were used: Nepsy II at time 1, Children's Memory Scale (Cohen, 1997),
at time 2

Laura, it appears that motor speed needed longer to recover than memory
functions.

In summary, Laura's memory functions showed a striking improvement,
particularly for her memory of faces and her delayed long-term memory. She
had continuing weaknesses in verbal working memory and her response speed.

Emotional and behavioural well-being

On the Strengths and Difficulties Questionnaire (SDQ, Goodman, Meltzer,
& Bailey, 1998), emotional symptoms continued to be a significant concern.
It was noted that Laura's social contact and participation in activities were less
than is typical for her age.

Impact on the family

There was a marked negative impact on the family's quality of life (Paediatric
Quality of Life Index, PedsQL, Varni et al., 2004). Parental scores on the Impact of Event scales increased at the time of the second assessment, reflecting
the ongoing and cumulative impact of the acute illness, ongoing challenges,
and uncertainty about the future.

Social participation

The scores on the Child and Adolescent Scale of Participation questionnaire (CASP, Bedell, 2009), at the second assessment, suggested that Laura's level of participation falls within the extremely low range. Her scores reflected a significant reduction in social life as this was too fatiguing and overwhelming for her, and her prioritisation of meeting educational goals. She had lost touch with her friends from her previous year group. Physical activity, which had been a large part of her life, had substantially reduced.

Neuropsychological rehabilitation

The intervention approach followed has been detailed elsewhere (Gracey et al., 2015), including a collaborative formulation process with the young person, family, and rehabilitation team members, followed by a mix of support and training for school and family, and selected psychoeducation, cognitive rehabilitation, and psychotherapeutic work with the young person.

Developing a shared understanding

In line with our service aims, Laura's physical and contextual strengths and areas of need were mapped out using the CCPNR interdisciplinary formulation based on the ICF model (Figure 9.2). This became a template to share her strengths and needs with herself, family, school, and other services in order to develop a shared understanding of her needs.

Further, 30 hours of community consultation and individual interventions were offered to provide:

- Access to local Child and Adolescent Mental Health Services (CAMHS) to address mood.
- Fatigue management interventions including support around activity pacing, fatigue, and sleep.
- Guidance to increase participation in independent living activities, including detailed task analysis and support to increase fluency of activities.
- Cognitive training and strategies to support attention, episodic memory, and face processing (to support her ability to recognise her friends) in addition to processing speed support.
- Communication support including offering choices, breaking down instructions, reducing background noise and distractions, simplifying and structuring conversations.
- Recommendations to support activities of daily living and self-care.
- Understanding brain injury training at school, including support with graded return to school/catch-up learning, exam access arrangements (extra time, rest breaks, use of a laptop word processor).

Interdisciplinary Formulation for Laura

School
Reported to be B grade student pre-injury. Will re-take this GCSEs this year, already sat mocks.
Worked hard; focused; pre-injury dyslexia: Access supports – laptop before injury.
Wants to go to university.
Reintegrating with new peer group (year below).

Early Development
Has known dyslexia (quite severe, difficulties with pronunciation of unfamiliar words). Reached motor skills milestones early (walk at 9 months); speech delayed but communication seemed good. SLT involved. Independent child

Injury: body process changes
Initial presentation behaving out of character. Referred to child and adolescent mental health service, psychotic episode diagnosed. Several weeks of attempted treatment for psychosis no response, sig. behavioural and functional impairment. EEG and tests – anti-NMDAR enc., steroids, plasma exchange, ICU.

Family
Mum, Dad, sister, cats. 3 close friends.

Family motto: Treat people as you want to be treated. To Laura always: Patience is a virtue.

Grandparents alive and supportive

Cognitive
General Intellectual Functioning: Very strong quantitative reasoning ability. General ability on domains of visual spatial, verbal and fluid reasoning are strong. Working memory and processing speed relative weaker areas.
Exec function: good verbal fluency, cognitive flexibility, inhibition. Observationally, good sustained attention.
Memory – Significant improvements and recovery to memory functions. Good memory for faces, stories and visual spatial information both immediately and following a long delay. Strong recognition memory. Verbal Working memory challenges –
stronger visual spatial working memory – span on both of 4.
Processing speed – Slower motor and information processing.
•**Attainments:** strong maths, ? generalising to school/exams. Continued phonological weaknesses, likely as part of a dyslexia profile

Communication
Speech much improved
Loss of confidence communicating socially, finds it difficult to follow conversations, cannot look at all the different people with the different noises. Used to be very sociable. Shuts down when feeling cannot follow conversation. Speech is monotone at the end of a day, when she is tired. Good vocab; some WFD.

Talking and TV is difficult. When out "I don't know what to say to people". Last 2 weeks better at picking up jokes and sarcasm.

Preinjury, 8/10 now 5/10 or 3/10 if tired. La Trobe self elevated for flow and focus. Mum: elevated for manner and focus.

Rehab goal: respond with practiced set phrase to someone in community, mum to wait in silence.

Emotion & Behaviour
Reported to always have independent person; laid back and a 'rounded' person.
Finds it difficult that needs quite a lot of supervision and help in areas of self care and mobility.
Mood swings severe after injury – was seen in CAMH due to overdose. Mum reported that things are better now.
Laura finds the situation very difficult, with her peers moving on and her having to repeat the year.
Anxious before seeing people, also friends. Feeling sad and worried in weekends +when tired. Can get stuck in feeling irritated about something.

Beck Youth Inventory– much below average self concept, mildly elevated anxiety. Average on dep, anger & disruptive behaviour scales
Adolescent Resilience Scale: Low social relatedness and mastery. Strength – low emotional reactivity.

Physical & Sensory-motor
Laura's mobility is improving; Local Physio and OT involved.
Mum reported ↓ tone and ↓confidence in physical ability. Has started swimming and really enjoyed this; can do exercises in the water and also did some lengths.
Hand tremors, especially when trying to eat or drink.
Cannot remember how to do breaststroke, swallow, walk stairs.
Used to do 7 hrs. of her main sport activity per week
Fatigue ++ → impact on self care + concentration/Attention
Sensory processing: Sensitive to noises - shuts down.
Sleep: takes hours to fall asleep; once asleep ok, but at times difficult to wake.
Sensorimotor: NEPSY Finger tapping – Extremely low score dominant and nondominant hands (slow, minor imprecision)

Participation
Home and family: Mum is currently at home to help/supervise/ plan the day. Activities of Daily Living: Now independent
School – pre-injury: popular with other girls; high targets for herself. Now: integrating back in slowly; re-doing academic year. Brain injury/illness training for teachers. School continues to be very supportive.
Community – cannot continue with her main sport activity at the moment; has started swimming. Hobbies, leisure activities
Community – peer relationships, was always very sociable, but now has lost confidence
Goals: **Laura**: Going back to school some time; starting up gymnastics again, to know more about anti-NMDAR Encephalitis, "getting back to normal" (make breakfast, walk to school, being more independent, get to places on my own).
Mum: *Immediate:* in school for short periods; being more independent in self care (showering, choosing what to wear), going out with friends. *Long term:* back to school full time, be able to sit exams and go on and back to a normal life, still be the same Laura, who is physically able.

Figure 9.2 Interdisciplinary shared formulation of Laura's strengths and needs at 11 months (including background information)

Post intervention school and family meeting to support school and exam access arrangements

Following the second assessment, Laura was seen at her school with her father and her teaching team to develop a shared understanding of Laura's needs and intervention approaches required. At that point, Laura was noted to have done well in her GCSE retakes, was making good progress at school, although working extremely hard. Fatigue was still a concern, particularly persisting tiredness at home, impacting homework and social participation. Provision to go to school learning support (to study) or the health centre (for rest and relaxation when fatigued) was put in place and relaxation of sixth form entry requirements was implemented.

Long-term outcome

Four years following her initial symptoms, Laura was reported to be well, and attending university. She was noted to have some persisting cognitive difficulties, despite reaching her overall goal to complete exams and attend university, although this was from self-report and we did not have formal as-sessment information to detail the nature of the residual difficulties. Further information on the impact of her difficulties on everyday life was also not provided during this final brief communication.

Conclusion

This chapter set out to describe anti-NMDAR encephalitis and highlight the challenges with accurate diagnosis at the acute stage and the importance of appropriate awareness of neuropsychological needs over the longer term, especially in children and young people. We described in brief the assessment and rehabilitation of Laura, a teenager who was participating in a range of activities to a high level and achieving well when she was faced with her illness. Not only did she have to navigate debilitating symptoms, but she also struggled with a three-month period before her condition was correctly identified and treated. Her neuropsychological profile was broadly consistent with what has been reported in the literature, with assessment findings con-firming that her cognition was markedly affected during her initial illness (five months post symptom onset), with an impressive, although incomplete recovery five months later (11 months post first presentation), with lingering speed and verbal memory difficulties noted. Community neuropsychological rehabilitation involving Laura, her family, and school assisted adaptation and achievement of goals with a good long-term outcome in terms of Laura's goal to attend university, despite self-reported ongoing residual cognitive issues.

The case that we present highlights the far-reaching impact of unusual or hard to diagnose conditions. For Laura and her family, there were several psychosocial challenges to her journey. Firstly, the path through acute health services was complicated, traumatic, and marked by an exacerbation of her condition. For many with anti-NMDAR encephalitis, it is not clear when or if a full recovery will occur. Secondly, the illness interrupted a key period of development, which, we hypothesised, reciprocally impacted her social tasks, neurodevelopment, milestone attainment, and her mood during her recovery. During this period of uncertainty, repeated testing and plotting of progress may serve to reassure and track response to treatment, recovery, or relapse risk.

Heine et al. (2017) were the first research group to highlight the need for repeated post-acute neuropsychological testing and dedicated cognitive rehabilitation. Few services are set up (or funded) for monitoring the long-term recovery of individuals with anti-NMDAR encephalitis. However, had this young person not had access to neuropsychological assessment and targeted support, her re-entry to education may have been less successful. Further, provision of early psychoeducation, support, and reassurance can facilitate emotional adaptation for the young person and family. Based on our service experience with individuals with autoimmune encephalitis, we have learnt that psychoeducation and putting in place a system of symptom monitoring (using standardised and bespoke visual rating scales) helps contain anxiety held by families, school, and broader systems. A detailed formulation, that can be flexibly updated as new information emerges, is perhaps key to developing understanding and managing anxiety in the context of uncertainty and sharing information across services.

The case also highlights the challenge of accurate monitoring of cognitive changes over time. In the acute stage, the individual may feel too distressed, or disabled by motor impairments to complete a full neuropsychological battery, so a briefer mapping of the cognitive profile may help to differentiate anti-NMDAR encephalitis from other psychiatric conditions. Consensus on the components included within a brief screen assessment, perhaps with an emphasis on verbal memory, face recognition, and motor skills whilst limiting fatigue or psychological distress, will be valuable to indicate relapse risk and measure long-term recovery. Further, early interventions can help reduce any secondary mental health consequences and the need for further child and adolescent mental health service (CAMHS) involvement, which has been our experience with other service users where prompt and intensive anti-NMDAR encephalitis treatment was not initiated. Consistent with Remy et al. (2017) we strongly advocate for a comprehensive rehabilitation package to improve long-term outcome that includes management of functional decline in motor skills and cognition, as soon as feasible to implement.

Whilst the focus of the literature on anti-NMDAR encephalitis highlights neurocognitive and psychiatric changes, this work emphasises the importance of also understanding the emotional impact on Laura, especially her social identity and goals as an adolescent, and the need for psychological support for family, and cognitive/learning support and psychoeducation for school. With early diagnosis and treatment, and community neuropsychological follow-up, there is potential for good outcomes to be achieved, despite some residual impairment.

Acknowledgements

We would like to acknowledge Laura and her family for consenting to sharing information so we could write this chapter to help raise awareness of anti-NMDAR encephalitis. We would also like to acknowledge the other young people we have seen with autoimmune encephalitis, to whom we are also indebted for our learning and awareness of this condition. Finally, we'd like to acknowledge the expertise of the wider clinical team who contributed to the clinical work described here.

References

Armangue, T., Petit-Pedrol, M., & Dalmau, J. (2012). Autoimmune encephalitis in children. *Journal of Child Neurology*, *27*(11), 1460–1469. https://doi.org/10.1177/0883073812448838

Barkus, C., McHugh, S. B., Sprengel, R., Seeburg, P.H., Rawlins, J. N., & Bannerman, D. M. (2010). Hippocampal NMDA receptors and anxiety: At the interface between cognition and emotion. *European Journal of Pharmacology*, *626*, 49–56.

Beck, A. T., Beck, J. S., Jolly, J., & Steer, R. (2005). *The Beck youth inventories*, 2nd ed. Pearson.

Bedell, G. (2009). Further validation of the Child and Adolescent Scale of Participation (CASP). *Developmental Neurorehabilitation*, *12*, 342–351.

Belanoff, J. K., Gross, K., Yager, A., & Schatzberg, A. F. (2001). Corticosteroids and cognition. *Journal of Psychiatric Research* 35, 127–145.

Blakemore, S.J. (2018) Inventing Ourselves: The Secret Life of the Teenage Brain. Transwold Publishers, London.

Brenton J. N., & Goodkin, H. P. (2016). Antibody-mediated autoimmune encephalitis in childhood. *Pediatric Neurology*, *60*, 13–23. https://doi.org/10.1016/j.pediatrneurol.2016.04.004

Cellucci, T., Van Mater, H., Graus, F., Muscal, E., Gallentine, W., Klein-Gitelman, M. S., Benseler, S. M., Frankovich, J., Gorman, M. P., Van Haren, K., Dalmau, J., & Dale, R. C. (2020). Clinical approach to the diagnosis of autoimmune encephalitis in the pediatric patient. *Neurology(R), Neuroimmunology and Neuroinflammation*, *7*(2), e663. https://doi.org/10.1212/NXI.0000000000000663

Cohen, M. J. (1997). *The children's memory scale*. Pearson.

Dalmau, J., Lancaster, E., Martinez-Hernandez, E., Rosenfeld, M. R., & Balice-Gordon, R. (2011). Clinical experience and laboratory investigations in patients with anti-NMDAR encephalitis. *The Lancet. Neurology*, *10*(1), 63–74. https://doi.org/10.1016/S1474-4422(10)70253-2

de Bruijn, M., Aarsen, F. K., van Oosterhout, M. P., van der Knoop, M. M., Catsman-Berrevoets, C. E., Schreurs, M., Bastiaansen, D., Sillevis Smitt, P., Neuteboom, R. F., Titulaer, M. J., & CHANCE Study Group (2018). Long-term neuropsychological outcome following pediatric anti-NMDAR encephalitis. *Neurology*, *90*(22), e1997–e2005. https://doi.org/10.1212/WNL.0000000000005605

Delis, D. C., Kaplan E., & Kramer, J. H. (2001). *The Delis-Kaplan Executive Function System*™ *(D-KEFS*™*)*. The first nationally standardized set of tests to evaluate higher level cognitive functions in both children and adults. Pearson.

Finke, C., Kopp, U. A., Pajkert, A., Behrens, J. R., Leypoldt, F., Wuerfel, J. T., Ploner, C. J., Prüss, H., & Paul, F. (2016). Structural hippocampal damage following Anti-N-Methyl-D-Aspartate receptor encephalitis. *Biological Psychiatry, 79*(9), 727–734.

Gibson, L. L., McKeever, A., Coutinho, E., Finke, C., & Pollak, T. A. (2020). Cognitive impact of neuronal antibodies: encephalitis and beyond. *Translational Psychiatry, 10*(1), 304. https://doi.org/10.1038/s41398-020-00989-x

Gamino, J. F., Chapman, S. B., & Cook, L. G. (2009). Strategic learning in youth with traumatic brain injury: Evidence for stall in higher-order cognition. *Topics in Language Disorders, 29*(3), 224–235.

Goodman, R., Meltzer, H., & Bailey, V. (1998). The Strengths and Difficulties Questionnaire: A pilot study on the validity of the self-report version. *European Child & Adolescent Psychiatry, 7*(3), 125–130.

Gracey, F., Olsen, G., Austin, L., Watson, S., & Malley, D. (2015). Integrating psychological therapy into interdisciplinary child neuropsychological rehabilitation. In J. Reed, K. Byard, & H. Fine (Eds.), *Neuropsychological rehabilitation of childhood brain injury: A practical guide* (pp. 191–214). Palgrave Macmillan.

Graus, F., Titulaer, M. J., Balu, R., Benseler, S., Bien, C. G., Cellucci, T., Cortese, I., Dale, R. C., Gelfand, J. M., Geschwind, M., Glaser, C. A., Honnorat, J., Höftberger, R., Iizuka, T., Irani, S. R., Lancaster, E., Leypoldt, F., Prüss, H., Rae-Grant, A., Reindl, M., & Dalmau, J. (2016). A clinical approach to diagnosis of autoimmune encephalitis. *The Lancet. Neurology, 15*(4), 391–404. https://doi.org/10.1016/S1474-4422(15)00401-9

Heine, J., Kopp, U. A., Klag, J., Ploner, C. J., Prüss, H. and Finke, C. (2021). Long-term cognitive outcome in anti–N-methyl-D-aspartate receptor encephalitis. *Annals of Neurology, 90*(6), 949–961. https://doi.org/10.1002/ana.26241. Epub 2021 Oct 21. PMID: 34595771

Hinkle, C. D., Porter, J. N., Waldron, E. J., Klein, H., Tranel, D., & Heffelfinger, H. (2017). Neuropsychological characterization of three adolescent females with anti-NMDA receptor encephalitis in the acute, post-acute, and chronic phases: An inter-institutional case series. *The Clinical Neuropsychologist, 31*(1), 268–288. https://doi.org/10.1080/13854046.2016.1191676

Irani, S. R., & Vincent, A., (2011) NMDA receptor antibody encephalitis. *Current Neurology and Neuroscience Reports, 11*, 298–304.

Johnson, S., Blum, R., & Giedd, J. (2009) Adolescent maturity and the brain: The promise and pitfalls of neuroscience research in adolescent health policy. *Journal of Adolescent Health, 45*(3), 216–221.

Kolb, B., & Gibb, R. (2011). Brain plasticity and behaviour in the developing brain. *Journal of the Canadian Academy of Child and Adolescent Psychiatry, 20*(4), 265–276.

Korkman, M., Kirk, U., & Kemp, S. L. (2007). *NEPSY II. Administrative manual.* Psychological Corporation.

Lit, R. A., & Nation, K. (2014). The nature and specificity of paired associate learning deficits in children with dyslexia. *Journal of Memory and Language, 71*(1), 71–88.

Loughan, A. R., Allen, A., Perna R., & Malkin, M. G. (2016). Anti-N-methyl-D-aspartate receptor encephalitis: A review and neuropsychological case study. *The*

Clinical Neuropsychologist, 30(1), 150–163. https://doi.org/10.1080/13854046.2015.1132772

Lupien, S. J., & McEwen, B. S. (1997). The acute effects of corticosteroids on cognition: Integration of animal and human model studies. *Brain Research Reviews, 24,* 1–27.

McIvor, K. & Moore, P. (2017) Spontaneous recovery of memory functions in an untreated case of anti NMDAR encephalitis: A reason to maintain hope. *The Clinical Neuropsychologist, 31*(1), 289–300. https://doi.org/10.1080/13854046.2016.1245358

Moss, N.,. Petranovich, C.L., Parks, L., & Sherwood, A. (2018). Two case reports of neuropsychological outcomes following pediatric anti-N-methyl-D-aspartate receptor autoimmune encephalitis. *Developmental Neuropsychology, 43*(7), 656–668. https://doi.org/10.1080/87565641.2018.1506456

Naber, D., Sand, P., & Heigl, B. (1995). Psychopathological and neuropsychological effects of 8-days' corticosteroid treatment. A prospective study. *Psychoneuroendocrinology, 21*(1), 25–31.

Nicolle, D. C. M., & Moses, J. L. (2018). A systematic review of the neuropsychological sequelae of people diagnosed with anti-N-methyl-D-aspartate receptor encephalitis in the acute and chronic phases. *Archives of Clinical Neuropsychology, 33*(8), 964–983. https://doi.org/10.1093/arclin/acy005

Prince-Embury, S. (2007). *The resiliency scales for children and adolescents.* Harcourt Assessment.

Remy, K., Custer, J., Cappell, J., Foster, C., Garber, N., Walker, L., Simon, L., & Bagdure, D. (2017). Pediatric anti-N-methyl-D-aspartate receptor encephalitis: A review with pooled analysis and critical care emphasis. *Frontiers in Pediatrics, 5*(250), 1–8.

Rison, R. A., & Stanton, P. K. (1995) Long-term potentiation and N-methyl-D-aspartate receptors: Foundations of memory and neurologic disease? *Neuroscience and Behavioural Reviews, 19*(4), 533–552.

Rosenfeld, M. R. & Dalmau, J. (2011). Anti-NMDA-receptor encephalitis and other synaptic autoimmune disorders. *Current Treatment Option in Neurology, 13*(3), 324–332. https://doi.org/10.1007/s11940-011-0116-y; PMID: 21298406; PMCID: PMC3705219

Sherwood Brown, E., Woolston, D. J., Frol, A., Bobadilla, L., Khan, D., Hanczyc, M., Rush, A. J., Fleckenstein, J., Babcock, E., & Munro Cullum, C. (2004). Hippocampal volume, spectroscopy, cognition and mood in patients receiving corticosteroid therapy. *Biological Psychiatry, 55,* 538–545.

Steinberg, L. (2014). *Age of opportunity: Lessons from the new science of adolescence.* First Mariner Books.

Steiner, J., Prüss, H., Köhler, S., Frodl, T., Hasan, A., & Falkai, T. (2020). Autoimmune encephalitis with psychosis: Warning signs, step-by-step diagnostics and treatment. *The World Journal of Biological Psychiatry, 21*(4), 241–254. https://doi.org/10.1080/15622975.2018.1555376

Varni, J. W., Sherman, S. A., Burwinkle, T. M., Dickinson, P. E., & Dixon, P. (2004). The PedsQL™ family impact module: Preliminary reliability and validity. *Health and Quality of Life Outcomes, 2*(55), 1–6.

Vijayakumar, N., Op de Macks, Z., Shirtcliff, E. A., Pfeifer, J. H. (2018). Puberty and the human brain: Insights into adolescent development. *Neuroscience & Biobehavioral Reviews, 92,* 417–436. https://doi.org/10.1016/j.neubiorev.2018.06.004

Wright, S., Hacohen, Y., Jacobson, L., Agrawal, S., Gupta, R., Philip, S., Smith, M., Lim, M., Wassmer, E., & Vincent A. (2015). N-methyl-D-aspartate receptor antibody-mediated neurological disease: Results of a UK-based surveillance study in children. *Archives of Disease in Childhood, 100*(6), 521–526. https://doi.org/10.1136/archdischild-2014-306795; Epub 2015, January 30. PMID: 25637141; PMCID: PMC4453622

Weiss, D. S. (2007). The impact of event scale-revised. In J. P. Wilson, & T. M. Keane (Eds.), *Assessing psychological trauma and PTSD: A practitioner's handbook* (2nd ed., pp. 168–189). Guilford Press.

Wechsler, D. (2005). *Wechsler Individual Achievement Test*, 2nd ed. (WIAT II). The Psychological Corp.

Wechsler, D. (2014) *Wechsler Intelligence Scale for Children*, 5th ed. (WISC-V). Pearson.

Wilkinson-Smith, A. Blackwell, L. S., & Howarth, R. A. (2021). Neuropsychological outcomes in children and adolescents following anti-NMDA receptor encephalitis. *Child Neuropsychology, 28*(2), 212–223. https://doi.org/10.1080/09297049.2021.1965110; Epub 2021, August 26. PMID: 34435553

World Health Organization (2007). *International classification of functioning, disability and health: Children & youth version: ICF-CY.* World Health Organization.

Zandi, M. S., Irani, S. R., Lang, B., Waters, P., Jones, P. B., McKenna, P., Coles, A. J., Vincent, A., & Lennox, B. R. (2011). Disease-relevant autoantibodies in first episode schizophrenia. *Journal of Neurology, 258*, 686–688.

Part 2

Diagnostic challenges

10 Neuropsychological, neuropsychiatric, and functional neurological symptoms

The challenges of overlapping and evolving presentations

Alexandra E. Rose and Michael Dilley

Initial presentation

TM, a 30-year-old man described by his family as kind, social, and a nature lover; presented to his general practitioner (GP) following a period of self-reported deterioration in his memory, attention, and ability to multi-task. He did well at school and went on to complete a university degree and was successfully employed in the city. He thought that his memory had been getting worse since the age of 18 but had deteriorated further in his city job which he reported hating. He reported a history of episodes of depression associated with periods of stress. He had left the city job to work as a tree surgeon. His mother noticed that he had poor sleep hygiene, that he was either 'all go' or 'asleep', and that he was 'unreliable' when it came to attending appointments. He was referred to a neurologist by his GP for further investigations. His mother was particularly worried and felt he was getting worse. Neurological examination and investigations, including magnetic resonance imaging (MRI) and electroencephalography (EEG), were essentially normal. His neurologist requested assessment by a neuropsychologist.

Neuropsychological assessment

The authors were not involved in neuropsychological assessments in this case. The findings of the neuropsychological assessment showed that his estimated premorbid functioning was towards the high end of Average. Results on the Verbal Comprehension Index (VCI) and Working Memory Index (WMI) of the Weschler Adult Intelligence Scale (WAIS) were within the average range, and his Perceptual Reasoning Index (PRI) was within the low average range. His performance on the Processing Speed Index (PSI) was impaired. His full scale IQ was within the average range. On tests of memory he was impaired in immediate recall of visual and verbal information, with significant loss at delayed recall. His list learning fluctuated over five trials with multiple

DOI: 10.4324/9781003228226-12

intrusions and impaired ability on recognition trials. His visual perception, naming, and semantic fluency were all within the expected range of performance. He demonstrated slowed switching ability in executive functioning assessments and reduced performance in attention tasks when distractors were introduced.

Overall, he demonstrated mild intellectual under-functioning in non-verbal domains. He was impaired on verbal and visual memory tests as well as processing speed performance. It was noted by the assessor that he was self-critical of his performance, and he reported feeling nervous and embarrassed and often reported that the information was 'all gone' and that he could feel he was getting stressed out with himself. It was observed that he did slightly better on a recognition task as it progressed, and when he was receiving positive feedback and reassurance.

The assessor at the time thought that the presenting issue was psychological, in accordance with the lack of positive neurological findings (repeated volumetric imaging, EEG, and bloods being all normal) and their observations of anxiety in testing and on formal screens. They thought that TM had developed a pattern of being unable to attend to information when under stress, which affected his encoding and subsequent recall abilities. This was reflected in TMs own report of feeling under pressure and overloaded with information and that his symptoms worsened when he was stressed and improved when he was reassured and given time. Psychological intervention was recommended and reassessment if his memory difficulties did not improve. There was subsequently a referral to a neuropsychiatrist, clinical psychologist, and occupational therapist.

Community multidisciplinary assessment, formulation, and treatment

TM reported that he thought that his mood had deteriorated during the time he had been working in the city and that this was also associated with a lack of energy, poor self-esteem, and a sense of 'feeling dead to things'. After starting his tree surgery training, he had noticed an improvement in his mood and contingent improvement in his memory, although he had not returned to his normal self. He thought that the last time that his memory and thinking skills had been normal was in his first job in the city.

Neuropsychiatric assessment identified the following problems reported by TM:

1. Not trusting myself – 'I don't trust a thought coming into my head – I doubt things including my thinking skills and memory and I need information repeated'.
2. 'I overcomplicate things in my brain' – 'if I can't think I tend to panic and have "white noise" and find it even harder to think'.
3. I am either 'all or nothing' – in terms of thinking and activity.

4. I get anxious and panic when I am confronted by things and that makes
    them more likely to go wrong.

There was no family history of mental ill health or memory problems. TM
and his mother reported a normal neurodevelopmental history and a happy
early life. There was no significant past medical history.

   In assessing his mental state, TM noted a particular difference between
himself and others and a tendency to compare himself and subsequently,
ruminate about his self-esteem. He described low-level energy, apathy, and
poor motivation, with a tendency to 'dawdle around the flat' and needing
to prompt himself with alarms throughout the day to initiate activity. He
thought that if he did not start an activity from the beginning of the day, he
would tend to procrastinate about his plans, put them off and postpone doing anything, subsequently being stuck at home all day. He reported 'mental
panic', particularly in the context of concerns about his thinking skills and
memory function.

   TM found that he tended to 'beat himself up' if he got to the end of the
day and had not achieved what he had set out to do. He described ruminating
over his thoughts about self-worth, with a degree of guilt about the impact on
his family, and particularly his mother, in terms of their concerns for him. He
thought that he was 'anxious about anxiety' and described having a 'foggy
brain'. He denied any obsessional thoughts, features of post-traumatic stress,
psychotic symptoms, or generalised anxiety phenomena.

   Importantly, when considering his cognitive symptoms there were examples of inconsistency in function and variability of symptoms associated with
changes in mental state.

Formulation

The MDT developed a working formulation for TM that served as a way
to understand his presenting symptoms and how they were perpetuating his
anxiety, depressed mood, and functional cognitive symptoms.

   Firstly, his experience of memory failures when he first became low in
mood at work meant that he developed an assumption about his 'cognitive
abilities being impaired'. Consequently, in situations where he needed to
perform, he would worry about forgetting information or getting something
wrong, leading him to feeling anxious. As a result, he would pay less attention to what is happening in the moment because his attention was focused
on ruminative worry. This inattention then led to poor encoding of information, which he experienced as a memory failure, confirming his fear. His
anxiety was compounded by understandable concerns from his friends and
family, who had observed the significant change in his functioning.

   Secondly, TM's depressed mood resulted in lower motivation and less activity. As a result of this lowered level of activity, he was very critical of himself compared to his assumptions about what his work and social functioning

should be. This compounded his depressed mood, low self-confidence, and avoidance of engaging in meaningful work, through fear of failure and being a disappointment to his family.

It also became apparent that TM had several perfectionistic assumptions, as he tried to complete tasks and remember 'perfectly', and this meant that he tended to overthink the steps he needed to take, resulting in him being caught up in thinking rather than performing the actual task. This meant he did not get things done that he set out to do, but also in front of other people, he appeared slow in his movements or talking and came across as confused. He would become aware that he was not 'performing' and reported feeling anxious, amplifying his difficulty at getting a task done. His repeated 'failures' confirmed the negative beliefs he had formed about himself.

Neuropsychiatry

The neuropsychiatric treatment plan considered the multidisciplinary formulation and the key reversible factors where a neuropsychologically informed approach to prescribing could be taken. A trial of anxiety and mood treatment with citalopram was commenced and showed initial benefits, although after several months of treatment with a dose of 30mg, TM complained that he was experiencing significant itching which he attributed to the medication and wanted to stop treatment. After an interval without medication, and a self-reported deterioration in mood and anxiety, he was commenced on sertraline and the dose escalated to 100mg. Following this, in the context of ongoing anxiety and mood symptoms, it was recommended that his sertraline continue to be increased at 25mg increments to a maximum tolerable dose dependent on side effects and benefits. Later, after several months of treatment but persisting reports of mood and anxiety symptoms he was commenced on venlafaxine.

Neuropsychology

Multidisciplinary treatment with clinical psychology and occupational therapy was undertaken over several months, alongside family support sessions. Psychology sessions were structured around a cognitive-behavioural therapy (CBT) approach. The sessions explored the maintaining factors for his difficulties, supported him in making small goals around behavioural changes, and challenged his assumptions and predictions connected to his difficulties. The sessions also explored relevant links to his past experiences. In line with behavioural activation for depression, a strong focus was placed on activity scheduling. Treatment also explored his tendency to self-criticise and ruminate, and how this fed into his low motivation and low mood. He noticed that when he was more active during his day, his mood improved. Much of the work completed in sessions was formulation-based.

TM showed limited awareness of incidents, concerns, or family worries about his overall performance in all areas of activities and everyday life. He was often upbeat and positive at the start of sessions, reporting to having had a good week and feeling he was moving forward and being in control. Only by the second part of a session, through reflection of not completing homework tasks, testing memory of appointments attended, and not achieving the small goals set by the therapist from one week to the next, did he become more open and realistic about his challenges. As a session progressed he was able to talk more openly about his lack of drive, self-deprecation, and blaming and criticism of himself.

Occupational therapy

Time was spent assessing TM's self-management in areas of personal care and domestic activities, i.e., shopping, cooking, and laundry. He was able to function in all these areas but lacked initiation and motivation to participate routinely in his domestic tasks and personal care tasks, which became evident over the months of working with him when his appearance deteriorated, and he appeared to have limited awareness of this. He did not respond well to feedback and was embarrassed by his lack of awareness of his reduced self-care. Goals were reduced to a minimal level to support his morning routine, i.e., laying out his clothes the night before and washing his hair daily, attempting to use a tick box method, and photo recording. A rehabilitation assistant was introduced in the later part of the therapy intervention with the agreement of the family to support him with his planning and initiation. Their feedback was that he required maximum support to focus and engage in the process and was unable to carry over information planned from one session to the next.

TM attempted to introduce more routine into his week and increase the variety of activities he was engaged in. He had a gym membership which he reported attending; however, it became clear this was not happening, following feedback from family and requests to record activities with photos that did not transpire for discussion in therapy. TM started to identify places of interest, such as museums, that he would like to visit to help motivate him to get out of the flat.

When using smart phone strategies to set up alerts and support his organisation and memory, TM's overall attendance at sessions was more successful. If these strategies were not used consistently, he could not rely on himself to recall routinely booked sessions. A good example was his neuropsychology sessions, which were in the same location at the same time every week. He was not consistent in recalling this or able to carry over from one session to the next and needed to diarise and add prompts to successfully attend. As rehabilitation continued, even with the appointment diarised and alerts on, the increase in late attendance and even missed appointments was noticeable and it was noted that his mother was also contacting him to prompt him and ensure he attended.

During vocational work planning, he spent much time ruminating over the negatives in his career history and poor decision making around opportunities and choices he had made. TM remained motivated with a goal of arranging a part-time job but breaking this into manageable and achievable steps was difficult and often he was unable to initiate how to make this goal realistic. He was supported to consider volunteer work and required maximum support to find a potential opportunity with a horticultural organisation. During rehabilitation, it had been concluded that TM would not be able to achieve this goal without the support of a 'buddy'/rehabilitation assistant to support him to successfully attend the volunteer work programme and support with initiating the tasks of the role.

Following a three-month period of multidisciplinary rehabilitation, a second neuropsychiatry opinion and further neurological opinions were requested to make sure that an underlying condition was not being missed. Further neurological examination and investigations, including neuroimaging and autoantibodies, were all reportedly normal, three and a half years after the first presentation. A referral for inpatient neuropsychiatric rehabilitation was also requested.

Despite the lack of any further clarity from further opinions, TM's presentation deteriorated with worsening in his memory and day-to-day function and the onset of motor symptoms and hypersalivation. TM was subsequently referred in consideration for an inpatient neurorehabilitation admission.

Hospital admission

Whilst awaiting an inpatient bed, TM's condition continued to deteriorate and his behaviour became more erratic, finally culminating in his family taking him to hospital for further assessment. Following this steep decline in function, he was referred to the National Hospital for Neurology and Neurosurgery (NHNN), a quaternary service, for further specialist investigations.

TM, by this time 34 years old, presented with a five-year history of worsening cognitive impairment and a one-year history of deteriorating physical and functional abilities. Over the previous year he had started becoming 'unsteady on his feet' and started to display 'jerking movements' at rest as well as 'drooling a lot'. He continued to display memory difficulties, as well as changes in his speech pattern and apraxia. Repeat neuropsychology assessments showed a decline in his verbal and performance IQ as well as a deterioration in his recall and recognition of visual and verbal information, his attention was impaired, and he showed poor performance on executive functioning tasks (see Table 10.1). Epilepsy investigations were indicated and a working diagnosis of progressive myoclonic epilepsy with apraxia was given. His MRI at this stage, 18 months after the most recent scan to have been reported as normal, showed volume loss and increased metabolic activity in the medial frontal and medial temporal lobe structures on both sides of his brain. The cortical changes and volume loss in the temporal-medial region were thought to be in keeping with autoimmune encephalitis. EEGs showed abnormal activity that could have explained the myoclonic jerking. He was investigated with a number of blood tests, genetic testing, and imaging.

Neuropsychological assessments were repeated during this admission and showed further decline in his verbal IQ and memory and attention abilities (see Table 10.1 for comparison of neuropsychological test performance across the three assessment occasions).

Table 10.1 TM Neuropsychological assessments over four-year period, with all scores expressed as percentiles unless stated otherwise. Abbreviations: TOPF, Test of Premorbid Functioning; WAIS, Wechsler Adult Intelligence Scale; VCI, Verbal Comprehension Index; PRI, Perceptual Reasoning Index; WMI, Working Memory Index; PSI, Processing Speed Index; FSIQ, Full Scale Intelligence Quotient; BMIPB, The Brain Injury Rehabilitation Trust Memory and Information Processing Battery; RMT, Recognition Memory Test; VOSP, Visual Object and Space Perception Battery; DKEFS, Delis-Kaplan Executive Function System; TEA, Test of Everyday Attention.

	December 2015	*January 2019*	*March 2019*
TOPF	All WAIS-IV index scores estimated 50th-75th centile	–	–

	December 2015	*January 2019*	*March 2019*
Subtests	WAIS-IV	WAIS-III★	WAIS-III
Block Design	25th (Low average)	Impaired	Failure to score
Similarities	25–50th (Average)	Average	Low Average
Digit Span	50th (Average)	Impaired	Impaired
Matrix Reasoning	10–25th (Low average)	–	–
Vocabulary	75th (High average)	Average	Average
Arithmetic	25–50th (Average)	–	Impaired
Symbol Search	<5th (Impaired)	–	–
Coding	<5th (Impaired)	–	–
VCI	63rd (Average)	Verbal IQ: 88	Verbal IQ: 76
PRI	18th (Low average)	(Low average)	(Borderline)
WMI	42nd (Average)	Performance IQ:	Performance IQ: 52
PSI	2nd (Impaired)	54 (Impaired)	(Impaired)
FSIQ	21st (Borderline)		
BMIPB Story			
Immediate	2nd	–	–
Delayed	<2nd		
Retained	<2nd		
BMIPB Figure			
Copy	25th	–	–
Immediate	<2nd		
Delayed	<2nd		
Retained	<2nd		
BMIPB list learning		–	–
Total A1–A5	<2nd		
A6	<2nd		
B	2nd		
Intrusions	<2nd		
Total word recognition	5th		
Total list recognition	<2nd		

(Continued)

Table 10.1 Continued

	December 2015	January 2019	March 2019
BMIPB Design Learning		–	–
Total A1–A5	25–50th		
A6	10–25th		
B	25th		
Intrusions	50–75th		
Design recognition total	<2nd		
Design identification total	2–5th		
Short RMT words	<5th	<5th	<5th
RMT Faces	50th	10th	Pictorial RMT: <1st
Graded Naming Test	50–75th	50–75th	50th
VOSP			
Object Decision	>5th	–	>5th
Cube Analysis	>5th	–	>5th
		Incomplete letters: >5th	
DKEFS			
Trail Making	<5th	Unable to keep	
Letter sequencing	25th	to task on the	
Number-letter switching		Stroop Colour Word Test, discontinued	
Phonemic fluency – F	>95th	'S': 18–21st, with 6 repetitions;	–
Semantic fluency (animals)	>90th	Animals: <10th	
TEA	'normal'	*He lost track when*	
Elevator counting	10–25th	*reciting the months*	
Elevator counting (distraction)		*of year forwards*	
Weigl sorting test	–	2/2	Unable to complete
Cognitive estimates	–	–	1–5th
Speed of processing	–	Cancelling 0s <1st	Counting backwards from 32; <1st

*   WAIS-III reported (not directly compared to WAIS-IV); Table reported according to referral reports received by author (AR).

At the time of discharge from NHNN he did not have a clear diagnosis and was being treated for his presenting symptoms. He had a working diagnosis of autoimmune encephalitis, progressive myoclonic syndrome with epileptiform activity, with further investigations being required (PET amyloid scans and genetic testing).

Disability management

Following his six-month assessment at NHNN and without a clear diagnosis, TM's family came to a local neuro-disability long-term care facility to look for support. The doctors and therapists at this facility felt that a period of disability management on their rehabilitation ward was warranted. By this stage his gait was ataxic, with a wide base and his upper body leaning back significantly; he had hypersalivation as he was not automatically swallowing; he was confused and disorientated with regard to time, and place; and his speech was dysarthric. Although the treating team still did not have a diagnosis for his condition, they were able to state with confidence that it was progressively getting worse, was clearly neurological in nature, and likely degenerative.

Orientation, awareness, and management of distress

It was discussed with TM whenever he became upset or distressed or asked, 'why am I here?' that there was something wrong with his brain and everyone was there to help him. He was unable to encode and retain this information and required others to continually remind him what was happening. He displayed agitation towards staff when they offered assistance, as he had no insight that he required help and found it confusing and threatening when apparent strangers tried to assist him. Due to his poor gait and lack of awareness of his impairments he had multiple falls when attempting to complete tasks, with no insight into the risks or his impairments. He had an episode of choking which required suctioning and back slaps, which understandably he found distressing.

Due to the severity of his presentation as well as his distress when he was confused, it was decided not to be in his best interests to repeat further formal assessments. In function, TM had cognitive communication impairments, which impacted his understanding of instructions and left his speech content vague and empty. He was able to follow basic commands and could make simple choices when provided with options. His previously learnt knowledge about his family, experiences, and preferences remained intact; however, he could not relate this knowledge to his current experience as he was unable to retain information about where he was or what was going on around him. He did not demonstrate the ability to learn new information, places, or routines. He had difficulties initiating tasks, required supervision and prompting for daily activities of living, and he was unable to consistently identify risks even with prompting from others.

TM had lucid periods throughout the day where he would become quite distressed and need others to reassure him. His family were crucial in providing emotional support and reassurance as well as continued social engagement.

Risk reduction and future planning

Due to the severity of his cognitive impairment, TM was assessed to lack capacity to consent to his placement and treatment and a Deprivation of Liberty Safeguards (DoLS) application was made. This included use of an alarm system and bed and chair sensors to alert staff when TM was getting up or had left the ward in order to provide distant supervision for his safety. TM was assessed to lack capacity to make decisions around eating and drinking in the context of his deteriorating swallow. A best interest meeting was required to discuss risk feeding as well as whether a percutaneous endoscopic gastrostomy (PEG) should be inserted. It was decided that TM should continue to have as high quality of life as possible. As he continued to enjoy eating and drinking, it was considered in his best interest that he continued with feeding, with foods being modified to reduce risk where possible. A PEG was discussed with TM and although he knew what it was, he was horrified when asked whether he should have one inserted and did not understand why we would do this to him as he had no issues. A decision was made, taking in TM's distress and confusion as well as the family's strong views that quality of life was more valuable than quantity of time and that TM would not have wanted to prolong his current state if he were not to recover; a decision was made not to insert a PEG.

TM's admission on the rehabilitation ward remained focused on disability management and quality of life. He was provided with comfortable seating and a wheelchair for longer distance mobility. He attended a concert with his family and had multiple trips to the park. His family, along with their dog, visited daily.

Diagnosis of very early onset Alzheimer's disease

Towards the end of his rehabilitation admission, TM's genetic testing results were received, and showed mutation of the gene Presenelin 1 (*PSEN-1*). Without a positive family history, this was a de novo mutation (meaning he was the first in his family to exhibit this mutation). The loss of Presenelin causes incomplete digestion of amyloid and is thought to contribute to an increased vulnerability of the brain and the development of early onset Alzheimer's disease. Very early onset Alzheimer's disease (VEOAD) can present with atypical features and reported cases of VEOAD are reportedly associated with *PSEN1* mutations (Filley et al., 2007).

End of life

TM's family were understandably devastated but also relieved to know the diagnosis and expected trajectory of his disease. He remained at the local neuro-disability long-term care facility where therapists and ward staff worked with his family to create an end-of-life care plan. The focus remained on quality of life, family contact, outings to local pubs and green spaces, and enjoyable social contact. Family and medical staff agreed that there would be a ceiling on care and that, when the time came that his swallow failed or he no longer took in food and fluids, that subcutaneous fluids would not be used. TM would be kept comfortable and pain free and, importantly, family would be present as TM would not have wanted to be alone.

In 2020, the COVID-19 pandemic meant that visitors were not permitted in to care homes. Exceptional circumstances were granted in TM's case for quality of life and because he was continuing to deteriorate. TM died in December 2020, five years after his assessment and one year after receiving his VEOAD diagnosis. He was comfortable and pain free and surrounded by his family and familiar carers at the end of his life. TM's mother donated his brain and spinal cord to NHNN brain trust after death, to advance scientific understanding of VEOAD.

Family

TM's family, particularly his mother, were incredibly devoted to him and the care he received. His mother remained actively involved in all decisions alongside TM's siblings and his father's side of the family. His mother has copious notes on the process of her son's deterioration, being the one to first notice that there was an issue. Within the cycle of her son becoming 'different' in her eyes (but perhaps without clinical symptoms) to her son getting a diagnosis of VEOAD, she had to deal with multiple professionals and both private and public services. She particularly struggled with the concept of 'it all being in (TM's) head'. She thought that the diagnosis of functional cognitive symptoms, depression, and anxiety meant that there was nothing wrong with her son, and that there was a degree of volition in his presentation which, alongside a continued deterioration of function, did not make sense to her and made her distrust professionals. From the professionals' perspective, TM had not shown evidence of a neurodegenerative illness initially and had a complex interplay of what was later established to be a prodrome of neuropsychiatric, neuropsychological, and functional cognitive symptoms that became more demonstrably neurological as the illness progressed.

Discussion

On reflection, a lack of integrated services, as well as splitting of neurological, neuropsychiatric, functional, and psychological diagnoses, leads to undue distress for our patients and their families. The perception that psychological and mental health problems do not have a neurological basis is common and is not always a helpful one. It can leave patients and families with unhelpful perspectives such as self-blame, that they should do better, or that they are not coping due to issues within their control. Language used with families can be empowering but can also reinforce dualistic models where the interface between the brain and the mind can be lost. If we use mutually exclusive diagnostic views, we can alienate patients and create further disintegration between services such as neurology, neuropsychiatry, and neuropsychology. Instead, a formulation-based approach including the neurological, neuropsychological, and neuropsychiatric factors and clearly illustrating how these are connected, related, and interacting, will help patients understand their condition and how an integrated rehabilitation approach to this can have an impact on disability management and independence.

This case demonstrates several of the challenges in unusual presentations that cross the traditional boundaries between neuropsychological, neuropsychiatric, and neurological symptoms. Our patients and their families tell us how difficult it is to access services for their mental health when they have neurological conditions. Equally, according to the Neurological Alliance (2021), not being asked about mental health and well-being in neurology services is extremely common. The overlap between psychological, psychiatric, and neurological conditions is perhaps unsurprising, as arguably they all arise from the same organ. Psychological upset can present with neurological symptoms, neurological illness can present with psychological symptoms, and neurological disease can cause psychiatric illness (Stone et al., 2005). The division between mind and brain in our conceptualisation of neurological illness has been written about many times before but remains challenging for our patients and their families not only because of the societal acceptance of dualism, but also the stigma and understanding of mental illness and functional symptoms over neurological and structural manifestations of illness. With this backdrop to our discussion, we have considered the key themes that arise from this case history.

TM presented initially with cognitive symptoms on an historical background of recurrent depressive disorder and intercurrent anxiety symptoms affecting cognitive performance. His cognitive symptoms early in his presentation were variable and sometimes inconsistent but became more consistent alongside a deterioration in his day-to-day functioning, as well as a deterioration in his mood and anxiety as time progressed. In considering their aetiology, this case highlights the challenge to clinicians in differentiating early neurodegeneration from psychiatric illness and functional cognitive disorders.

Cognitive impairment in depression and anxiety

The cognitive presentation of mood and anxiety disorders is well recognised within the literature but, perhaps surprisingly, not as commonly considered as affective disturbance in clinical encounters. There is increasingly convincing evidence that cognition is an important target for treatment in depression (Miskowiak et al., 2016).

In their systematic review and meta-analysis of cognitive impairment in depression, Rock et al. (2014) identified significant, moderate impairment in executive function, memory, and attention in people with depression compared to controls. The executive and attention deficits were shown to persist despite remission of mood symptoms after treatment.

Castaneda et al. (2008), in their review that focused on younger people with anxiety and depression, highlight the prevalence of executive function impairment in this group, alongside attentional deficits, short-term and working memory impairment in verbal and visual tasks, and psychomotor impairments. They note that cognitive impairment is more severe in those with psychotic depression and recurrent depressive disorder, and that cognitive symptoms persist even after a remission of mood symptoms in younger people as well. In comparison, anxiety disorders have been described to impact divided attention and short-term verbal memory with fewer reports of executive impairment. In contrast, obsessional compulsive disorder (OCD) has been associated with impairments in executive impairment, long- and short-term visual memory, attention, and processing speed.

Depression and anxiety as predictors for dementia

Considering the presentation of anxiety and depression in mild cognitive impairment (MCI), much of the literature relates to older adults. Subjective cognitive decline (SCD) is commonly described and increases with age (Mitchell, 2008). A meta-analysis completed by Mitchell et al. (2008) identified that individuals with SCD were up to twice as likely to develop dementia as those without SCD. Buckley and colleagues established that those with greater beta amyloid burden and SCD had a fivefold elevated risk of developing dementia (Buckley et al., 2016).

Whilst a continuum from SCD to MCI to dementia has been suggested (Cheng et al., 2017), not all individuals with SCD develop MCI, with reports of conversion rates being as low as 14% (Hessen et al., 2017). The heterogeneity of underlying factors for SCD, including personality, mood, and functional symptoms, mean that its predictive validity for MCI is poor. Nonetheless, depression has been identified as a risk factor for developing dementia in older populations (Livingston et al., 2020), and the same authors also highlight the potential for a reduction in dementia of 4% if depression were eradicated in older age groups. In a systematic review and meta-analysis, Desai et al. (2021) identified that whilst higher depressive symptoms did not increase the risk of progression to MCI or dementia, anxiety or SCD-related worry increased the risk of progression to cognitive impairment by 40%. A population-based study of the progression to dementia from MCI over a seven-year period identified that 53% continued to present as MCI cases and 35% returned to having normal cognition (Ganguli et al., 2019). There have been further reports associating anxiety and post-traumatic stress disorder with dementia risk, with one meta-analysis reporting an increased risk of 57% (Gulpers et al., 2016).

Functional cognitive symptoms

Functional cognitive disorders have received increasing interest in recent years. It is recognised that a significant number of cognitive symptom presentations have a functional cause characteristically clinically internally inconsistent and not better explained by another condition (Ball et al., 2020).

The way that this diagnosis is explained and understood by patients and their families is critical to successful treatment of functional cognitive symptoms and clinicians should identify that functional cognitive symptoms are common, amenable to treatment, and are significantly disabling, rather than malingered or exaggerated. The diagnostic criteria for functional cognitive disorder (FCD) have been defined by Ball and colleagues as:

1. One or more symptoms of impaired cognitive function.
2. Clinical evidence of internal inconsistency.
3. Symptoms or deficit that are not better explained by another medical or psychiatric disorder.
4. Symptoms or deficit that cause clinically significant distress or impairment in social, occupational, or other important areas of functioning, or warrants medical evaluation.

Conclusion

It is important to recognise that people may have comorbid medical, neuropsychiatric, and indeed neurodegenerative conditions alongside functional symptoms and that it is not unusual for there to be a neuropsychiatric or behavioural prodrome before the clear identification of neurodegenerative illness.

The complex interplay and evolution of people's presentations over time require our reappraisal of the formulation at intervals and especially when there are new symptoms.

The authors consider that integrated, multidisciplinary formulation and neuropsychologically informed prescribing are vital in the process of differential diagnosis as well as treatment and rehabilitation. Moving toward integrated neurological, neuropsychological, and neuropsychiatric approaches recognises the needs of our patients and their families and the false dichotomy between the brain and mind that only serves as a barrier to excellent patient-centred care.

References

Ball, H. A., McWhirter, L., Ballard, C., Bhome, R., Blackburn, D. J., Edwards, M. J., Fleming, S. M., Fox, N. C., Howard, R., Huntley, J., Isaacs, J. D., Larner, A. J., Nicholson, T. R., Pennington, C. M., Poole, N., Price, G., Price, J. P., Reuber, M., Ritchie, C., Rossor, M. N., Schott, J. M., Teodoro, T., Venneri, A., Stone, J., & Carson, A. J. (2020). Functional cognitive disorder: Dementia's blind spot. *Brain*, *143*(10), 2895–2903. https://doi.org/10.1093/brain/awaa224

Buckley, R. F., Maruff, P., Ames, D., Bourgeat, P., Martins, R. N., Masters, C. L., Rainey- Smith, S., Lautenschlager, N., Rowe, C. C., Savage, G., Villemagne, V. L., & Ellis, K. A. (2016). Subjective memory decline predicts greater rates of clinical progression in preclinical Alzheimer's disease. *Alzheimer's & Dementia*, *12*, 796–804. https://doi.org/ 10.1016/j.jalz.2015.12.013

Castaneda, A. E., Tuulio-Henriksson, A., Marttunen, M., Suvisaari, J., & Lönnqvist, J. (2008). A review on cognitive impairments in depressive and anxiety disorders with a focus on young adults. *Journal of Affective Disorders, 106*(1–2), 1–27. https:// doi.org/ 10.1016/j.jad.2007.06.006

Cheng, Y. W., Chen, T. F., & Chiu, M. J. (2017). From mild cognitive impairment to subjective cognitive decline: Conceptual and methodological evolution. *Neuropsychiatric Disease and Treatment, 13*, 491–498. https://doi.org/10.2147/NDT.S123428

Desai, R., Whitfield, T., Said, G., John, A., Saunders, R., Marchant, N. L., & Stott, J. (2021). Affective symptoms and risk of progression to mild cognitive impairment or dementia in subjective cognitive decline: A systematic review and meta-analysis. *Ageing Research Reviews.* Article 101419. https://doi.org/10.1016/j. arr.2021.101419

Filley, C. M., Rollins, Y. D., Alan A. C., Arciniegas, D. B, Howard, K. L., Murrell, J. R., Boyer, P. J., Kleinschmidt-DeMasters, B. K., & Ghetti, B. (2007). The genetics of very early onset alzheimer disease. *Cognitive and Behavioral Neurology, 20*(3), 149–156. https://doi.org/10.1097/WNN.0b013e318145a8c8

Ganguli, M., Jia, Y., Hughes, T. F., Snitz, B. E., Chang, C. C., & Berman, S. B. (2019). Mild cognitive impairment that does not progress to dementia: A population-based study. *Journal of the American Geriatric Society, 67*, 232–238.

Gulpers, B., Ramakers, I., Hamel, R., K¨ohler, S., Oude Voshaar, R., & Verhey, F. (2016). Anxiety as a predictor for cognitive decline and dementia: A systematic review and meta-analysis. *American Journal of Geriatric Psychiatry, 24*, 823–842. https://doi.org/10.1016/j. jagp.2016.05.015.

Hessen, E., Eckerström, M., Nordlund, A., Selseth Almdahl, I., Stålhammar, J., Bjerke, M., Eckerström, C., Göthlin, M., Fladby, T., Reinvang, I., & Wallin, A. (2017). Subjective cognitive impairment is a predominantly benign condition in memory clinic patients followed for 6 years: The Gothenburg-Oslo MCI Study. *Dementia and Geriatric Cognitive Disorders Extra, 7*, 1–14. https://doi.org/10.1159/000454676

Livingston, G., Huntley, J., Sommerlad, A., Ames, D., Ballard, C., Banerjee, S., Brayne, C., Burns, A., Cohen-Mansfield, J., Cooper, C., Costafreda, S. G., Dias, A., Fox, N., Gitlin, L. N., Howard, R., Kales, H. C., Kivimaki, M., Larson, E. B., Ogunniyi, A., Orgeta, V., Ritchie, K., Rockwood, K., Sampson, E. L., Samus, Q., Schneider, L. S., Selbæk, G., Teri, L., & Mukadam, N. (2020). Dementia prevention, intervention, and care: 2020 report of the Lancet Commission. *Lancet, 396*, 413–446. https://doi.org/10.1016/S0140-6736(20)30367-6

Miskowiak, K. W., Ott, C. V., Petersen, J. Z., & Kessing, L. V. (2016). Systematic review of randomized controlled trials of candidate treatments for cognitive impairment in depression and methodological challenges in the field. *European Neuropsychopharmacology, 26*(12), 1845–1867. https://doi.org/10.1016/j.euroneuro.2016.09.641.

Mitchell, A. J. (2008). Is it time to separate subjective cognitive complaints from the diagnosis of mild cognitive impairment? *Age Ageing, 37*, 497–499. https://doi.org/ 10.1093/ageing/afn147

Mitchell, A. J., Beaumont, H., Ferguson, D., Yadegarfar, M., & Stubbs, B. (2014). Risk of dementia and mild cognitive impairment in older people with subjective memory complaints: Meta-analysis. *Acta Psychiatrica Scandinavica, 130*, 439–451. https://doi.org/ 10.1111/acps.12336

Neurological Alliance (2021). *NeuroLife now.* https://neurolifenow.org/wp-content/ uploads/2022/01/NLN-report_NovDec-FINAL.pdf

Rock, P., Roiser, J., Riedel, W., & Blackwell, A. (2014). Cognitive impairment in depression: A systematic review and meta-analysis. *Psychological Medicine*, *44*(10), 2029–2040. https://doi.org/10.1017/S0033291713002535

Stone, J., Carson, A., & Sharpe, M. (2005). Functional symptoms and signs in neurology: Assessment and diagnosis. *Journal of Neurology, Neurosurgery & Psychiatry*, *76*, i2–i12. https://doi.org/10.1136/jnnp.2004.061655

11 Factitious disorder after severe head injury

Andrew Worthington

Introduction

Factitious disorder is characterised by the falsification of physical or psychological signs or symptoms as a form of deception. Since the first formal psychiatric recognition in DSM III the condition has been controversial; it remains poorly articulated theoretically and is often misunderstood clinically. Factitious disorders have historically been regarded as occupying a middle ground between hysterical, conversion, or somatoform disorders and outright malingering. Tracing the origins of the term, Kanaan and Wessely (2010) suggested that it came about in part to meet a need from doctors, 'adapting to the changes in their relationship with their patients: a diagnosis without the condemnation of malingering and without the sanction of hysteria' (p. 80).

In contrast to somatoform presentations, in factitious disorder symptoms are wilfully (consciously) generated but unlike malingering there is no obvious goal except to embrace a 'sick role' so the underlying motives remain internal (unconscious) rather than external (see Table 11.1). Conventionally the person with a somatoform disorder genuinely believes they are ill whereas factitious disorder is a deliberate deception. This may extend to the tampering with evidence or sabotage of investigations that underpins the most well-known form of factitious disorder, Munchausen's syndrome.[1] This is an over-simplification however: there is no reliable empirical basis to determine motive; factitious disorder may also reflect underlying illness (or illness behaviour) and can occur in the context of demonstrable pathology. Moreover, the presence of an external incentive does not exclude the existence of internal motivators for deception and involvement in litigation is not necessarily the main driver underlying such behaviour (Eisendrath & McNiel, 2002).

This chapter presents an unusual case of factitious disorder following severe brain injury. It illustrates the challenges of identifying factitious behaviour, reaching a theoretical understanding, formulating a case clinically and providing appropriate therapeutic intervention. The fact that it occurred against a background of civil litigation for compensation adds a further layer of complexity for formulation and therapy.

DOI: 10.4324/9781003228226-13

Table 11.1 Conventional distinction between types of illness behaviour, adapted from Slick et al. (1999) and Zeshan et al. (2018)

Diagnosis	Mechanism of illness behaviour	Motivation for illness behaviour	Types of incentive
Somatoform disorder	Unconscious	Unconscious	Reduce intrapsychic conflict or stress
Factitious disorder	Conscious	Unconscious	Play sick role Seek attention, Manage stress Escape from responsibility
Malingering	Conscious	Conscious	Financial gain Avoidance of military duty or criminal punishment

Case presentation

At 45 years of age NP sustained a very severe traumatic brain injury in a road accident (GCS 3, cerebral haemorrhage, PTA lasting several weeks). A CT scan two years after the accident showed atrophy of the left frontal lobe and both temporal lobes in keeping with the severity of the injury. After a period of acute hospital treatment she was discharged home to the care of her long-term partner. As a result of the circumstances of her brain injury, NP was involved in a personal injury claim, brought on her behalf by her partner who married her several years after her accident during the course of her claim. He described her as previously vibrant, spontaneous, and with a strong-willed personality. After her brain injury, however, NP received 24-hour support at home. She demonstrated significant disability in day to day activities with problems of mobility, communication, and self-care, requiring supervision. She needed assistance with more complex tasks such as preparing meals. Her cognitive presentation, which was initially considered to be in keeping with the severity of injury, became more puzzling when subject to closer scrutiny and formal neuropsychological evaluation. The nature of her condition and the likely motivational drivers beyond the obvious financial benefit became more apparent over time although not without debate amongst her treating clinicians and medical experts.

Achieving a consensus about her condition and motivations for behaviour was essential for providing effective therapy and support and in assessing damages for her personal injury claim (especially care costs). As is often the case in factitious disorder where the underlying behaviour is to some degree under voluntary control, the question of motivation is crucial and in a litigation context malingering has to be considered as an alternative explanation. Yet a very severe brain injury may well impair the insight and self-control necessary for simulation and the brain injury alone was sufficiently severe to warrant substantial support. Finally, where a person exhibits a factitious disorder alongside a genuine brain injury, they should not be penalised for the former if this can be shown to have been caused by their injuries, as it represents an additional psychological consequence of the incident.

Critical to an understanding of NP's presentation was the psychosocial context in which her brain injury was sustained and the changing family dynamics that followed. Premorbidly, her husband (then her partner) spent much of his time working away including periods abroad; there were signs from comments by family that NP was very unhappy with the arrangement. It was possible that the marriage was on the verge of breakdown although this could not be confirmed. Following her brain injury, he gave up work and reported that he felt obliged to marry her. He cared for her almost single-handedly around the clock, at significant cost to his own lifestyle. Despite his professed desire to return to work and resurrect his own life, he was reluctant to engage with therapy and support for his wife and exerted a considerable degree of control over her contacts, frustrating efforts at rehabilitation and in effect reinforcing her illness behaviour.

Neuropsychological assessment

Neuropsychological input was requested by a private brain injury case manager to carry out an initial assessment with a view to formulating an intervention programme. At interview, NP presented as flat in affect, speaking in a monotone, and making little eye contact or spontaneous conversation, though she could be roused to anger. She complained of an emptiness of mental content because there was much that she could not remember. She said, 'I can remember what I did yesterday, nothing after that, I'm stuck'. Interestingly, the level of anterograde memory impairment she showed on formal testing when she would not recall material after half an hour would have made it unlikely that she could recall anything of the previous day's events. This illustrates a disconnection between the person's understanding of the processes underlying cognitive testing and their reported symptoms. One of the most striking aspects of interaction with NP was her apparent severe retrograde amnesia for her pre-injury life, stating that she did not recognise herself from old photographs. This too was explored during the assessment.

Cognitive testing

On formal neuropsychological tests her performance was characterised by numerous abnormal and inconsistent features. She scored at little above chance on the Benton Visual Form Discrimination test and on a Dot Counting task (VOSP battery) she appeared unable to count stimuli, scoring one out of five items correctly. She could count up to six on the faces of a die but could not count out three blocks on a table or when asked to count aloud.

Her digit span on the WAIS III was limited to a single digit (asked to repeat the sequence 6 – 3 she answered 6 – 7). Yet she could repeat a complex question verbatim: 'is there anything that I'd like to be doing that I'm not doing at the moment?' On the Information subtest, asked how many months were in a year she asked if she could guess and answered six. On the Comprehension subtest she could not state what people used money for. Expressive vocabulary was implausibly poor: she was unable to define the word *ship*, stating she had never heard of it. On the Similarities test she could not draw any similarity between *red* and *green* despite multiple prompts and examples. When asked to copy a basic two-block design of one red and one white block she produced the same pattern in reverse with the blocks the other way around.

She showed an extremely low level of performance with scores at floor level on most cognitive tests. Her Index scores on the WAIS III battery are shown in Table 11.2.

She was unable to complete psychomotor speed tasks, seemingly due to problems with manual dexterity. She appeared to be unable to reproduce simple designs from the Benton Visual Retention Test. On a design learning test (BMIPB) her total score of 6 was well below the 2nd percentile cut-off score of 19, and design recognition was severely impaired (scoring 28 out of 40). She professed to be guessing as she had forgotten the stimuli. She recalled meagre fragments from a short spoken story (BMIPB) representing about 7% of the total content, where 98% of people her age would recall at least 30% of the information. She could recall nothing of the story after 30 minutes. Given a 15-item word list her scores across five trials were: 2 – 3 – 3 – 2 – 3 with no evidence of explicit learning. Her total score of 13 was well below the total score of 32 achieved by at least 98% of her peers. Recognition memory for words in the list was at chance level (16/30).

Autobiographical Memory Interview

With assistance from her husband to corroborate information, NP completed the Autobiographical Memory Interview (Kopelman et al., 1989), with

Table 11.2 NP's IQ scores on WAIS III

WAIS III scale	Score
Verbal IQ	48
Performance IQ	53
Full scale IQ	46

Table 11.3 NP's scores on the Autobiographical Memory Interview

	Personal semantics	Autobiographical incidents
Childhood	0 / 21	0 / 9
Early adult life	0 / 21	1 / 9
Recent life	8 / 21	3 / 9
Totals	8 / 63	4 / 27

results shown in Table 11.3 indicating an unusual temporal gradient poorest in more distant time and encompassing sematic and episodic memory in equal measure.

Memory for famous faces

NP was shown 90 photographs of celebrities from the worlds of politics, sport, film, television, and music and was asked in each case, (i) if she knew their name, (ii) whether she knew what they were famous for, and (iii) whether she had even a vague recollection she had seen them somewhere before. She failed to name any face and recognised only one from television (an actor from her favourite TV programme). She 'failed' to recognise diverse public figures such as Queen Elizabeth, Elvis Presley, Prince Charles, Margaret Thatcher, Marilyn Monroe, and Diana Princess of Wales.

Memory for famous names

She was shown the names of 50 celebrities from the 1950s to 2000s, including film stars, pop stars, and politicians. Each of which was presented with two similar but non-celebrity names and NP was asked to indicate which name she thought might represent someone famous. She scored 15 correct out of 50, slightly but not significantly below chance and reported she was guessing as she did not recognise any of the names.

Memory for public events

She was shown 20 news photographs illustrating four key world events from the 1950s to the 1990s. These included the Queen's coronation, the moon landing, the wedding of Prince Charles and Lady Diana and the release from prison of Nelson Mandela. NP stated she had not seen any of the iconic images previously and did not recognise any of the events depicted.

Performance and symptom validity tests

Factitious memory complaints provide the basis for some of the earliest examples of validity testing (Binder & Pankratz, 1987). NP completed the Memory Complaints Inventory (MCI) a 58-item computer administered self-report measure comprising nine domains of memory problems. She endorsed extremely high levels of symptomatology on six of the scales. On the Word Memory Test (WMT) her results are all highly abnormal as shown in Table 11.4. Her responses were extremely slow and despite scoring around chance level, at the end of the test she said, 'I enjoyed that, it was good'. In addition, she also failed the less sensitive coin-in-the-hand test and Rey-15 item test.

Table 11.4 Word Memory Test scores

Immediate recall	Delayed recall	Consistency	Multiple choice	Paired associates	Free recall
48%	46%	52%	25%	25%	15%

In light of her abnormal performance on measures of performance validity, the results of other conventional cognitive tests could not be considered valid, despite a recognised severe brain injury. There were other signs that NP's flatlining on testing was not genuine. For example, whilst she claimed lack of memory for common words and recent events in a semi-structured clinical interview, her conversation outside of formal sessions, though stilted, demonstrated that she was capable of using vocabulary appropriately and accessing general world knowledge. She would complain about her carers, the house being too small and having a lawyer managing her affairs. In daily life, though passive and willing to have people do things for her, there were moments of adaptive behaviour in context: she was able to make a cup of tea for the neuropsychologist, showing ability to recall where each item was located in the kitchen and remember whether milk or sugar was required.

Intervention

In factitious disorder the notion of therapy or treatment is particularly challenging. Clinicians are frequently unsure about appropriate objectives and the means of achieving them. Due to the difficulties recognising illness behaviours and underlying motives which are by definition non-conscious, as well as the opprobrium associated with the label of factitious disorder, sharing a formulation as a precursor to intervention also presents difficulties. Direct confrontation is risky. Evidence that confronting examinees about insufficient testing effort can lead to valid performance going forward (Suchy et al., 2012) may not apply to factitious disorders. Feldman (2004) notes one study where 12 individuals were confronted about their behaviour and only one admitted to wilful deception, but five others ceased to produce symptoms. Most research, however, suggests this is counter-productive and angry, defensive confrontations may exacerbate the behaviour. Where protective defences are suspected, a process of supportive but firm disclosure can be helpful, along the lines of 'we recognise you have a genuine problem but it is not the problem you have been communicating to us'. Krahn et al. (2003) advocate gradually developing an empathetic relationship that induces the person to give up the maladaptive behaviours. Zeshan et al. (2018) recommended showing disinterest in the fabrication but maintaining interest in the patient. In general, the aim is to identify the likely drivers to behaviour in order to allow the person a means to change their behaviour and save face at the same time.

By its very nature, factitious disorder does not lend itself to easy identification, especially when there is also a recognised health condition as in NP's case. Professionals tend to take people at face value and when taking a history, people with factitious disorder may be guarded about their past. Documentary evidence may be contradictory. Therefore, what might be termed a panoramic approach to management is required. It is only by piecing together disparate threads of evidence from multiple sources that a threadbare tapestry emerges, which the therapist can then begin to weave into an integrated picture.

Consequently, information was obtained from a range of interested parties on a one-to-one basis to derive a picture of NP's interactions in different contexts, including NP's husband and children, her physiotherapist, occupational therapist and carers. In addition to revealing information about consistency of her clinical presentation, this also provided opportunity to consider attitudes and behaviour of key personnel who might influence NP's condition. A provisional formulation was shared with the multidisciplinary team and each member considered the implications for their own role. Key to the formulation was recognising the complex dynamic between NP and her husband. NP's illness behaviour was hypothesised to be motivated by dual motives, (i) to disrupt her partner's future plans and punish his indiscretions on the one hand, and (ii) self-protection to keep the family together as she struggled to adjust to the very real consequences of a serious brain injury. For his part her husband repeatedly claimed he was only remaining in the relationship under duress and would eventually leave (thereby reinforcing NP's illness behaviour), whilst simultaneously controlling her life and undermining efforts at rehabilitation, seemingly unwilling to support measures that would facilitate her independence (and thereby provide a rationale for his eventual departure due to carer burnout).

A three-stage plan for neuropsychological intervention was outlined:

1. Initial phase – building trust and rapport within the family, through a series of low-key covert assessments and structured activities.
2. Challenging phase – setting small cognitively challenging functional goals in liaison with other therapists, using behavioural and motivational strategies to encourage engagement without directly confronting the underlying emotional motives.
3. Generalisation/resolution phase – supporting NP to understand her capabilities and develop her role and identity within the family.

Though difficult to predict progress, each stage was planned to take up to three months, comprising weekly or two-weekly neuropsychology sessions of one to two hours taking place at NP's home or the local community. In practice, neuropsychology input continued for two years and was to be carried out alongside formal physiotherapy and occupational therapy and in the context of numerous daily activities intended to be facilitated by a professional carer or her husband. All interventions were normalised as everyday activities so as far as possible NP felt she was living her life with a brain injury rather than undergoing therapy, reflected in NP suggesting on one occasion that it would be good to meet her neuropsychologist over lunch in the community, whereas initially she had presented as a highly dependent and passive recipient of therapy at home.

Throughout the following months, interventions proved difficult to monitor and deliver consistently, frequently being interrupted or compromised by a variety of external factors. These included ill-health, financial difficulties, lost recording sheets, apparent communication breakdowns between therapists and family, and (instigated by her husband) dismissal of one therapist and introduction of a new physiotherapist not integrated within the wider multidisciplinary team and therefore not apprised of the broader context of rehabilitation.

Through experience, it was established that the following were helpful:

- Adopting a non-judgemental approach even when NP failed to carry out a task considered within her capabilities, showing unconditional support.
- Incorporating tasks into daily life without identifying them as rehabilitation activities.
- Incorporating paradoxical statements such as 'this may be too difficult for you but …'.
- Communicating a belief in her right to autonomy, including setting goals and taking responsibility for rehabilitation.
- Reinforcing her ability to choose who she wanted to be (Wagner & Sanchez, 2002).
- At the same time, commenting how important it was to show she did not need residential care (such comments having been shown to improve her communication and initiative).

Conversely the following was not helpful:

- Raising expectations of her performance at the outset of a task.
- Asking how hard she was trying or any references to effort.
- Avoiding too much overt praise and suggestions she was becoming 'independent'.
- Overt outcome measurement.

Guidance for carers was also prepared to support engagement in everyday activities. This centred on providing gentle encouragement, subtle memory cues, and informal prompting, recognising she was likely to have genuine neuropsychological difficulties, and avoiding references to formal therapy such as goals or targets. Examples of guidance in activity included:

- If she is having difficulty remembering a recent event, it may help if you talk about something that happened around the same time that she can recall.
- If there is a natural break in an activity, casually ask if she is ok to carry on:

- That's that done. Do you feel ok to try the next bit?'.
- If she seems tired you might gently suggest a break, for example, 'Would you like a rest now; I reckon you deserve one?'.

Advice on dealing with agitation and distress included:

- Acknowledging distress: 'I can really see how important/frustrating that is for you'.
- Action planning: 'I will certainly raise that with X/let X know how strongly you feel …'.
- Distraction: 'Before you mentioned that, you were starting to tell me about …'.
- Reinforcing the distraction: 'You know it's funny you should say that because …'.

Ultimately intervention was only partially successful. After two years the psychology input came to an end as a result of a combination of having gone as far as was possible, consequent end of funding for support, and her husband's desire to bring all therapies to a close. Ensuring consistency across carers and therapists was difficult as was the indirect way of working, which was contrary to many clinicians' established practice and intuitive responses. Consolidating fragile therapy gains in the context of delicate family dynamics was a constant challenge, with the medicolegal compensation case in the background adding further complexity. In addition, all therapists had to work around her fatigue and the cognitive and physical constraints of her brain injury. Nevertheless, with sensitive support, NP was able to carry out most aspects of washing and dressing and partake in meal preparation, shopping, and limited social interaction, which she had been unable to do prior to intervention.

Conclusion

Factitious disorder is a complex condition, often assumed to be synonymous with Munchausen's syndrome and one that cannot be considered in the presence of an obvious external incentive like a compensation claim because of the difficulties of excluding financial gain as the incentivising force. Yet any disability may incur entitlements to state aid so this seems an unnecessary restriction and ultimately could lead to genuine needs being dismissed as malingering. Behaviour may be feigned for more than one reason and notions of what is conscious or not are speculative at best. Patients with factitious complaints may become involved in litigation, sometimes to sue medical staff. Eisendrath and McNeil (2002) suggested it may be driven not by desire for money per se (as in malingering) but as positive reinforcement for illness behaviour and validation of their difficulties in life. Factitious disorder is often presented as occurring in the absence of organic pathology (unless it leads to self-harm), as exemplified in a recent systematic review (Yates & Feldman, 2016). This is especially problematic if the factitious symptoms are cognitive or psychological, leading Rogers et al. (1989) to complain, 'The diagnosis of factitious disorder with psychological symptoms appears to be based on the tenuous logic that if you want to be a patient badly enough, then you are mentally ill' (p. 1312).

For neuropsychologists, cases like NP present many challenges such as how such cases should be evaluated, how test results and formulation can be effectively communicated without jeopardising the therapeutic relationship, and what treatments are available. They also raise questions about motives for behaviour, levels of awareness, and notions of agency and volition. The role of clinical neuropsychologists in somatoform disorders is increasingly recognised (Lamberty, 2008) and is likely to be equally important in factitious presentations, not least in the use of validity measures (Chafetz et al., 2020).

A diagnosis or label of factious disorder is a hypothesis about behaviour that has no identifiable organic basis being driven by underlying emotional motives of which the person is only partially, if at all, aware. A proper formulation that goes beyond diagnosis is necessary for understanding the illness behaviour and its limits where there is also genuine pathology as in the severe brain injury sustained by NP. Bass and Halligan (2016) suggested the WHO ICF framework provides a more useful framework than a traditional biomedical model for conceptualising factitious disorder as it highlights the role of the person when defining illness (and also emphasises the importance of environmental factors). Hamilton et al. (2008) suggest that taking a broad biopsychosocial perspective in which physical and psychological factors combine to affect health outcomes may allow a person to engage in psychosocial interventions without their sick role being threatened. A biopsychosocial perspective also encourages the psychologist to consider the role of agency in factitious disorder in terms of exercise of power (Bolton & Gillett, 2019) – perhaps there is a sense in which NP was demonstrating her autonomy by not fulfilling her recovery potential. Exploring power relations in people who adopt a sick role as an antidote to the more typical blame and criticism that illness deception generates may improve understanding and treatment. The management of NP pre-dates but resonates with the Power, Threat, Meaning Framework in clinical psychology (Johnstone & Boyle, 2018), the key message of which has been summarised as,

> You are experiencing a normal reaction to abnormal circumstances. Anyone else who had been through the same events might well have ended up reacting in the same way. However, these survival strategies may no longer be needed or useful. With the right kind of support, you may be able to leave them behind.
>
> (p. 18)

In the context of neurological disability, it is incumbent on clinicians to consider the negative consequences of recovery as well as the presumed benefits. Eisendrath et al. (1996) argued that unlike malingerers, for people with factitious disorder,

> the apparent secondary costs are usually greater than the secondary gain. What ignites the factitious disorder, then, is the primary gain of gratifying a psychological need. The gain for the individual, however, is not usually apparent to an outside observer.
>
> (p. 76)

These authors reported a case of a woman suing for a factitious blindness which was not motivated by desire for financial gain but induced by fear of losing her husband following an accident. In NP's case there was also a fear of losing her partner as well as a hypothesised motive for disrupting his life plans. Her husband had his own motives for ensuring she remained in a state of significant disability which were considered to provide a justification to end the relationship (after a suitable period of dutiful caring to establish his loyalty). Her illness behaviour was described by one neurologist who examined her as being in part promoted by her husband to the extent that she believed herself to have a major disability. This raises questions as to the motivations of both parties in the relationship. As Lipsitt (1996) noted, 'the diagnosis of factitious disorder often hinges upon who is the deceiver and who is the deceived'. It highlights the need to consider factitious disorder not as a stable condition but as a fluid behavioural response to an evolving transactional dynamic.

In this regard, Rashidi et al. (2006) attempted to model the interactions between a doctor and a patient with factitious disorder from a game theory perspective, but little attention has been given to potential gains and losses within families of the kind illustrated in NP's case. Given the challenges such interpersonal conflicts present for therapy, this could well prove a fruitful avenue for further research and greater comprehension of illness behaviour and ultimately more effective interventions. Finally, whether there is any inherent difference between factitious disorder occurring in isolation and when comorbid with genuine physical (including neurological) pathology has not been systematically investigated. The impact of brain injury on self-awareness and behavioural control may have implications for factitious symptoms, one recent single-case study raising frontal lobe damage as a possible risk factor (Coebergh et al., 2021), suggesting that neuropsychological insights may also have much to contribute to understanding these complex behaviours.

Note

1 The outlandish reminiscences of Baron Hieronymous Karl Friedrich von Munchausen, a former soldier, were intended not to deceive but to ridicule a growing public credulity. He did not take kindly to Rudolf Erich Raspe's (1785) fictionalised character that he inspired and initiated legal action (Kareem, 2012).

References

Bass, C., & Halligan, P. (2016). Factitious disorders and malingering in relation to functional neurologic disorders. In M. Hallett, J. Stone, & A. Carson, (Eds.), *Handbook of clinical neurology, vol. 139: Functional neurological disorders, 3rd series* (pp. 509–520). Elsevier.

Binder, L. M., & Pankratz, L. (1987). Neuropsychological evidence of a factitious memory complaint. *Journal of Clinical and Experimental Neuropsychology, 9*(2), 167–171.

Bolton, D., & Gillett, G. (2019). *The biopsychosocial model of heath and disease: New philosophical and scientific developments.* eBook: Palgrave Macmillan, 149 pp.

Chafetz, M. D., Bauer, R. M., & Haley, P. S. (2020). The other face of illness-deception: Diagnostic criteria for factitious disorder with proposed standards for clinical practice and research. *The Clinical Neuropsychologist, 34*(3), 454–476.

Coebergh, J. A., Amlani, A., Edwards, M., Mah, T., & Agrawal, N. (2021). A brain origin for factitious disorder (Munchausen's) with malingering? A single case with an old frontal lobe lesion. *Neurocase, 27*(1), 8–11.

Eisendrath, S. J., & McNiel, D. E. (2002). Factitious disorders in civil litigation: Twenty cases illustrating the spectrum of abnormal illness-affirming behaviour. *Journal of the American Academy of Psychiatry and Law, 30*, 391–399.

Eisendrath, S. J., Rand, S. C., & Feldman, M. D. (1996). Factitious disorders and litigation. In M. C. Feldman & S. J. Eisendrath (Eds), *The spectrum of factitious disorders* (pp. 65–81). American Psychiatric Press.

Feldman, M. C. (2004). *Playing sick? Untangling the web of Munchausen syndrome, Munchausen by proxy, malingering and factitious disorder.* Routledge.

Hamilton, J. C., Feldman, M. D., & Cunnien, A. J. (2008). Factitious disorder in medical and psychiatric practices. In R. Rogers (Ed.), *Clinical assessment of malingering and deception* (3rd ed., pp. 128–144). The Guilford Press.

Johnstone, L., & Boyle, M. with Cromby, J., Dillon, J., Harper, D., Kinderman, P., Longden, E., Pilgrim, D. & Read, J. (2018). *The power threat meaning framework: Towards the identification of patterns in emotional distress, unusual experiences and troubled or troubling behaviour, as an alternative to functional psychiatric diagnosis.* British Psychological Society.

Kanaan, R. A. A., & Wessely, S. C. (2010). The origins of factitious disorder. *History of the Human Sciences, 23*(2), 68–85.

Kareem, S. T. (2012). Fictions, lies and Baron Munchausen's narrative. *Modern Philology, 109*(4), 483–509.

Kopelman, M. D., Wilson, B. A., & Baddeley, A. D. (1989). The Autobiographical Interview: A new assessment of autobiographical and personal semantic memory in amnesic patients. *Journal of Clinical and Experimental Neuropsychology, 11*(5), 724–744.

Krahn, L. E., Hongshe, L., O'Conner, M. K. (2003). Patients who strive to be ill: Factitious disorder with physical symptoms. *American Journal of Psychiatry, 160*, 1163–1168.

Lamberty, G. L. (2008). *Understanding somatization in the practice of clinical neuropsychology.* Oxford University Press.

Lipsitt, D. (1996). Introduction. In M. D. Feldman & S. J. Eisendrath (Eds.), *The Spectrum of Factitious Disorders* (pp. xix–xxviii). American Psychiatric Press.

Rashidi, A., Khodarahmi, L., & Feldman, M. D. (2006). Mathematical modelling of the course and prognosis of factitious disorders: A game-theoretic approach. *Journal of Theoretical Biology, 240,* 48–53.

Rogers, R., Bagby, R. M., & Rector, N. (1989). Diagnostic legitimacy of factitious disorder. *American Journal of Psychiatry, 146,* 1312–1314.

Slick, D. J., Sherman, E. M. S., & Iverson G. L. (1999). Diagnostic criteria for malingered neurocognitive dysfunction: Proposed standards for clinical practice and research. *The Clinical Neuropsychologist, 13,* 545–561.

Suchy, Y., Chelune, G., Franchow, E., & Thorgusen, R. (2012). Confronting patients about insufficient effort: The impact on subsequent symptom validity and memory performance. *The Clinical Neuropsychologist, 26*(8), 1296–1311.

Wagner, C. C., & Sanchez, F. P. (2002). The role of values in motivational interviewing. In W. R. Miller & S. Rollnick (Eds.), *Motivational interviewing: Preparing people for change* (2nd ed., pp. 284–298). The Guilford Press.

Yates, G. P., & Feldman, M. D. (2016) Factitious disorder: A systematic review of 455 cases in the professional literature. *General Hospital Psychiatry, 41,* 20–28.

Zeshan, M., Cheema, R., & Manocha, P. (2018) Challenges in diagnosing factitious disorder. *The American Journal of Psychiatry Residents Journal, 13*(9), 6–8.

12 Deafness or brain injury?

Diagnostic overshadowing in a deaf person with bilateral temporal lobe damage and visual agnosia

Joanna Atkinson and Darren Townsend-Handscomb

Introduction

The assessment of prelingually deaf people is particularly challenging for clinical neuropsychologists. Overshadowing of cognitive impairments is common in deaf people because clinicians are unfamiliar with what 'normal' or 'impaired' cognition typically look like in a deaf person, and means that acquired brain injuries may go unrecognised. Clinicians who lack familiarity with healthy deaf people, and do not share a language with their client, will struggle to identify abnormalities. The term 'overshadowing' is used to describe the underdiagnosis of physical or mental conditions in people with whom clinicians struggle to communicate. Symptoms are missed or misattributed to mental illness, learning disability, deafness, or cultural differences. Working with interpreters does not solve this problem. Communication is a primary tool of the neuropsychologist's trade. Clinicians usually rely extensively on verbal and nonverbal cues during the clinical interview. The way that a person describes their symptoms provides information about many areas of cognition – language, memory, executive function, speed of information processing. These clues to cognition are often lost when using an interpreter. Unless the interpreter is specifically trained to work in neuropsychology settings, they may inadvertently 'assist' answers, by scaffolding responses, or providing choices and examples to facilitate the deaf person's understanding. Sign language interpreters are trained to find the meaning in a British Sign Language (BSL) utterance and to render the equivalent meaning in spoken English. They may inadvertently 'repair' impaired communication and make it more coherent in their translated version. They are not trained clinicians so these 'repairs' may mask aspects of communication that clinical neuropsychologists and other professionals are looking out for to inform their assessment. Significant neurological dysfunction can easily be masked during the clinical interaction, as communication takes place in a different modality with space, movement, facial expressions, and handshape used to convey grammatical meaning in BSL. An interpreter's translation of test items and responses involves not only translation between languages, but

DOI: 10.4324/9781003228226-14

also between visual and auditory modalities. This can create unrecognised disadvantages or advantages that distort the assessment of a person's cognitive abilities (M. J. Harris et al., 2020).

This chapter tells the journey of Lydia Handscomb, a deaf actor, from the perspective of her son, Darren, and her neuropsychologist, Jo, as Lydia struggled for nearly seven decades with perplexing symptoms before finally getting confirmation of a brain injury. This was most likely caused by encephalitis or meningo–encephalitis in early childhood which also resulted in profound deafness. Dr Jo Atkinson is currently the only deaf neuropsychologist in the United Kingdom and her research provided the neuropsychological tools to enable the establishment of the UK's first cognitive disorders clinic for deaf patients at the National Hospital for Neurology and Neurosurgery in London. Lydia finally received a diagnosis for her lifelong difficulties after just two sessions at the specialist deaf neurology clinic, where neuropsychological assessment and history-taking were conducted in BSL using cognitive tests developed directly in British Sign Language with norms for deaf people (Atkinson et al., 2015; Denmark et al., 2016), and the neurologist's examination was conducted in English with BSL translation to ensure that Lydia's deaf cultural and language needs underpinned the entire diagnostic process.

DARREN: The assessment at the Deaf clinic was a remarkably different experience for us. Previously we had always seen professionals who had no understanding of deafness, Deaf culture, or BSL. Mum was an accomplished and respected deaf actress: one of the first deaf people to obtain an Equity card. But she had to make use of inventive strategies to learn her lines and then suffered weeks of fatigue and burnout. Throughout her life, she experienced unexplained 'fits', an exaggerated response to physical stimulus, brain fog, sight issues, severe mood swings, body pains, and gastric symptoms, among other symptoms.

The problem was that the clinicians could not communicate directly with her or see beyond her deafness, so they struggled to understand the meaning of Mum's difficulties. Many were unable to see past their negative assumptions of what it meant to be a deaf person, including assuming low intelligence or that her cognitive and reading difficulties were simply caused by her deafness, and consequently, Mum was given inaccurate diagnoses and ineffective treatment.

I often had to challenge the use of assessments that were inappropriate for a Deaf person, or a non-English speaker, or where the norms being judged against were those of hearing populations, that may or may not have had any relevance to my mother's results.

In comparison, this team were fully Deaf aware. Not just at a surface level, but in understanding what it meant to be a functional, articulate Deaf person who uses BSL. For the first time in her life, Mum was assessed as a whole person, not simply as someone who was deaf. This was particularly striking in the clinical assessments, conducted in BSL, measured against norms from Deaf populations (where possible). After 25 years of visiting doctor after doctor, and a multitude of diagnoses, we finally received a neurological diagnosis that provided the missing piece of the jigsaw. Suddenly things made perfect sense. My mum had a brain injury, and her experience and symptoms could be explained. It was a huge relief for us both and transformed our experience of the last years of her life.

Before my mother died, of unrelated causes, she said that she wanted her story to be published, with her real name and photographs, with the hope of spreading awareness of the experiences of deaf people with unusual brains, and to help demonstrate the need for improvements in future provision. In my work, as a BSL-English interpreter, I regularly come across other deaf people who, like Mum, seem to be living with undetected cognitive problems. There are other deaf people living their whole lives not knowing that they are living with a serious brain injury or cognitive disability. My mother's story is just the tip of an iceberg of hidden impairments in deaf people.

Clinical interview and history

When Lydia walked into the room, one of the first things she signed was, 'My brain hurts. I would like a new brain. I just want to be free'. She appeared anxious to get across the extent of her difficulties, which had previously been

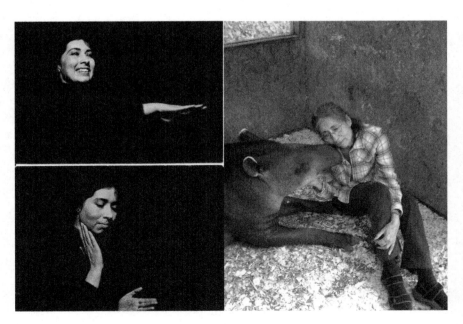

Figure 12.1 Photos show Lydia as a young actress and making friends with a tapir

put down to her deafness or to mental health difficulties. The referral letter from the GP stated, 'Thank you for seeing this 70-year-old lady who is deaf since childhood as a result of meningitis at the age of 2 years and uses sign language. She came with her son recently, who says she is suffering with considerable memory problems. She lives alone and is finding it difficult to look after herself adequately and is constantly leaving herself notes. She is also under Moorfields eye hospital with a visual problem'. This was not an unusual referral letter, as we typically would assess deaf people with neurodegenerative conditions where memory and difficulty coping at home were the chief complaints. However, a very thick folder containing historical notes from the medical archives of many London hospitals had landed on the neurologist's desk, indicating long-standing concerns. The notes included investigations by psychiatrists for unspecified mental health difficulties, ophthalmological tests ruling out primary visual impairment, and a diagnosis of ME in 1989 due to severe fatigue. It was clear that Lydia and Darren had spent 50 years looking for answers, attending one frustrating medical appointment after another, without finding any real answers, at great expense to the NHS and their own well-being. Lydia's voluminous medical records were a testimony to this but lacked any clear explanation for her symptoms.

Lydia was expressive and keen to tell her story. She had written notes to help her memory. Her sign language was rapid, circuitous, and hard to follow. Her meaning was not always clear because she did not provide explanatory context, and frequently changed the topic without giving all the information that others would need to understand her meaning. Darren confirmed that her communication had been like this for as long as he could remember.

Main concerns

During our consultation, Lydia's main concern was forgetting conversations, the names of people and places, and struggling to find things in her home or groceries in the supermarket. 'I cannot find what I'm looking for even when it is right in front of me'. She spent hours struggling to find things, to focus, to organise her home, to remember information, and to make plans. She felt overwhelmed and would spend her days writing lists repeatedly, trying to make sense of things. Lydia was a creative person who had tried lots of strategies. She used brightly coloured post-it notes to remind herself to do household tasks but still failed to see these. Lydia and Darren had noticed worsening ability to cope after she was knocked over by a motorcycle four years previously, during which she sustained a head injury without loss of consciousness, a pelvic injury requiring surgery, and permanent loss of her sense of smell and taste.

Reported visuoperceptual difficulties flagged further assessment of visual agnosia and prosopagnosia

Lydia did not see the motorbike before her accident, despite looking straight at it, and she believed that there was something wrong with her eyes. She had bought herself a white symbol cane to use while crossing the road so that drivers would realise that she could not see them. She was frustrated that despite her experience she had received no ophthalmologic diagnosis. Eye tests had shown no primary visual difficulties with acuity or visual fields.

DARREN: Mum had lots of strange 'visual' problems such as being unable to see notices on a crowded pinboard, a face in a crowd, or pick out objects from a busy visual scene. I always wore red to make it easier for her to spot me! She had difficulties with judging distances such as being unaware of personal space, not seeing a bicycle on the pavement until it was near, or the opposite, jumping as if a bike was about to hit her even though it was some distance away. She had difficulty recognising objects such as keys when she was looking for them, and so would keep a single object on a table to ensure that she could find it, but still often could not.

People in the Deaf community often thought she was ignoring them because she had not seen them wave to attract her attention or was unable to recognise their faces. Sometimes she would not see or respond to people even when she was looking straight at them.

Unusual features affecting communication in BSL

Lydia showed some unusual features while communicating in BSL which would not have impacted a hearing person using spoken language. These features would have been easily missed by a clinician who is not fluent in sign language, as sign language interpreters are not trained to pick up these subtle neuropsychological symptoms.

1)   *Observed difficulties with facial grammar in sign language indicated need for detailed assessment of face processing*

Lydia's use of British Sign Language had some unusual features. Even though it was clear that she did not have a primary language impairment as her signing was grammatical with no apparent aphasia or sign-finding difficulties, she had subtle difficulties with the use of the face in BSL. Some types of BSL grammar can be conveyed on the face. During BSL conversation, one way to convey negation or adverbs, or to mark the topic, is to use a facial expression such as a furrowed brow, raised eyebrows, or puffed cheeks. Lydia did not make much use of these linguistic face expressions; instead she conveyed the same message by using lexicalised manual signs or more English-based sign order. Signers often switch between these methods for conveying grammatical meaning in BSL, so Lydia's signing did not appear atypical unless she was specifically asked to use linguistic face expressions and then she struggled. What was more striking was that Lydia asked me *not* to use grammatical face expressions, as deaf BSL users would typically have no trouble with understanding facial grammar. This inability could not be explained by lack of exposure or fluency because Lydia had lived very much within the Deaf Community since early childhood; instead this seemed to point to a specific difficulty with face processing. Understanding BSL facial grammar requires intact right-hemisphere ability to process dynamic facial actions (Atkinson et al., 2004).

DARREN: Mum would often misunderstand what was signed to her, for example, understanding that someone wanted her to do something when they were actually asking her not to. If she noticed someone using facial grammar she would get cross, and would mimic the facial grammar in an exaggerated way. I certainly couldn't sign with her fluently and expect her to understand, as she would say it was too fast and too complicated. All of these are examples of frequent sources of frustration and conflict that the neurological diagnosis ameliorated.

2) *Perceptual difficulties understanding sign language flagged further assessment of visual agnosia*

Another unusual feature was that Lydia could not understand sign language on a screen, unless the person was looking directly into the camera. During face-to face conversation she found it disorientating if her conversation partner looked away and then back again. This was not something I had ever come across, even among signers with impaired vision, who sometimes struggle with understanding BSL from a side view, but do not generally report an issue with having to recalibrate each time the person turned their head. This observation led to further assessment of visuoperception and agnosia, particularly as Lydia said that she could not recognise objects that were crowded by other objects, or from certain angles.

DARREN: Mum struggled to understand me on video calls. She just could not understand me signing in 2D at all, no matter how slowly I signed. In the end we just gave up trying to communicate this way.

Semantic and reading difficulties

Prelingually deaf people often have poor literacy due to reduced access to spoken English and ineffective literacy teaching for deaf sign language users (Harris et al., 2017). However, Lydia made semantic errors while reading and showed surface-level difficulties such as visual crowding, which are not typical of deaf readers, even those with poor literacy. Dyslexia was suggested by an adult education tutor but had never been formally assessed.

DARREN: I would often write notes to help Mum remember something, but she had difficulties with reading. I would have to use as few words as possible, in short sentences with wide spaces between them, use of highlighting and bold etc. However, Mum would then often not be able to find the note in order to remind herself. When she sent me text messages, Mum made mistakes with meaning such as typing 'red car' for 'bus' or reading 'bee' as 'wasp' which made decoding them a frustrating puzzle.

Disinhibition and masking strategies in a Deaf cultural context

Learning about Lydia's difficulties made me think back to when I had briefly met her before. The Deaf community is small and our paths had briefly crossed occasionally at deaf events. Lydia would not recognise me until I told her my name, and then she greeted me warmly and laughed it off in a theatrical way by doing an impression of a dog that was pleased to see me. With hindsight, this appeared to function as a well-practised strategy to mask her difficulties with recognising people, but at that time it did not seem particularly socially inappropriate to me in the Deaf cultural context. Behaviour that perhaps might more readily be seen as socially disinhibited in a hearing person might not raise particular concern because her behaviour fitted with the visual humour that is widely used in the Deaf Community, the role-play aspects of BSL where the signer can embody another character, and the expectation that a deaf actor would have these skills. However, with the full history, it became clear that Lydia was sometimes socially disinhibited.

DARREN: Sometimes Mum would break into a signed song and dance routine in the street, or bark at hearing people in public places and act like an excited dog. This usually confused people at first – which she did not notice, although they generally made some sense of it in the end, and she got away with it.

The general public might attribute similar behaviour to eccentricity or misattribute it to disability or deafness. Thus, this is a nice example of how overshadowing of social disinhibition can occur in a deaf person, which may be difficult to spot in both deaf and hearing contexts, but with careful questioning and cultural insight might come to be understood as a feature of brain injury.

Hypersensitivity and interoception

Hypersensitivity may manifest differently in a deaf person because of their reliance on vision and vibrotactile senses rather than hearing. The usual and culturally appropriate way to attract a deaf person's attention is by waving, tapping on their arm, flashing the lights, or banging on the table or the floor to create a vibration.

DARREN: My mum was over-sensitive to lots of stimuli and it was a real struggle to get her attention without scaring her. She often could not see me waving, and if I banged on the table or touched her to get her attention she would often jump or scream, even when she could see the source of the touch. She was so easily startled by vibrations or touch that I often resorted to blowing gently towards her to attract her attention.

Other features seemed to relate to interoception, the ability to monitor and respond to internal signals from within the body, which may have contributed to her sense of unreality or not really being present.

DARREN: Mum didn't notice when she was thirsty. She had to eat meals routinely rather than rely on what her body was telling her about needing food, and would leave notes for herself to have a drink. She always complained about a sensation of feeling bloated for which no medical explanation was found. Mum had an incredibly strong reaction to pain, repeatedly experiencing a pain as if for the first time, which frightened her, and sometimes triggered fainting or seizures for which we never found an explanation. She described a sense of not being present, of being with people but feeling 'that I am not there' or 'not alive'. This worsened after she lost her sense of smell and taste which, for her as a deaf person, compounded her sense of not really being present.

Neuroimaging

The MRI scan showed significant bilateral damage to the anterior temporal lobes including volume loss and hyperintensities. The damage to the right side was greater than to the left side, with additional marked atrophy of the right parahippocampal and fusiform gyri, volume loss in the right amygdala and associated ex vacuo dilation of the temporal pole of the lateral ventricle.

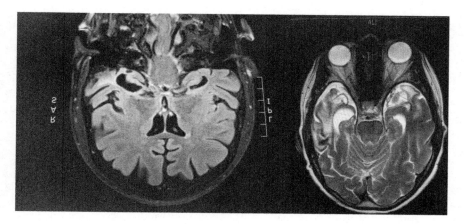

Figure 12.2 MRI scans showing bilateral atrophy to the anterior temporal lobes which is more severe in the right hemisphere

A further scan after 12 months showed no evidence of progression and attributed the damage as likely to be secondary to a former undiagnosed herpes encephalitis infection.

Background literature

Deafness

Neurological conditions in deaf people are often identified late – when difficulties become obvious – or not at all (Atkinson & Woll, 2012). There is a lack of specialist provision and most deaf people are assessed in their local services by psychologists who cannot communicate directly in their own language. When seen in standard clinics, deaf patients and their families often have a poor experience, and often express a lack of trust that they will receive an accurate assessment (Smith, 2010).

There are high levels of undiagnosed neurological conditions in the Deaf Community. Research by Atkinson et al. (2015) showed that among those aged 50–59 years, attending a holiday camp for deaf adults aged 50+, there was a bimodal distribution of nonverbal cognitive ability, as measured by WASI Matrix Reasoning, with a second hump of low ability showing on the distribution graph. All of the participants had been screened to exclude those with brain disorders or intellectual disability, yet we picked up people with substantial, undiagnosed cognitive impairments.

There are many factors that make it difficult for clinicians without specialist experience to conduct accurate assessments. Deaf people are highly heterogeneous in terms of their early development, which is shaped by many factors, including: whether they had exposure to fully accessible, fluent language as infants, for example, learning BSL from deaf parents or an older sibling; whether language milestones were achieved at the expected age; degree and age of onset of hearing loss; effectiveness of auditory aids or cochlear implants in enabling access to spoken language development; age of exposure to an accessible first language; extent of communication deprivation and language delay, particularly where families and/or educators did not use sign language, or lacked fluency (see Maller & Braden, 2012 for a review). There are neuroplastic effects of early deafness (Simon et al., 2020), and the use of a visuomotor rather than a spoken language has subtle influences on cognition, meaning that normative performance may differ for some cognitive tasks (e.g. Emmorey et al., 1993). Cultural and linguistic differences pose further difficulties in using cognitive tests designed for hearing people (Atkinson et al., 2015). Verbal tests, in particular, lack validity when used with deaf people (Braden, 1994), particularly tests of language, naming, verbal reasoning, verbal memory, and tests of executive function that rely on measurement in the verbal modality. Prelingually deaf people consistently show weaker serial memory than hearing people (see Keehner & Atkinson, 2006 for a review). Reference to deaf norms is essential but these are often not available.

The neuropsychologist assessing a deaf person has to be alert to possible causes of prelingual deafness that may also cause neurological disorder such as CNS infections during gestation (e.g. maternal rubella or cytomegalovirus) or early childhood (e.g. meningitis), or mitochondrial disorders. In this case, the cause of the comorbid deafness and brain injury is thought to be encephalitis, but it is possible it could have been meningo-encephalitis or an outside possibility that two separate periods of illness caused the deafness (meningitis) and brain injury (encephalitis). Profound bilateral deafness and brain damage has been documented following encephalitis and meningo-encephalitis (e.g. Rabinstein et al., 2001).

Encephalitis

Encephalitis is inflammation of brain tissues, causes of which can include viral infection. Herpes simplex is the most common such virus, which can cause bilateral tissue degeneration, specifically within the temporal lobes and limbic system (Barnett et al., 1994). It results in death, seizures, or neuropsychological impairment in up to one-third of cases (McGrath et al., 1997). There are high levels of fatigue, distress, anxiety, depression, anger, frustration, and obsessive-compulsive symptoms in survivors of encephalitis (Dowell et al., 2000).

Hallmarks of encephalitis are amnestic, semantic, and executive dysfunctions (Kapur et al., 1994) but exact symptoms depend on the location and extent of tissue damage, and the type of virus. Herpes simplex-type encephalitis was suspected from neuroimaging, which usually spreads along the trigeminal ganglion and fibres innervating the meninges of the anterior and middle cranial fossa, often resulting in bilateral damage to specific areas often including the anterior and medial temporal lobes, deep temporal lobe structures, the insular cortex, and the basal and orbital parts of the frontal lobe (Theil et al., 2003).

This pattern of bilateral damage of corticolimbic temporal and frontal systems leads to a characteristic cognitive profile:

- Severe memory difficulties and amnesia (McGrath et al., 1997).
- Typically affecting anterograde and autobiographical memory (Pewter et al., 2007).
- Semantic association deficits (Borgo & Shallice, 2001).
- Category specific anomia (Utley et al., 1997).
- Impairments to executive functioning, language, and sometimes, visuospatial functioning (Harris et al., 2020).
- Visual agnosia sometimes occurs in encephalitis patients (Borgo et al., 2000).

Anterior temporal lobe function

Research into brain conditions where there is specific damage to the anterior temporal lobe (ATL), such as encephalitis, stroke, surgery for tumours, epilepsy, and frontotemporal dementia, provide further insight into ATL function. Damage to the left ATL causes difficulties with auditory and verbal perception, language comprehension impairments, verbal and visual memory impairments, and difficulties with learning and retention. Damage to the right ATL causes impaired memory for faces and places, impaired face recognition and emotion recognition, and disinhibited social behaviour (see Bonner & Price, 2013; Rice et al., 2015). The ventral temporal cortices are involved in high-level visual processing of complex stimuli such as faces, words, and scenes. Damage to the right fusiform gyrus causes prosopagnosia (inability to recognise faces) and pure word blindness (inability to recognise words). Damage to the right parahippocampal gyrus causes difficulty with remembering and processing visual scenes and backgrounds (Mégevand et al., 2014). The anterior ventral stream areas are involved in object perception and recognition with damage causing associative visual agnosia (De Renzi, 2000).

The anterior temporal lobes are often conceptualised as amodal hubs for the relay of semantic information to other areas of the brain (Bonner & Price, 2013) used for both language and visual processing. The lateralisation and precise location of lesions within the ATLs will determine whether linguistic processing (lateral ATL) or visual object processing (ventral ATL) is more affected (Visser et al., 2010). Bilateral ATL damage can cause semantic language impairment including proper names for people and places and poor organisation of verbal material (Hodges & Patterson, 2007). Damage to the left ATL can selectively impair naming categories such as people, animals, or tools (Noppeney et al., 2007). Right ATL damage will affect semantic knowledge about object properties, conceptual information about social rules, semantic knowledge about people we know, famous or familiar faces, and semantic knowledge that allows us to infer mental states and emotions in others (Rice et al., 2015).

Right hippocampal and fusiform areas

Lydia's brain scan showed damage to the right parahippocampal and fusiform areas. These are adjacent to the occipital lobes and form part of the visual association cortex. Their general function is the higher-order processing of visual information for faces, memory, and text. Difficulty recognising faces is caused by right parahippocampal damage that impairs access to stored semantic knowledge about face identity (associative prosopagnosia). This region also plays an important role in topological processing and memory for environmental scenes such as landscapes, cityscapes, room layouts, or backgrounds (Mégevand et al., 2014). Damage to the right fusiform gyrus is also associated with dyslexia (Liu et al., 2021).

Agnosia

Associative visual agnosia is caused by damage to the visual association area. This is the inability to identify objects caused by impaired access to the stored semantic information necessary for differentiating similar objects. Orientation agnosia occurs when someone can recognise a canonical view of objects or faces but has lost associative knowledge about what they look like in different orientations, causing them to struggle when viewed from different angles (Biran & Coslett, 2003). It is caused by loss of semantic access to multiple view-dependent representations of an object (Harris et al., 2001). Simultanagnosia is the inability to rapidly recognise multiple objects in a visual scene at the same time and arises from damage to the left temporo-occipital regions (Farah, 1990). All objects can be seen but must be recognised one by one. People with simultanagnosia can experience visual crowding while reading so need the text spread out and use a letter-by-letter reading strategy.

Interoception

The deep temporal lobe structures and connections, particularly the frontal-temporal sides of the right insula, regulate a person's sensitivity to internal interoceptive bodily signals (Critchley et al., 2004), somatic states, and their evaluation of pain intensity (Kong et al., 2006). The insula is thought to underpin the sense of interoception, or the ability to identify, access, understand, and respond appropriately to the patterns of internal bodily signals (Craig, 2002). Damage to this system is a possible explanation for many of medically unexplained symptoms such as hypersensitivity to pain, lack of recognition of thirst or hunger, and an increased sensation of bloating (Ladabaum et al., 2001; Mayer, 2011). Interoception has also been found to be dysregulated in ME and chronic fatigue syndrome (Sharp et al., 2021), for which Lydia had received a diagnosis. Damage to these areas can also cause disruption to coenesthesic awareness, which is the combined organic sensations that give a person a sense of their bodily existence, which may result in a feeling of unreality (see Tran The et al., 2021 for a review).

Socioemotional aspects

The insula plays an additional role in empathy and metacognitive emotional abilities, such as awareness of emotions in others (Mutschler et al., 2013). It is strongly connected to the amygdala which regulates emotional responses to sensory stimuli. Damage to these paralimbic structures and connections might explain Lydia's extreme emotional reactions to pain, vibrations, or to being touched. The amygdala also plays a vital role in facial recognition, processing emotion on faces, and making social judgements (Baxter & Croxson, 2012). These structures are intimately connected with the frontal lobes allowing emotions and social judgements to be weighed up in decision-making (Baeken et al., 2010). Damage to paralimbic areas might account for the difficulties with interoception, socio-emotional processing, and decisiveness.

Neuropsychological assessment

This was conducted in two stages. Neuropsychology screening using a routine battery for deaf patients took place before a more extensive history was taken by the neurologist, with the neuropsychologist in attendance. The battery included the BSL Cognitive Screening Test (Atkinson et al., 2015) and BSL Verbal Learning and Memory Test (Denmark et al., 2016), developed and normed for deaf BSL users. After realising the extent of the visual difficulties and receiving the scan report, areas of cognition indicated by anterior temporal lobe damage and ventral stream damage were assessed in more depth, including visuospatial processing, visual memory, visual attention, face processing, semantic knowledge, executive function, and reading.

Observations

During the interview and testing, Lydia often had to close her eyes as she reported finding it difficult to think with her eyes open. During face processing tasks she used a painstakingly slow, local feature-based strategy. For example, on the Benton she spent a long time matching up the eyebrows to decide if two pictures showed the same person. This mirrored everyday situations when she relied on what a person is wearing or idiosyncratic individual facial features as a clue to a person's identity.

Table 12.1 shows the tests and results for each domain of cognitive function. Table 12.2 shows the results of the assessment of reading.

Results

Prior and current intellectual function

It is difficult to reliably establish estimates of premorbid function in deaf signers as conventional tests are unsuitable. It also may not be appropriate in a case where a brain injury was sustained during infancy. Nonetheless, measures of predicted and current intellectual ability were useful to rule out a pervasive intellectual disability. Crawford's demographic equation (CDE) produced an estimated *average* performance IQ (25th–75th percentile) (Crawford et al., 2001). However, it should be borne in mind that the correlational relationship between IQ and years of education and occupation may not hold true for deaf people, who typically experience poorer access to education and employment. This caveat means that we should always take estimates as the minimum level of the deaf person's true ability. Interestingly, a measure of current non-verbal reasoning, WAIS Matrix Reasoning, showed that Lydia performed at a higher level than suggested by the CDE. Her score was within the *Superior* range (95th percentile). Matrix reasoning is often used as a measure of general non-verbal intellectual ability in deafness research because it is a 'hold' test as one of the WAIS subtests least affected by brain damage

Table 12.1 Tests, results and interpretation (citations are provided for tests that are not commercially available or widely used)

Domain	Test	Scores/ Standardised scores	Interpretation
General cognitive screen	BSL Cognitive Screening Test (Atkinson et al., 2015)★	40th percentile (Dropped points on visual attention, working memory, executive tasks, visual errors on picture naming)	Normal range but below expected
Non-verbal intellectual function	WAIS III Matrix Reasoning★	95th percentile	Superior range
Processing speed	WAIS III Symbol Search★	15th percentile	Reduced but in normal range
Verbal memory and learning (BSL)	BSL Verbal Memory and Learning Test (Denmark et al., 2016)★	Trial 5th percentile	Borderline impairment in immediate recall but learning over time, encoding and recognition was reduced but in normal range
		Trial 10th	
		Trial 20–30th	
		Delayed recall: 40th	
		Recognition: 10th–20th	
Integrity of posterior visuospatial analysis	Visual Object and Space Perception Battery (VOSP) Cube analysis	4/10	Impaired spatial analysis and object decision
		Cut off is 6	
		Cumulative frequency 1.0%	
	VOSP Object Decision	12/20	
		Cut off is 14–15	
		Cumulative frequency 1.6%	
	Rey-Osterrieth Complex Figure (copying)	90th percentile	Intact visuospatial copying
Visual attention and speed	WAIS III Digit Symbol Colour Trails Test 1★	5th percentile	Impaired visual attention and processing speed
Visual memory (*The Camden Memory Tests*, 1996)	Rey-Osterrieth Complex Figure	<1st percentile	visuospatial memory
	Camden Pictorial Recognition memory (Warrington, 1996)	Immediate recall 9th percentile	Borderline
	Camden Topographic Recognition Memory	25/30 cumulative frequency 1.6%	Impaired visual memory
		Completely unable. Performance at floor	Impaired topographic (location) memory

(Continued)

Table 12.1 Continued

Domain	Test	Scores/ Standardised scores	Interpretation
Memory for faces	Camden Recognition Memory for Faces	Completely unable. Performance at floor	*Impaired memory for faces*
Face recognition	Benton Test of Face Recognition (Benton et al., 1983)	Short form 19/27 Long form conversion 43/54 (<40 is the cut-off for impairment) Extremely slow, effortful local-feature strategy (e.g. eyebrows)	Score is in *normal* range but qualitatively, performance is markedly *impaired* Inability to globally recognise faces and reliance on local features = *Impaired face recognition ability*
Judgement of facial affect	Visual sorting of emotional faces into emotion categories using Ekman faces (Ekman & Friesen, 1971) – a bespoke test with a low ceiling and no norms	Happy – 11/11 Angry – 5/6 Fear – 6/7 Disgust – 8/10 Sad –11/18 Surprise – 8/13	*Impaired* emotion recognition and judgement of emotion
Grammatical face processing in British Sign Language	Test of BSL Negation★	Positive 15/16 Negation on hands 15/16 Negation on face 7/16 Clinical cut-off is >1 error	*Impaired* comprehension of BSL grammar (negation) expressed solely on face. Extremely slow responses. Lack of automatic processing which will adversely impact her communication in BSL
	Test of BSL adverbials★ (Denmark et al., 2023)	Size and shape Specifiers expressed on: hands and face 16/17 face only 4/20	*Impaired* comprehension of BSL grammar (adverbials) expressed solely on face
Famous faces	BSL Famous Faces Test (Atkinson, unpublished)★	Naming 4/12 Semantic info 4/12 <1st percentile	*Impaired recognition/ semantic associations for familiar faces*
Semantic relationships	Visual semantics using pictorial: Pyramid and Palm trees	Score 47/52 (90%) 90% cut-off for impairment	90% is *borderline* for a hearing person The cut-off is unknown for a deaf person

Size and weight attribution test (SWAT, pictorial) (Warrington & Crutch, 2007)	SWAT Animals (visual) largest 13/15 smallest 12/15 heaviest 6/8 lightest 5/8 TOTAL 36/46 (78%)	No deaf norms are available. However, it is expected that healthy hearing person would make <2 errors on this easy test. This score represents a *semantic impairment*
Verbal semantics SWAT (written word) (Warrington & Crutch, 2007)	Heaviest 4/7 Lightest 5/7 TOTAL 9/14 (64%)	*As above. Semantic impairment*
Cambridge semantic category fluency (Adlam et al., 2010)	Animals 19 Fruits 10 Birds 10 Household items 9 Vehicles 9 Tools 3	Age-related norms are not available for deaf people except for animals (Atkinson, unpublished research) 19 animals = 80–90th centile. There is discrepancy between categories, and a *category specific semantic impairment for tools*
Semantic knowledge about visual world/ apperceptive deficits: Usual and Unusual Views Test (Warrington & Taylor, 1973)	9/20 for unusual views 20/20 for usual views	*Impaired visual perception of objects in unusual views indicative of orientation agnosia*
Executive function		
Nelson Card Sorting Test (cognitive flexibility) (Nelson, 1976) ★	47 Responses, 6 categories, 5 perseverative errors, 5 non-perseverative errors, 10 total errors.	*Normal range for deaf signers aged 70–79 years*
Delis Kaplan Executive Function System (DKEFS) Tower test (planning ability)★	Achievement score 1st percentile Rule violations: 2nd percentile Time per move: 0.1st percentile	*Impaired ability to plan*
DKEFS Design Fluency (ability to generate novel visuospatial designs) ★	Total correct 37th percentile Design accuracy: 2nd percentile	*Normal range but impaired design accuracy due to rule violations*
Colour Trails 2 (Measure of visual scanning, speed and cognitive flexibility)★	8th percentile	*Borderline impaired*

★ Asterisk denotes tests for which deaf norms were available.

Table 12.2 Findings of the reading assessment

PALPA	Test	Impairment
Whole paragraph reading	Completely unable to do this.	*Impaired*
Phonological reading	PALPA Rhyme identification task 23/30 PALPA Reading task – Do these words have the same sound? 26/30 She made some errors which would be typical of a deaf person. However, her score is well above 50% chance level which suggests she does possess reasonable phonological decoding skills	Evidence of phonological reading skills.
Visual errors with letters/groups of letters	PALPA Letter identification task 18/18 PALPA Reading decision task – decide if two items have the same letters (mixed upper and lower case) 30/30	No visual errors or letter reversals detected in single letter or word reading.
Pronunciation of irregular words	Unable to assess as a deaf person	n/a
Homophone reading	PALPA Homophone 'Define-then-Read' task 8/10 regular 5/10 irregular She was able to read and define in BSL most regularly spelled words (the exceptions being 'gait' and 'haul' which are likely to be outside her vocabulary). By contrast, for irregularly spelled words she only got 50% correct and made visual errors that suggested impaired visual reading strategy ('pear' for bear, 'hire' for heir).	Regular >irregular implying difficulties with visual reading strategies
Homophone judgement	PALPA homophone identification task 33/60 Performance just above chance level. Unable to assemble phonology of irregular words. This fits with surface dyslexia although caution is needed because deaf people would also be likely to have reduced scores on this test.	*Impaired*

(Donders et al., 2001), but it may still be reduced if underpinning cognitive abilities are affected so should not be wholly relied upon. Furthermore, clinical judgement from my own familiarity with deaf people led me to consider that without a brain injury Lydia would most likely have had above-average intellectual ability.

Cognitive testing

General cognitive screening using a BSL test did not detect any cognitive impairment. This basic screening tool is designed to detect dementia and neurodegeneration in BSL users (akin to the ACE III) and does not contain items screening for agnosia or face processing, or more complex executive or memory tasks. This shows how significant brain injuries can easily be overlooked without comprehensive testing.

There was reduced processing speed on WAIS Symbol Search, and visual attention problems on Colour Trails 1. There was no global amnesia. Immediate verbal memory was borderline impaired but with evidence of learning over time and normal recognition ability. Visual memory was worse than verbal memory. There was borderline impaired visual memory for recalling a complex design (Rey-Osterrieth) and picture recognition (Warrington's), and a total inability to remember topographic scenes or faces (Warrington's).

Basic visuospatial abilities were preserved as Lydia was able to copy a complicated spatial design (Rey-Osterrieth), but her higher-order spatial analysis was impaired, indicating difficulties generating or rotating internal visual imagery (VOSP Cube Analysis). Visual agnosia was indicated by poor object decision (VOSP) and orientation agnosia by poor recognition of objects in unusual views (see Figure 12.3a and 12.3b). Lydia had prosopagnosia which was apparent on tests requiring the recognition of famous faces (these were normed with deaf BSL users to ensure cultural familiarity), and the recognition of unfamiliar faces from different angles (Benton). She was also unable to judge emotion on faces (Ekman's) or to understand BSL grammar expressed by the face. She performed poorly on tests of BSL negatives and adverbs if grammatical information was presented only on the face but was unimpaired if an additional channel of information was presented on the hands, in the form of a lexical sign.

There were semantic deficits on picture and word matching tests that required knowledge about how objects or concepts were related (Pyramids and Palm Trees) or whether they were bigger or heavier (Size and Weight Attribute Test). Lydia displayed a strong dissociation in semantic category fluency with excellent fluency for animals but impaired tool naming. This category-specific dysfluency selectively affecting tools supports the notion of impaired access to semantic information about objects impacting both language (naming) and visual processing (agnosia).

Some aspects of executive functioning were impaired although she retained some ability to be flexible in her thinking, she showed severe difficulties with

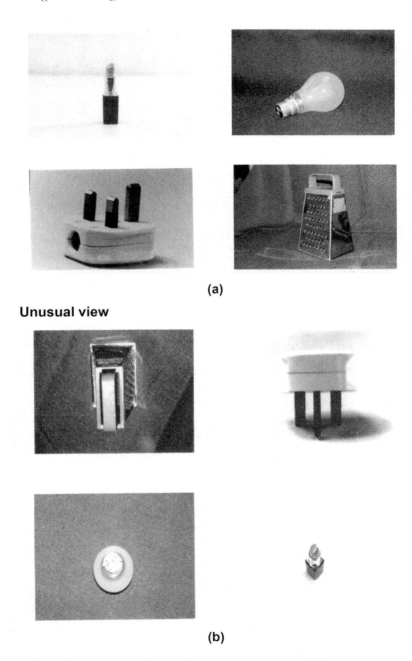

(a)

Unusual view

(b)

Figure 12.3a Usual views of objects (Warrington & Taylor, 1973)

Figure 12.3b Unusual views of objects (Warrington & Taylor, 1973)

planning on the DKEFS Tower Task, which fits with her reported everyday problems with organising her flat and making decisions.

Assessment of reading

Lydia's reading was assessed using the PALPA in conjunction with a Speech and Language therapist familiar with deaf BSL users. The PALPA is used to assess surface dyslexia following anterior temporal lobe damage in hearing people. Much of PALPA presupposes a person's English phonology and vocabulary were excellent before, which is a problem for assessing prelingually deaf people who typically have reduced phonological knowledge and English vocabulary because of lack of access to the spoken word and suitable education. Poor literacy is common in deaf people. Deaf readers show great variability in their ability to use a phonological route to reading and some may rely more on visual strategies and whole-word reading rather than sounding out phonemes (Rowley, 2018). This means that a deaf reader with surface dyslexia may be more disabled by it than a hearing person because they may be less able to use phonological strategies as an alternative pathway to word recognition. They may also be reliant on reading to access subtitles on television or to communicate via written notes with hearing people in their community.

Hearing individuals with anterior temporal lobe damage typically show surface dyslexia, which means they are unable to use a visual route or to read words by sight. Instead, they must sound words out to understand them. A person with surface dyslexia would:

- Skip letters or paragraphs.
- Be unable to keep place in the text.
- Need to sound out letters (phonological strategy) and be unable to use a visual strategy in reading.
- Fail to match homophones like 'doe' and 'dough' because they cannot assemble the phonology of the irregular word 'dough'.
- Make mistakes pronouncing irregularly spelled words but still understand meaning.

Summary of reading findings

Lydia's reading ability showed many of the features of surface dyslexia. She experienced visual crowding and was completely unable to read paragraphs. She could only read single words and short sentences, and her single-word reading showed errors indicative of surface-level difficulties. Figure 12.4 provides an example of a note that Lydia wrote and kept in her coffee jar to remind herself how Darren liked his coffee made. She wrote it on double-spaced lines and still had trouble reading it, so she annotated it, the red dots show her letter–by–letter reading strategy, and the arrows were used to direct her attention to each word because she would often miss a word or part of it.

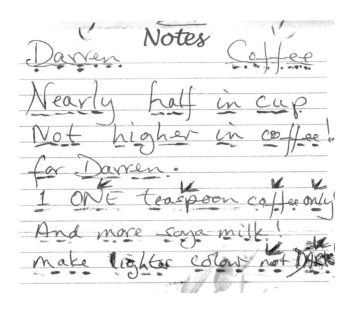

Figure 12.4 An example of one of Lydia's notes with her markings that show her reading strategies

The results show that despite her deafness, Lydia had reasonably well-developed phonological skills for reading single words, which stood in contrast to her difficulties with irregularly spelt words. This dissociation between regular and irregular words is not a typical feature of poor deaf readers (Wass et al., 2019). Irregular words must be read or spelt using a visual strategy, and Lydia struggled with this. Her difficulties were opposite to the pattern shown by skilled deaf readers who may prefer a visual strategy over a phonological one (Costello et al., 2021). It is clear that Lydia did experience a substantial reading impairment and that was over and above the reading difficulties typically experienced by those prelingually deaf people who struggle with literacy. It was our opinion that there was sufficient evidence to suggest that neurological damage had caused surface dyslexia. However, without research identifying patterns of surface dyslexia in deaf readers, it was hard to be clinically certain.

Summary of findings

Finally, we had some answers to share with Lydia and Darren that explained her puzzling symptoms. Lydia had sustained a brain injury probably during toddlerhood as a result of herpes simplex encephalitis or meningo-encephalitis which also caused her to lose her hearing. The pattern of her cognitive impairments mirrors those found in hearing people with bilateral damage to the anterior temporal lobes. She had impairments in autobiographical memory; complex visuospatial processing; visual memory; visual attention; face processing; recognition and memory for faces; semantic knowledge; planning; reading; socioemotional judgement and inhibition. She had feelings of unreality, hypersensitivity to sensory stimuli and unexplained pain, which have been reported in other people with damage to this area of the brain. She did not show the global anterograde amnesia that can be characteristic of bilateral temporal damage, but she did have very impaired visual memory for faces, topographic layouts and scenes, and lesser problems with verbal memory that fits with the lesions shown on the scan, which is more severe on the right side than the left. The pattern of the visual findings also fitted with this more extensive damage within the right ATL, extending into the visual association areas of the ventral stream. She showed orientation agnosia with difficulties with recognising objects from unusual angles and simultanagnosia with ability to distinguish objects within scenes and backgrounds or to recognise more than one object at a time. She had prosopagnosia and struggled to recognise familiar, unfamiliar and famous faces. This was worsened with a change in face orientation.

There were two key ways that her experience of these symptoms differs from hearing people. Firstly, as a deaf person, she was not hypersensitive to sound but to visual stimuli and vibrations. Secondly, her difficulties with visuospatial imagery, agnosia, and face processing had a detrimental impact on communication through sign language in ways that would not be true for spoken languages. These caused a subtle cognitive-communication (cog-com) disorder in BSL that is markedly different in nature to BSL aphasia that would result from damage to the left perisylvian language cortex. Cog-com disorders are communication impairments where the cognitive deficit is the cause, rather than a primary language disorder. Lydia did not show the errors with sign meanings or handshapes, jargon signs or absence of grammar that would be seen in a primary left hemisphere aphasia; instead, she presented more like signers with stroke who have right hemisphere damage (Atkinson et al., 2005), where they have more subtle difficulties with BSL that are secondary to visuospatial or face processing impairments. Her poor spatial analysis caused problems using and understanding more complex aspects of BSL grammar, which employs the use of topographical signing space to express real-world relations or the use of spatial verbs and classifier constructions using handshape and movement within the signing space to convey linguistic meaning (Atkinson et al., 2002). While this did not disrupt sign language to the extent that a primary language impairment or aphasia would, it meant that Lydia showed a preference for aspects of BSL grammar that did not rely on space.

Lydia's emotion and face processing impairments meant that she was unable to pick up on emotional and grammatical meanings conveyed solely by the face in BSL (e.g. affect, negation, adverbials, manner). This inability would not be immediately apparent to a conversation partner but led to communication breakdowns and frustration for Lydia during social interactions.

Lydia showed evidence of simultanagnosia and orientation agnosia with severe difficulties distinguishing objects from their visual background, more than one object at a time, or recognising objects seen from a non-typical angle. This also affected her perception of sign language. She struggled to see signing against a cluttered background or if her conversation partner was not orientated head-on, and had to stop and recalibrate if they turned their head while communicating. She also could not understand signing on a flat-screen. These are highly unusual features that have not, to our knowledge, been previously documented.

DARREN: Finally after diagnosis and explanation from Jo and the team, Mum's strange symptoms made sense. The sense of relief was enormous. For the last two years of her life, we were able to stop tilting at windmills, stop wasting precious time trying to solve things that were unsolvable, and instead put time and energy into the things that we maybe could do something about. And perhaps more importantly I could understand and accept why Mum was the way she was, and not get so frustrated. When things got tough, we could get back to a calmer place; stop forever looking for answers and instead enjoy life in the moment. If this service had been available previously, and this diagnosis made earlier, the NHS would have saved massive costs, as well as saving us the years of profound difficulty, doubt, and confusion.

Conclusions

It was a testament to Lydia's resilience, resourcefulness, and coping strategies (and the support she received from Darren) that she lived with a serious hidden brain injury for nearly 70 years. Too often her bewildering symptoms were simply put down to her deafness, and other possible causes were overlooked or attributed to mental illness. Lydia and Darren's experience poignantly illustrates diagnostic overshadowing, the highly specialist nature of accurate neuropsychological assessment in deaf people who use sign language, and the lack of services equipped to meet their needs. High levels of bilingual and bicultural cross-language competency are essential. It is insufficient to rely on translators; instead, specialist services are needed for deaf sign language users, as subtle interactions between brain injury and communication will be missed by hearing clinicians using sign language interpreters. We need more clinicians who are fluent in sign languages and understand how brain injury intersects with visuospatial languages like BSL, and how hallmark features may often be quite different from how symptoms manifest in spoken language users. Just as diagnosticians should not overlook how symptoms may manifest differently in people of varying language or cultural backgrounds, neuropsychologists must not overlook the impact of language modality on psychology assessment if we are to reduce diagnostic overshadowing in deaf people who use visual rather than auditory language.

Transferable learning

The spotlight on the Deaf Community flags up challenges inherent in neuropsychological provision for other minority language, culture, and disability groups. Diagnostic overshadowing is an issue for those from different cultural backgrounds or relying on spoken language interpreters; also for blind, visually impaired, or physically disabled people, people with learning disabilities, neurodiversity, mental health conditions or poor literacy, or other marginalised populations such as homeless people and traveller communities. Neuropsychology faces challenges in developing better awareness, access to services, tests and norms for these groups. It is not enough to have good intentions and to simply hope that translation or crude test modifications are a panacea to our lack of specialist services or tests for these groups. We must become more aware of our blind spots as a profession. A one-size-fits-all approach will not provide an equitable and timely service for all demographic groups. Differences in language, culture, and ability must not just be a footnote in our reports but should be driving the profession towards new models of measurement, assessment, and formulation of neuropsychological disorders that are not just based on a monoculture of white western non-disabled users of spoken languages, but which are fit for assessing brain conditions in diverse humanity. Better use of technology and neuroimaging hold some promise. Until we broaden our thinking and tools, diagnostic overshadowing is likely to remain an intractable problem for the neuropsychology profession. Until we achieve this, we need to recognise that each clinician is limited in their amount of specialist cultural, language, and disability competence. It is not possible to know everything. Therefore we should have specialist neuropsychology services for hard-to-serve populations such as people with congenital sensory impairments that impact cognitive development, services for acquired brain conditions in people with congenital intellectual disability, or services for people using a particular language, or within a particular culture. Remote technology will be particularly beneficial in allowing neuropsychologists with specialist skills to reach geographically dispersed populations.

We need to develop greater awareness of how different disabilities intersect in neuropsychological presentations. Lydia's case shows how certain neurological disabilities, in her case visual agnosia and difficulties with visuospatial cognition and faces, may be more disabling for a deaf person reliant on visual language, and manifest differently in their communication and behaviour. As a profession, we must pay greater attention to the intersectional nature of neurological disability and how different culture, language, and disability groups experience brain injuries and display neurological symptoms in very different ways.

Acknowledgements

With special thanks to Dr Cath Mummery, Consultant Neurologist, and Katy Judd, Consultant Nurse, Dementia Research Centre, UCL and National Hospital of Neurology and Neurosurgery.

In memory of Lydia Handscomb. For mum, whose amazing brain made the impossible possible.

References

Adlam, A.-L. R., Patterson, K., Bozeat, S., & Hodges, J. R. (2010). The Cambridge Semantic Memory Test Battery: Detection of semantic deficits in semantic dementia and Alzheimer's disease. *Neurocase*, *16*(3), 193–207. https://doi.org/10.1080/13554790903405693

Atkinson, J. (unpublished). BSL Famous Faces Test for British deaf older adults.

Atkinson, J., Campbell, R., Marshall, J., Thacker, A., & Woll, B. (2004). Understanding 'not': Neuropsychological dissociations between hand and head markers of negation in BSL. *Neuropsychologia*, *42*(2), 214–229.

Atkinson, J., Denmark, T., Marshall, J., Mummery, C., & Woll, B. (2015). Detecting Cognitive Impairment and Dementia in Deaf People: The British Sign Language Cognitive Screening Test. *Archives of Clinical Neuropsychology: The Official Journal of the National Academy of Neuropsychologists*, acv042-. https://doi.org/10.1093/arclin/acv042

Atkinson, J., Marshall, J., Woll, B., & Thacker, A. (2005). Testing comprehension abilities in users of British Sign Language following CVA. *Brain and Language*, *94*(2), 233–248.

Atkinson, J. R., Woll, B., & Gathercole, S. (2002). The impact of developmental visuospatial learning difficulties on British Sign Language. *Neurocase*, *8*(6), 424–441.

Atkinson, J., & Woll, B. (2012). The health of deaf people. *The Lancet*, *379*(9833), 2239. https://doi.org/10.1016/S0140-6736(12)60974-X

Baeken, C., De Raedt, R., Van Schuerbeek, P., Vanderhasselt, M. A., De Mey, J., Bossuyt, A., & Luypaert, R. (2010). Right prefrontal HF-rTMS attenuates right amygdala processing of negatively valenced emotional stimuli in healthy females. *Behavioural Brain Research*, *214*(2), 450–455. https://doi.org/10.1016/j.bbr.2010.06.029

Barnett, E. M., Jacobsen, G., Evans, G., Cassell, M., & Perlman, S. (1994). Herpes simplex encephalitis in the temporal cortex and limbic system after trigeminal nerve inoculation. *The Journal of Infectious Diseases*, *169*(4), 782–786. https://doi.org/10.1093/infdis/169.4.782

Baxter, M. G., & Croxson, P. L. (2012). Facing the role of the amygdala in emotional information processing. *Proceedings of the National Academy of Sciences*, *109*(52), 21180–21181. https://doi.org/10.1073/pnas.1219167110

Benton, A., Hamsher, K., Varney, N., & Spreen, O. (1983). *Contributions to neuropsychological assessment: A clinical manual*. Oxford University Press.

Biran, I., & Coslett, H. B. (2003). Visual agnosia. *Current Neurology and Neuroscience Reports*, *3*(6), 508–512. https://doi.org/10.1007/s11910-003-0055-4

Bonner, M. F., & Price, A. R. (2013). Where is the anterior temporal lobe and what does it do? *Journal of Neuroscience*, *33*(10), 4213–4215. https://doi.org/10.1523/JNEUROSCI.0041-13.2013

Borgo, F., Sgaramella, T. M., Penello, B., L'Erario, R., & Toso, V. (2000). A componential analysis of visual object recognition deficits in patients with herpes simplex virus encephalitis. *Brain and Cognition*, *43*(1–3), 53–56.

Borgo, F., & Shallice, T. (2001). When living things and other 'sensory quality' categories behave in the same fashion: A novel category specificity effect. *Neurocase*, 7(3), 201–220. https://doi.org/10.1093/neucas/7.3.201

Braden, J. P. (1994). *Deafness, deprivation, and IQ*. Springer. http://books.google.com/books?id=9u2t-nrEIIsC&pgis=1

Costello, B., Caffarra, S., Fariña, N., Duñabeitia, J. A., & Carreiras, M. (2021). Reading without phonology: ERP evidence from skilled deaf readers of Spanish. *Scientific Reports*, 11(1), 5202. https://doi.org/10.1038/s41598-021-84490-5

Craig, A. D. (2002). How do you feel? Interoception: The sense of the physiological condition of the body. *Nature Reviews. Neuroscience*, 3(8), 655–666. https://doi.org/10.1038/nrn894

Crawford, J. R., Millar, J., & Milne, A. B. (2001). Estimating premorbid IQ from demographic variables: A comparison of a regression equation vs. clinical judgement. *The British Journal of Clinical Psychology*, 40(1), 97–105. https://doi.org/10.1348/014466501163517

Critchley, H. D., Wiens, S., Rotshtein, P., Ohman, A., & Dolan, R. J. (2004). Neural systems supporting interoceptive awareness. *Nature Neuroscience*, 7(2), 189–195. https://doi.org/10.1038/nn1176

De Renzi, E. (2000). Disorders of visual recognition. *Seminars in Neurology*, 20(4), 479–485. https://doi.org/10.1055/s-2000-13181

Denmark, T., Marshall, J., Mummery, C., Roy, P., Woll, B., & Atkinson, J. (2016). Detecting memory impairment in deaf people: A new test of verbal learning and memory in British Sign Language. *Archives of Clinical Neuropsychology*, 31(8), 855–867. https://doi.org/10.1093/arclin/acw032

Denmark, T., Swettenham, J., Campbell, R., & Atkinson, J. (2023). The processing of facial actions in deaf children with autism who use British Sign Language (BSL) [Faces em Questão: o não-manual nas línguas de sinais]. *Revista Inclusão & Sociedade*, UFABC, Brazil.

Donders, J., Tulsky, D. S., & Zhu, J. (2001). Criterion validity of new WAIS-III subtest scores after traumatic brain injury. *Journal of the International Neuropsychological Society*, 7(7), 892–898. https://doi.org/10.1017/S1355617701246153

Dowell, E., Easton, A., & Solomon, T. (2000). *Consequences of encephalitis*. Encephalitis Society.

Ekman, P., & Friesen, W. V. (1971). Constants across cultures in the face and emotion. *Journal of Personality and Social Psychology*, 17(2), 124–129. https://doi.org/10.1037/h0030377

Emmorey, K., Kosslyn, S. M., & Bellugi, U. (1993). Visual imagery and visual-spatial language: Enhanced imagery abilities in deaf and hearing ASL signers. *Cognition*, 46(2), 139–181. https://doi.org/10.1016/0010-0277(93)90017-P

Farah, M. J. (1990). *Visual Agnosia: Disorders of Object Recognition and What They Tell Us about Normal Vision*. The MIT Press.

Harris, I., Harris, J., & Caine, D. (2001). Object orientation agnosia: A failure to find the axis? *Journal of Cognitive Neuroscience*, 13, 800–812. https://doi.org/10.1162/08989290152541467

Harris, L., Griem, J., Gummery, A., Marsh, L., Defres, S., Bhojak, M., Das, K., Easton, A., Solomon, T., Kopelman, M., Barlow, G., Beeching, N., Blanchard, T., Body, R., Boyd, G., Cebria-Prejan, L., Chadwick, D., Cooke, R., Crawford, P., ... Warlow, C. (2020). Neuropsychological and psychiatric outcomes in encephalitis: A multi-centre case-control study. *PLoS ONE, 15*(3). https://doi.org/10.1371/JOURNAL.PONE.0230436

Harris, M. J., Atkinson, J. R., Judd, K., Bergson, M., & Mummery, C. J. (2020). Assessing Deaf patients in the neurology clinic. *Practical Neurology, 20*(2). https://doi.org/10.1136/practneurol-2019-002422

Harris, M., Terlektsi, E., & Kyle, F. E. (2017). Concurrent and longitudinal predictors of reading for deaf and hearing children in primary school. *Journal of Deaf Studies and Deaf Education, 22*(2), 233–242. https://doi.org/10.1093/deafed/enw101

Hodges, J. R., & Patterson, K. (2007). Semantic dementia: A unique clinicopathological syndrome. *The Lancet Neurology, 6*(11), 1004–1014. https://doi.org/10.1016/S1474-4422(07)70266-1

Kapur, N., Barker, S., Burrows, E. H., Ellison, D., Brice, J., Illis, L. S., Scholey, K., Colbourn, C., Wilson, B., & Loates, M. (1994). Herpes simplex encephalitis: Long term magnetic resonance imaging and neuropsychological profile. *Journal of Neurology, Neurosurgery, and Psychiatry, 57*(11), 1334–1342.

Keehner, M., & Atkinson, J. R. (2006). Working memory and deafness: Implications for cognitive development and functioning. In S. Pickering (Ed.), *Working memory and education* (pp. 189–214). Academic Press.

Kong, J., White, N. S., Kwong, K. K., Vangel, M. G., Rosman, I. S., Gracely, R. H., & Gollub, R. L. (2006). Using fMRI to dissociate sensory encoding from cognitive evaluation of heat pain intensity. *Human Brain Mapping, 27*(9), 715–721. https://doi.org/10.1002/hbm.20213

Ladabaum, U., Minoshima, S., Hasler, W. L., Cross, D., Chey, W. D., & Owyang, C. (2001). Gastric distention correlates with activation of multiple cortical and subcortical regions. *Gastroenterology, 120*(2), 369–376. https://doi.org/10.1053/gast.2001.21201

Liu, T., Thiebaut de Schotten, M., Altarelli, I., Ramus, F., & Zhao, J. (2021). Maladaptive compensation of right fusiform gyrus in developmental dyslexia: A hub-based white matter network analysis. *Cortex, 145*, 57–66. https://doi.org/10.1016/j.cortex.2021.07.016

Maller, S., & Braden, J. P. (2012). Intellectual assessment of deaf people: A critical review of core concepts and issues. *The Oxford Handbook of Deaf Studies, Language, and Education: Second Edition, 1*. Oxford Academic. https://doi.org/10.1093/oxfordhb/9780199750986.013.0033

Mayer, E. A. (2011). Gut feelings: The emerging biology of gut–brain communication. *Nature Reviews Neuroscience, 12*(8), 453–466. https://doi.org/10.1038/nrn3071

McGrath, N., Anderson, N. E., Croxson, M. C., & Powell, K. F. (1997). Herpes simplex encephalitis treated with acyclovir: Diagnosis and long term outcome. *Journal of Neurology, Neurosurgery, and Psychiatry, 63*(3), 321–326. https://doi.org/10.1136/jnnp.63.3.321

Mégevand, P., Groppe, D. M., Goldfinger, M. S., Hwang, S. T., Kingsley, P. B., Davidesco, I., & Mehta, A. D. (2014). Seeing scenes: Topographic visual hallucinations evoked by direct electrical stimulation of the parahippocampal place area. *The Journal of Neuroscience: The Official Journal of the Society for Neuroscience, 34*(16), 5399–5405. https://doi.org/10.1523/JNEUROSCI.5202-13.2014

Mutschler, I., Reinbold, C., Wankerl, J., Seifritz, E., & Ball, T. (2013). Structural basis of empathy and the domain general region in the anterior insular cortex. *Frontiers in Human Neuroscience, 7*. www.frontiersin.org/article/10.3389/fnhum.2013.00177

Nelson, H. E. (1976). A modified card sorting test sensitive to frontal lobe defects. *Cortex; a Journal Devoted to the Study of the Nervous System and Behavior, 12*, 313–324. https://doi.org/10.1016/S0010-9452(76)80035-4

Noppeney, U., Patterson, K., Tyler, L. K., Moss, H., Stamatakis, E. A., Bright, P., Mummery, C., & Price, C. J. (2007). Temporal lobe lesions and semantic impairment: A comparison of herpes simplex virus encephalitis and semantic dementia. *Brain, 130*(4), 1138–1147. https://doi.org/10.1093/BRAIN/AWL344

Pewter, S. M., Williams, W. H., Haslam, C., & Kay, J. M. (2007). Neuropsychological and psychiatric profiles in acute encephalitis in adults. *Neuropsychological Rehabilitation, 17*(4–5), 478–505. https://doi.org/10.1080/096020107012 02238

Rabinstein, A., Jerry, J., Saraf–Lavi, E., Sklar, E., & Bradley, W. G. (2001). Sudden sensorineural hearing loss associated with herpes simplex virus type 1 infection. *Neurology, 56*(4), 571–572. https://doi.org/10.1212/WNL.56.4.571

Rice, G. E., Lambon Ralph, M. A., & Hoffman, P. (2015). The roles of left versus right anterior temporal lobes in conceptual knowledge: An ALE meta-analysis of 97 functional neuroimaging studies. *Cerebral Cortex (New York, NY), 25*(11), 4374–4391. https://doi.org/10.1093/cercor/bhv024

Rowley, K. E. (2018). Visual word recognition in deaf readers: The interplay between orthographic, semantic and phonological information. (Doctoral dissertation). University College London.

Sharp, H., Themelis, K., Amato, M., Barritt, A., Davies, K., Harrison, N., Critchley, H., Garfinkel, S., & Eccles, J. (2021). The role of interoception in the mechanism of pain and fatigue in fibromyalgia and myalgic encephalomyelitis/chronic fatigue syndrome (ME/CFS). *European Psychiatry, 64*(S1), S139–S139. https://doi.org/10.1192/J.EURPSY.2021.382

Simon, M., Campbell, E., Genest, F., MacLean, M. W., Champoux, F., & Lepore, F. (2020). The impact of early deafness on brain plasticity: A systematic review of the white and gray matter changes. *Frontiers in Neuroscience, 14*, 206. https://doi.org/10.3389/fnins.2020.00206

Smith, T. (2010). Neuropsychological assessment of deaf adults: Cross cultural validity. Unpublished doctoral thesis, University of East London.

The Camden Memory Tests: Topographical Recognition Memory Test. (n.d.). Routledge & CRC Press. Retrieved 19 July 2022, from https://www.routledge.com/The-Camden-Memory-Tests-Topographical-Recognition-Memory-Test/Warrington/p/book/9780863774270

Theil, D., Derfuss, T., Paripovic, I., Herberger, S., Meinl, E., Schueler, O., Strupp, M., Arbusow, V., & Brandt, T. (2003). Latent herpesvirus infection in human trigeminal ganglia causes chronic immune response. *The American Journal of Pathology, 163*(6), 2179. https://doi.org/10.1016/S0002-9440(10)63575-4

Tran The, J., Magistretti, P. J., & Ansermet, F. (2021). Interoception disorder and insular cortex abnormalities in schizophrenia: A new perspective between psychoanalysis and neuroscience. *Frontiers in Psychology, 12*, 628355. https://doi.org/10.3389/FPSYG.2021.628355

Utley, T. F., Ogden, J. A., Gibb, A., McGrath, N., & Anderson, N. E. (1997). The long-term neuropsychological outcome of herpes simplex encephalitis in a series of unselected survivors. *Neuropsychiatry, Neuropsychology, and Behavioral Neurology, 10*(3), 180–189.

Visser, M., Jefferies, E., & Lambon Ralph, M. A. (2010). Semantic processing in the anterior temporal lobes: A meta-analysis of the functional neuroimaging literature. *Journal of Cognitive Neuroscience, 22*(6), 1083–1094. https://doi.org/10.1162/jocn.2009.21309

Warrington, E. K. (1996). *The Camden Memory Test Battery*, Psychology Press.

Warrington, E. K., & Crutch, S. J. (2007). A within-modality test of semantic knowledge: The Size/Weight Attribute Test. *Neuropsychology, 21*(6), 803–811. https://doi.org/10.1037/0894-4105.21.6.803

Warrington, E. K., & Taylor, A. M. (1973). The contribution of the right parietal lobe to object recognition. *Cortex: a Journal Devoted to the Study of the Nervous System and Behavior, 9*(2), 152–164. https://doi.org/10.1016/s0010-9452(73)80024-3

Wass, M., Ching, T. Y. C., Cupples, L., Wang, H.-C., Lyxell, B., Martin, L., Button, L., Gunnourie, M., Boisvert, I., McMahon, C., & Castles, A. (2019). Orthographic learning in children who are deaf or hard of hearing. *Language, Speech, and Hearing Services in Schools, 50*(1), 99–112. https://doi.org/10.1044/2018_LSHSS-17-0146

13 Aerotoxic syndrome

Are passengers and aircrew breathing toxic cabin air?

Sarah Mackenzie Ross

Introduction

The list of substances that can damage brain tissue is vast, yet few healthcare professionals in the United Kingdom receive training in toxicology unless they specialise in occupational medicine. This means neurotoxic conditions are frequently misdiagnosed or not diagnosed at all, which can be disastrous for the patient because successful treatment of chemical poisoning requires early diagnosis and cessation of exposure. Failure to diagnose results in patients being referred to multiple specialists (often over many years), based on symptom clusters rather than a clear diagnosis; and the lack of a clear diagnosis makes it difficult for patients to access appropriate treatment, decide whether it is safe to return to work, claim health insurance, and/or retire on ill health grounds.

There is an urgent need for increased awareness and understanding of neurotoxic conditions and neuropsychologists have an important role to play in both clinical and research settings in detecting and evaluating the effects of toxic substances. Indeed, neuropsychological assessment has been described by Muriel Lezak as the most sensitive means of examining the effects of toxic exposure, of monitoring for industrial safety, and of understanding the complaints and psychosocial problems of persons exposed to toxins (Lezak, 1984; Bowler & Lezak, 2015). Although there have been advances in neuroimaging over the last two decades, there hasn't been a concomitant increase in imaging studies of persons exposed to toxic substances. There are a number of reasons why this might be the case including the fact that many neurotoxicants have a short half-life and can't be detected in the brain once excreted, even though brain damage may have occurred. Neurotoxic substances do not necessarily cause structural brain damage, but can alter brain function, which means functional brain scans are often more appropriate than standard MRI and CT, but functional imaging is not routinely offered in healthcare settings for diagnostic purposes. The mechanism of action of many toxic substances is unknown, making it difficult to determine the location or type of damage expected and therefore the type of imaging required. Furthermore, brain imaging doesn't reveal the neurobehavioural consequences of exposure

DOI: 10.4324/9781003228226-15

to toxic substances or enable clinicians to document the profile of cognitive and emotional sequalae, undertake differential diagnosis, plan rehabilitation, or determine the degree of progression or remission of symptoms. Some psychometric tests are considered more sensitive to neurotoxic effects than others, e.g. processing speed and reaction time tasks, memory and working memory tests, dexterity and aiming tests, executive tests (Bowler & Lezak, 2015; Hartman, 1995).

The manufacture and use of industrial chemicals increased more than 15-fold in the past 70 years and concern has been growing about the impact on human health. Indeed, some researchers attribute the rise in neurodevelopmental and neurodegenerative disorders to exposure to neurotoxic substances as common targets, and pathways underlying exposure to certain chemicals and neurodegeneration have been noted (Grandjean & Landrigan 2014). The capacity of industry to produce new chemicals outstrips our capacity to research the health effects and few chemicals are subjected to neurotoxic or behavioural analysis prior to regulation and sale. Furthermore, there is almost no research undertaken on the effects of chemical mixtures which can be additive, synergistic, antagonistic or completely novel in their neurotoxic effect (Hartman, 1995).

People can be exposed to toxic substances through food, water, skin contact, and inhalation, which is generally considered to be the most dangerous route of exposure; and in different settings such as homes, schools, and the workplace. Exposure may be high level and brief (in the case of accidental release of chemicals) or cumulative over time and the latter may not result in observable effects initially. Symptoms may differ depending on duration, frequency, and level of exposure; and some people are known to be more sensitive and vulnerable to chemical insults because of their age, gender, health status, or because of genetic differences in the ability to metabolise specific substances. To confuse matters further neurotoxic effects can take time to evolve and may not be seen until after exposure has ceased (e.g. manganese, methyl iodide, carbon monoxide poisoning) and few healthcare professionals appreciate the latter, and assume a toxic cause for a person's presentation is unlikely if their symptoms worsen over time (Mackenzie Ross, 2016).

Diagnostic issues

Lack of awareness regarding the toxicity of chemical substances means neither patient nor doctor may consider a toxic cause for their symptoms. In many cases patients present long after exposure has ceased (having not previously considered a toxic cause for their symptoms), by which time there is no biomarker of exposure or means of gauging the level/dose, intensity, or duration of exposure other than from self-report, which can be unreliable. Symptoms of neurotoxic exposure can be so non-specific and varied that they are mistaken for other conditions such as a virus, chronic fatigue syndrome, multiple sclerosis, a psychiatric problem, or a psychogenic or functional disorder. Even when patients are evaluated by a medical expert, routine medical and neurological tests including brain imaging are frequently normal. There are many reasons why this may happen such as lack of knowledge as to the mechanism by which certain chemicals damage the body, which results in the wrong tests being undertaken (e.g. structural vs functional brain imaging); or because of subclinical toxicity where signs of poisoning are invisible initially but develop over time until a threshold is reached, with or without further exposure.

Controversy

Neurotoxic conditions often attract considerable controversy because exposure frequently occurs in the workplace, where people may be using chemicals approved by regulatory authorities; or health and safety breaches may result in accidental exposure; or manufacturers may dispose of chemicals in a way that leads to contamination of groundwater, air, or food chains. People can struggle to get a diagnosis if an admission of chemical poisoning might have health and safety implications for the employer and result in litigation. Those who work in toxicology often find themselves in a world where the interests of science, industry, politics, and the law conflict. Several neurotoxic syndromes have resulted in considerable debate and controversy over the last three decades such as the Camelford Water disaster, Gulf War syndrome, and Aerotoxic syndrome. In this chapter I will discuss the case of an airline pilot who reports ill health and cognitive impairment following alleged exposure to contaminated air whilst flying aircraft, to highlight the role of the neuropsychologist in evaluating neurotoxic conditions, and discuss the diagnostic challenges and controversies inherent in this type of work.

Aerotoxic syndrome

The term 'Aerotoxic syndrome' was coined by two toxicologists in 2000 to refer to a constellation of neurological, respiratory, cardiovascular, gastrointestinal, eye, nose and throat irritation, dermatological, and systemic symptoms (fatigue, arthralgias) reported by aircrew, which are thought to be caused by exposure to toxic substances in cabin air (Winder & Balouet, 2000). The primary route of exposure in this case is presumed to be inhalation but can also involve skin contact.

Cabin air is a mixture of outside air and recirculated air which is introduced into the aircraft in different ways depending on whether the aircraft is in flight or on the ground. On the ground the air supply is provided by Auxiliary Power Units which draw air from a vent at the back of the aircraft. During flight (on most commercial aircraft types), outside air is drawn into the aircraft and circulated around the engine where it is heated and pressurised to a breathable level. This air is then 'bled off' and pumped into the cabin. Cabin air can be contaminated by a large number of toxic substances such as ingestion of exhaust from other aircraft, engine oil and hydraulic fluid leaks, application of de-icing fluids, and combusted and pyrolised materials (e.g. carbon monoxide). Contamination can occur in two ways: (1) chronic repeated low-level exposure due to jet aircraft design, which allows continuous leaking of oil past wet-oil seals, (2) acute high-level exposure (referred to as 'fume events') associated with odours and sometimes a visible haze, caused by general system failures such as seal bearing failure, worn seals, overfilling of oil and hydraulic reservoirs (Howard et al., 2017). Commercial aircraft do not have air quality monitoring systems on board so the full spectrum of contaminants and levels in bleed air are poorly understood. Synthetic jet engine oils contain a large number of chemicals, some of which are irritating and sensitising and some of which are neurotoxic (e.g. toluene, xylenes, organophosphates), and aircrew have expressed particular concern about the presence of organophosphate compounds in engine oil, which are known to be neurotoxic (Winder & Balouet, 2002).

Aircrew and some passengers around the world have been reporting ill health following exposure to contaminated air events for many years and immediate symptoms include eye irritation, respiratory problems, headache, skin problems, nausea, dizziness, fatigue, and cognitive impairment. These symptoms often recede following cessation of exposure, but many individuals report persistent chronic ill health including fatigue, gastrointestinal problems, respiratory difficulties, palpitations, muscle pain/weakness, immunosuppression, and neurological problems such as headache, parasthesias, and cognitive impairment. Work incapacity may be as high as 35% (Mackenzie Ross et al., 2006).

A small number of cabin air quality studies have been undertaken over the last two decades, primarily focused on levels of organophosphate compounds in cabin air, but a few other chemicals have also been measured including volatile organic compounds (VOCS), carbon dioxide, carbon monoxide, and ozone. Results indicate that during routine flight, air pollutant levels in aircraft cabins are similar to those found in other indoor environments (e.g. offices) and seldom exceed exposure levels permitted in buildings (Chen et al., 2021). Airlines and Regulatory Authorities have concluded from these findings that the health risk of exposure to chemical contaminants in cabin air is negligible and that other factors are to blame for 'Aerotoxic syndrome' such as hyperventilation, the nocebo effect, or some other aspect of flying (EASA, 2014). Unions and legal firms representing aircrew and many other scientists disagree and argue that firm conclusions cannot be drawn from air quality studies undertaken to date because all are flawed by methodological and procedural issues such as failure to measure the full spectrum of contaminants that may be found on aircraft, failure to mimic flight conditions, inadequate sample volumes, collection times, sampling methods and analytical techniques, inappropriate use of exposure standards, failure to consider synergistic effects between contaminants or to consider the synergistic impact of hypoxia and altitude; and most importantly of all, failure to capture a fume event of sufficient severity to trigger formal reporting procedures, or to consider the impact of low level cumulative exposure over a prolonged period of time (Howard, 2020). Hence the debate and controversy surrounding Aerotoxic syndrome continues.

Case presentation

A 45-year-old airline pilot was referred for neuropsychological assessment by his neurologist as he was suffering from an array of different symptoms including neurological problems and cognitive impairment, which he attributed to exposure to contaminated cabin air. His licence to fly had been suspended nine months prior to the neuropsychological assessment.

Exposure history

For the first ten years of his career, the pilot was employed by a European airline and then a chartered airline group and flew ATR 72s, Boeing 757s, and Airbus aircraft types. He reports being in relatively good health during this time, apart from an eight-month period in which he lost his medical licence because he was suffering dizzy spells. He recovered and secured a job managing aircraft on behalf of wealthy businessmen and companies, during which time he flew the Learjet 45 and the Dassault Falcon 900 for the first four years, then the Falcon 7X aircraft type for the next three years. The latter job involved flying a client to business meetings around the world and the pilot's work schedule was punishing in terms of the number of hours flown a year (circa 850) and the intensity (12–14 hours flying at a time, 40–50 hours per week), with minimal rest periods. It was during this time that his health dramatically deteriorated.

The pilot informed me that there were known issues with the Falcon X aircraft, regarding suspected APU oil leaks resulting in fumes entering the cabin. Oil leaks had been reported on the Falcon X the pilot was allocated and the APU was being monitored as it was showing signs of depreciation and was not functioning properly. Aircrew on this aircraft had repeatedly complained of oil smells and at one point the client's wife commissioned air quality analysis as she had noticed strange smells on board the aircraft and her husband had been diagnosed with a rare form of lung cancer (not related to smoking) and she thought there might be a connection between these factors. The analysis found high concentrations of volatile organic compounds (mainly solvents found in fuels) and the APU was subsequently replaced on the aircraft.

Symptom onset

Initial symptoms experienced by the pilot after he began flying the Falcon X aircraft included the sudden onset of a chesty cough and altered sense of taste, which lasted 4–5 days, and fatigue, and the pilot had to stay in bed for two days. A year later the pilot developed pins and needles in his hands and feet and a stabbing pain in his right foot and groin and he was referred to a neurologist by his GP for further evaluation. Nerve conduction studies did not reveal any abnormalities and although MRI revealed cervical stenosis at C3–C5, this was not thought to account for his symptoms. A month after consulting his GP about parasthesias in his limbs, the pilot consulted his GP because he was suffering from fever, sweating, headache, diarrhoea, fatigue, and shortness of breath. His GP suspected he might have a urinary infection or malaria, but both were ruled out. His symptoms persisted for several weeks, and he was referred to a specialist in tropical diseases who told the pilot his symptoms were similar to pneumonia but were not diagnostic of pneumonia and he asked the pilot if he had been exposed to toxic chemicals. The pilot eventually responded to antibiotic treatment but went on to suffer three more bouts of bronchitis over the ensuing year.

In the 18 months before the pilot lost his licence, he felt progressively more run down, his eyesight deteriorated, and he suffered intermittent pins and needles and shooting pains and recurrent groin pain. He also noticed that his client, whom he was flying for, was unusually moody and abusive and later admitted to suffering periods of confusion, insomnia, mood swings, and intolerance to alcohol which he attributed to medication or flying; and aircrew on the aircraft also developed strange symptoms. One colleague developed pins and needles in their feet and suffered an episode of anaphylaxis; another colleague developed cognitive impairment, headaches, and visual problems; a third colleague developed nausea and balance problems and a fourth colleague developed haematuria and coughs. In addition, a flight attendant developed severe mood swings and irritability and was subsequently fired as she was a flight safety risk

The pilot attributed his own deteriorating health to work stress and exhaustion. The pilot subsequently went on leave when the aircraft's APU was replaced but continued to feel exhausted and asked if his hours could be reduced when he returned to work. He flew on five more occasions and following his last flight he felt cognitively impaired and found simple tasks like driving a car or operating a supermarket checkout very difficult, which alarmed him. He then collapsed in bed and slept for 15 hours and remained unwell for several weeks. He developed an irregular heartbeat, elevated blood pressure, persistent sweats, and went on to suffer another bout of 'flu'. He spent most of his time in bed, but doctors were unable to identify a cause for his symptoms.

The pilot's symptoms gradually improved over a three-month period, and he decided to attend a training course in another country, but by the time he got there his pins and needles and dizziness returned and he found it increasingly difficult to walk over ensuing days. He attended a local emergency department, but they were unable to identify the cause of his symptoms, suggesting it may be a post-viral infection and once he got home his GP referred him back to neurology for further investigations. MRI of his spine and brain did not reveal any abnormalities. Soon after a colleague contacted the pilot and told him about Aerotoxic syndrome and recommended he pay for specialist tests in Europe.

Specialist tests

The pilot underwent a series of specialist tests. Genetic testing revealed slightly decreased activity of enzymes purported to be involved in the metabolism of organophosphate compounds; CAPS balance testing revealed impaired balance; autoantibodies to nervous system proteins were detected in blood serum, indicative of nervous system injury; quantitative EEG was reported as showing disconcerting features in brain wave activity in visual and parietal brain cortices; and psychometric testing of attention was reported to show impaired sustained attention. The pilot was then referred to a Medical Toxicology Unit in the UK but clinical examination was unremarkable. The toxicologist who examined him told him his symptoms were suggestive of peripheral neuropathy, but no objective evidence of this could be found. He recommended the pilot undergo brain MRI, psychiatric, and neuropsychological assessment. Meanwhile, the pilot's client died from lung cancer.

Neuropsychological assessment

Subjective complaints

The pilot complained of the following symptoms when assessed in 2015: fatigue, headaches, pins and needles in hands and feet, dizziness and vertigo, tinnitus, muscle pain, poor eyesight, multiple chemical sensitivity, memory problems, concentration difficulties, arithmetical problems, executive problems, irritability, and mood swings. His flying licence had been suspended and he no longer had an income and was forced to sell his house and various investments and his financial concerns had a great impact on his children and partner. His partner described him as struggling to cope with basic tasks because he had difficulty processing information and working methodically through the various steps involved in completing a task, he appeared unable to process and retain the amount of information he used to absorb before falling ill, and he was chronically fatigued. The pilot described himself as an optimistic, friendly, kind, humorous person prior to falling ill, but now suffers mood swings and worries about his health, finances, and future career prospects, and feels frustrated a diagnosis has not been forthcoming nor any treatment offered.

Medical and educational background

The pilot did not have a significant past medical or psychiatric history prior to his recent illness. He was not on any medication and did not consume any alcohol at this time. In terms of his educational history, he left school with five 'O' levels and a few CSEs and chose not to stay on and do 'A' levels as he was keen to secure work to pay for flying training. He worked in conveyancing for three years, then the meteorological office, following which he qualified as an Air Traffic Controller and then a Commercial Airline Pilot.

Psychometric testing in 2015

Neuropsychological assessment did not find evidence of generalised intellectual decline, but did reveal subtle, patchy under-functioning on tests of processing speed, auditory memory, and executive function (see Table 13.1).

Premorbid IQ was estimated to be in the high average range (FSIQ 111). Overall current IQ was also in the high average range (FSIQ 112, GAI 115) and the pilot's nonverbal reasoning abilities were better developed than his verbal reasoning abilities (PRI 121, VCI 107). Although individuals often show differences in terms of their performance on verbal vs non-verbal tasks, a discrepancy of the magnitude observed in this case is rather unusual and seen in only 15% of the normative sample. Working memory was in the superior range (WMI 122). In contrast, performance on processing speed tests was in the low average range (PSI 89) and significantly lower than expected, given his estimated premorbid IQ and his overall level of current intellectual functioning (base rate 1.7–13.6% depending on the specific index score PSI is compared with).

Performance on memory tests was variable. Auditory memory was lower than expected, given his overall level of intellectual functioning, with lower performance on the story recall task compared to the list learning task (AMI 100 vs GAI 115), but a discrepancy of this size is not rare in comparison to his peers (base rate >25%). Nevertheless, this may reflect a subtle deterioration in functioning, given his subjective reports of memory difficulties in everyday life. Performance on visual memory tests was in the average range (VMI 108) and comparable to his overall level of intellectual functioning, but performance on visual working memory tests (VWMI 103) was lower than expected, given his level of perceptual reasoning (PRI 121) and his superior auditory working memory, and may reflect a subtle deterioration in functioning. Immediate and delayed memory was comparable (IMI 105, DMI 106) and consistent with his general intellectual functioning, so there was no evidence of retention difficulties.

Performance on tests of executive function was lower than expected. Performance on a standalone performance validity test was satisfactory as was performance on several other embedded measures of effort (Reliable Digit Span, recognition memory trials from the WMS-IV), so there was nothing to suggest malingering or exaggeration of symptoms.

Scores on questionnaire measures of anxiety and depression revealed mildly elevated levels of emotional distress, but the pilot did not meet criteria (DSM-V) for a formal diagnosis of major depressive disorder, generalised

Table 13.1 Neuropsychological test results

Psychometric Test	Standardised scores	Qualitative description or percentile score
Premorbid IQ – TOPF		
Predicted Full Scale IQ	111.4	High average
Predicted VCI	110.4	High average
Predicted PRI	109.5	Average
Predicted WMI	113.2	High average
Predicted PSI	103.8	Average
Predicted IMI	110.4	High average
Predicted DMI	110.6	High average
Predicted VWMI	112.6	High average
Current IQ – WAIS-IV		
VCI	107	Average
PRI	121	Superior
WMI	122	Superior
PSI	89	Low average
FIQ	112	High average
GAI	115	High average
Scaled scores		
Vocab	10	Average
Similarities	10	Average
Information	14	High average
Arithmetic	15	Superior
Digit Span (DF9 DB6 DS6)	13	High average
Coding	7	Low average
Symbol search	9	Average
Block design	15	Superior
Matrix reasoning	13	High average
Visual puzzles	13	High average
Memory – WMS-IV		
Auditory memory	100	Average
Visual memory	108	Average
Visual working memory	103	Average
IMI	105	Average
DMI	106	Average
Scaled scores		
Logical memory 1	9	Average
Logical memory 2	9	Average
VPA 1	11	Average
VPA 2	11	Average
Designs 1	12	Average
Designs 2	13	High average
Visual rep 1	11	Average
Visual rep 2	10	Average
Symbol span	11	Average
Spatial addition	10	Average

(Continued)

Table 13.1 Continued

Psychometric Test	Standardised scores	Qualitative description or percentile score
Executive function		
Verbal fluency (FAS)	Scaled score 7	Low average
Stroop	Raw score = 103	32nd percentile
Symptom validity test		
MSVT		Pass
Mood		
HAD A (7 NS)	7	NS
BAI (15 Mild)	15	Mild
HAD D (10 Mild)	10	Mild
BDI-II (21 Moderate	21	Moderate

anxiety, or panic disorder. The pilot was also asked to complete a personality questionnaire (PAI; Morey, 1991) which includes four sets of scales: (1) clinical scales covering major categories of psychopathology corresponding to the Diagnostic and Statistical Manual of Mental Disorders nosology; (2) treatment scales relating to case management; (3) interpersonal scales; and (4) symptom validity indices which measure the degree to which a patient has been careful, consistent, and honest in responding to the test questions. Once again there was no evidence to suggest the pilot was motivated to portray himself in a more negative or pathological light than the clinical picture would warrant. In other words, there was nothing to suggest he was malingering or exaggerating symptoms. He reported marked concerns about his physical health and functioning and significant cognitive problems involving confusion, indecision, distractibility, difficulty concentrating, and the sense that his thoughts are somehow blocked or disrupted.

Follow-up interview 2021

I interviewed the pilot again in 2021 at which time he reported that his symptoms improved dramatically during 2017 and so he decided to consult an aviation medical examiner about whether he could regain his Class 1 medical certificate, needed to resume flying. He was referred for a repeat neuropsychological assessment in 2017, undertaken by a neuropsychologist in the NHS. Performance on neuropsychological tests was reported to be within the limits expected of a person with his level of intellectual functioning on all but one test. The pilot did not endorse any cognitive impairment or emotional distress at this consultation, but he continued to report fatigue which he was managing better so that it was less disabling. The NHS neuropsychologist used a different test battery, making direct comparison difficult; but of note is that performance on the story recall subtest from the

AMIPB was between the 50th and 75th percentile; performance on the Rey Figure Test and Recognition Memory Test for Faces was between the 50th and 99th percentile. Performance on a verbal fluency task (FAS) was at the 70th percentile; performance on processing speed tests (WAIS-IV coding and Trail Making A) was in the very superior range; and performance on tests of executive function was generally within the high average to very superior range. The psychologist concluded that there was no evidence of cognitive impairment and on the basis of his cognition alone, she could see no reason why the pilot should not regain his Class 1 medical. This gave the pilot the confidence to return to work.

The pilot regained his Class 1 medical and licence to fly and took a job with a regional airline in early 2018. However, he struggled to cope with the workload due to fatigue and he developed tingling in his lips, which he suspected was caused by exposure to fumes, so he stopped flying after a couple of months. He subsequently got a job as a private pilot in which he is paid full-time but only flies once or twice a month and this suits him much better, although he feels it is a lesser job. He loves flying and his mood has improved as a result. Although neuropsychological assessment did not find evidence of memory impairment, the pilot continues to report bouts of forgetfulness particularly when multi-tasking.

Conclusion

There is an urgent need for increased awareness and understanding of neurotoxic conditions and neuropsychologists have an important role to play in both clinical and research settings in detecting and evaluating the effects of toxic substances. The case presented in this chapter illustrates some of the diagnostic challenges inherent in this type of work, particularly when the condition, in this case 'Aerotoxic syndrome', is controversial.

Neurotoxic conditions are frequently misdiagnosed or not diagnosed at all, as few healthcare professionals in the UK receive training in toxicology; there is a lack of awareness amongst the public about the potential neurotoxicity of chemicals they work with or are exposed to in everyday life; and routine medical investigations frequently fail to identify abnormalities in neurotoxic conditions. In this case, neither the pilot nor his treating physicians considered a toxic cause for his symptoms, which meant evasive action was not taken (i.e. prevention of further exposure) and the pilot continued to fly for another 21 months. Furthermore, by the time a toxic cause was considered it was too late to perform blood tests to prove exposure, as these need to be undertaken within hours of exposure (i.e. there was no biomarker of exposure anymore).

Meanwhile the pilot consulted and was referred to multiple specialists, underwent numerous tests including nerve conduction tests, spine and brain MRI scans, but none identified abnormalities that could account for his symptoms. Doctors were unable to provide a clear diagnosis and only one expert questioned whether the pilot had been exposed to noxious chemicals.

It was not until other crew members and the pilot's client became ill that a link with noxious fumes on board the aircraft was considered. Air quality analysis subsequently revealed high concentrations of VOCs in the aircraft cabin and the APU, which had been faulty for months and was being monitored, and was subsequently replaced. The pilot resumed flying but continued to feel unwell and eventually collapsed a few months later and it was only after this that he encountered a colleague who told him about Aerotoxic syndrome. He was advised to pay for specialist tests, but unfortunately, these tests are not routinely used for diagnostic purposes in the health service and were dismissed by his treating physicians. It was at this point he was referred to neuropsychology.

Neuropsychological assessment did not find evidence of global intellectual decline, but did reveal subtle, patchy under-functioning on tests of processing speed, auditory memory, and executive function. Performance on memory test was variable and seemed to reflect reduced information processing/encoding rather than a memory problem per se. This illustrates the fact that neuropsychological assessment can detect abnormalities prior to the occurrence of other objective neurological sequelae and early testing can identify people who may need removing from a toxic environment to prevent lasting brain damage (Hartman, 1988). However, neuropsychologists have to consider the wide range of factors that can influence performance on psychometric testing which can complicate interpretation such as low effort, mood disorder, pain, fatigue, medication effects, chance factors, and base rates etc; and caution is advised when there is a lack of corroborating results from other medical disciplines and self-reported cognitive difficulties and neuropsychological test scores are the only data suggestive of brain damage.

What proved useful in this case was the application of Bradford Hill criteria (Fedak et al., 2015), a group of nine principles that can be useful in establishing a causal relationship between a presumed cause and an observed effect. These include the need to demonstrate a temporal relationship and strong association between cause and effect, a biological gradient (dose–response relationship), a plausible mechanism between cause and effect; and findings should be consistent with previous research. In addition to these criteria it is generally accepted in toxicology that a 'red flag sign' that noxious chemicals may be present is when other people and/or animals become ill at the same time as a given individual.

In this case, the pilot became ill when flying an aircraft with a faulty APU and known issues with oil leaks (*strength of association and temporal relationship*). At the same time other crew members became ill (*red flag*) and subsequent air quality analysis revealed high concentrations of VOCs in the cabin (*objective evidence of exposure*).

Furthermore, physical symptoms were *consistent with those reported in previous studies* of aircrew (Michaelis et al., 2017) as were the neuropsychological deficits identified. For example, Coxon examined eight Australian aircrew who had been exposed to oil emissions on board aircraft and found evidence of reduced information processing speed, reaction time, verbal memory, and fine motor skills in the majority of cases (Coxon, 2002). In 2006 I published a single case study involving a pilot who presented with a nine-month history of cognitive impairment and a ten-year history of gastrointestinal and skin problems, which he attributed to exposure to oily fumes while flying and he obtained scores lower than premorbid estimates on tests of information processing speed, attention, verbal memory, and executive functioning (Mackenzie Ross et al., 2006). In 2008 I published the findings of a case series of 27 UK pilots (self-selected) who reported ill health following alleged exposure to contaminated air, who reported alarming cognitive failures at work and showed evidence of reduced information processing speed, attention, verbal memory, and executive function relative to controls; and number of years/hours spent flying correlated with lowered scores on neuropsychological tests (Mackenzie Ross, 2008). In 2011, colleagues and I published the findings from a study of 22 pilots (randomly selected) with a history of exposure to contaminated air events and found reduced performance on tests of information processing speed in 32% of pilots and reduced performance on tests of attention and executive function in 18% of pilots (Mackenzie Ross et al., 2011).

Finally, the nature of the cognitive deficits identified in these studies is consistent with what would be expected following exposure to solvents, which target fat rich neuronal tissue such as white matter, i.e. response slowing, reduced working memory/attention, and memory problems secondary to reduced processing rather than forgetting, implying a *biologically plausible* mechanism (Lezak et al., 2004).

Key themes and learning points highlighted by this case include:

- The need for healthcare professionals to consider the possibility toxic exposure could account for an individual's symptoms.
- The importance of taking a detailed occupational history as opposed to simply noting a person's occupation and the need to construct a timeline of events to determine whether exposure to noxious substances is likely.
- Healthcare professionals need to avoid making assumptions, particularly given how little training they receive in toxicology. Common myths include the idea that toxic exposure is rare, that symptoms will resolve following cessation of exposure, that if routine medical tests fail to identify pathology, then the patient must be suffering from a psychological disorder, and an over-reliance on 'safe exposure standards', many of which are based on weak or flawed data.
- Physical symptoms that follow exposure to toxic substances can be so non-specific and varied they can be mistaken for many other conditions, both medical and psychological; and the absence of neurological signs on routine examination can lead to misdiagnosis.
- The usefulness of neuropsychological assessment because of its ability to detect abnormalities prior to the occurrence of other objective

neurological sequelae and also because it is relatively cheap and non-invasive. However, the limits of neuropsychological assessment are also apparent in this case in terms of how far neuropsychology can go in terms of diagnosis and establishing causation without information derived from other sources and input from other medical specialities. In this case the clinical history suggested a toxic cause for the pilot's symptoms which was supported by air quality analysis, as opposed to there being a unique, diagnostic neuropsychological profile; and criteria derived from epidemiology were used to assist interpretation.

- Some psychometric tests are more sensitive to neurotoxic effects than others, e.g. coding, symbol search, digit span backwards, reaction time, memory tests, dexterity and aiming tests, and executive tests.
- Deficits may be subtle but even small degrees of CNS dysfunction, fatiguability, lethargy, slowed reaction times are dangerous in certain occupations such as aviation.
- There are limited treatment options available to those who suffer chronic ill health following exposure to toxic substances and few follow-up studies are available to determine prognosis.
- The impact of neurotoxic conditions extends beyond the patient and includes the family, particularly when ongoing controversy prevents a person receiving a diagnosis and the financial consequences of this in terms of not being able to apply for state benefits, income protection insurance, critical illness cover, or determine whether it is safe to resume work.

Fortunately, the pilot described in this chapter recovered over time and was able to obtain his Class 1 medical and resume flying. However, fatigue continues to limit what he can do and how many hours he can work, and he feels he has no choice but to accept a 'lesser' job than the one he had before. He also feels frustrated and upset by the way he was treated by some healthcare professionals who dismissed his complaints or charged him large sums of money for tests that were not useful to him in the end; and for the financial losses he sustained and the impact of this on his partner and children.

References

Bowler, R.M, & Lezak, M.D. (2015). Neuropsychological evaluation and exposure to neurotoxicants. In M. Lotti & M. L. Bleecker (Eds.), *Handbook of clinical neurology 131* (pp. 23–45). Elsevier.

Chen, R., Fang, L., Liu, J., Herbig, B., Norrefeldt, V., Mayer, F., Fox, R., & Wargocki, P. (2021). Cabin air quality on non-smoking commercial flights: A review of published data on airbourne pollutants. *Indoor Air, 31*, 926–957.

Coxon, L. (2002). Neuropsychological assessment of a group of Bae146 aircraft crew members exposed to jet engine oil emissions. *Journal of Occupational Health & Safety: Australia, New Zealand, 18*(4), 313–319.

European Aviation Safety Agency (2014). *Final report*. Research project: CAQ Preliminary cabin air quality measurement campaign. EASA.

Fedak, K. M, Bernal, A., Capshaw, Z. A., & Gross, S. (2015). Applying the Bradford Hill criteria in the 21st century: How data integration has changed causal inference in molecular epidemiology. *Emerging Themes in Epidemiology*, 12(14). https://doi.org/10.1186/s12982-015-0037-4. PMID: 26425136; PMCID: PMC4589117.

Grandjean, P., & Landrigan, P. L. (2014). Neurobehavioural effects of developmental toxicity. *Lancet Neurology*, 13, 330–338.

Hartman, D. E. (1988). *Neuropsychological toxicology: Identification and assessment of human neurotoxic syndromes*. Plenum Press.

Hartman, D. E. (1995). *Neuropsychological toxicology: Identification and assessment of human neurotoxic syndromes* (2nd ed.). Plenum Press.

Howard, C. V. (2020) Inappropriate use of risk assessment in addressing health hazards posed by civil aircraft cabin air. *Open Access Journal of Toxicology*, 4(2), 555–634. https://doi.org/10.19080/OAJT.2020.04.555634

Howard, C. V., Michaelis, S., & Watterson, A. (2017). The aetiology of Aerotoxic syndrome: A toxico-pathological viewpoint. *Open Access Journal of Toxicology*, 1(5), 555–575. https://doi.org/10.19080/OAJT.2017.01.555575.

Lezak, M. D, Howieson, D. B., & Loring, D. W. (2004). *Neuropsychological assessment* (4th ed.). Oxford University Press.

Lezak, M. D. (1984). Neuropsychological assessment in behavioral toxicology: Developing techniques and interpretative issues. *Scandinavian Journal of Work, Environment & Health*, 10, 25–29. www.jstor.org/stable/40965024

Mackenzie Ross, S. (2008). Cognitive function following exposure to contaminated air on commercial aircraft: A case series of 27 pilots seen for clinical purposes. *Journal of Nutritional Environmental Medicine*, 17, 111–126.

Mackenzie Ross, S (2016). Delayed cognitive and psychiatric symptoms following methyl iodide and manganese poisoning: Potential for misdiagnosis. *Cortex*, 74, 427–439.

Mackenzie Ross, S., Harper, A., & Burdon, J. (2006). Ill health following exposure to contaminated aircraft air: Psychosomatic disorder or neurological injury? *Journal of Occupational Health and Safety (Australia & New Zealand)*, 22, 521–528.

Mackenzie Ross, S., Harrison, V., Madeley, L., Davis, K., Abraham-Smith, K., Hughes, T., & Mason, O. (2011). Cognitive function following reported exposure to contaminated air on commercial aircraft: Methodological considerations for future researchers. *Journal of Biological Physics and Chemistry*, 11(4), 180–191.

Michaelis, S., Burdon, J., & Howard, C. V. (2017). Aerotoxic syndrome: A new occupational disease. *Public Health Panorama*, 3(1), 141–356.

Morey, L.C. (1991). Personality Assessment Inventory. Pearson Assessment.

Winder, C., & Balouet, J. C. (2000). Aerotoxic syndrome: Adverse health effects following exposure to jet oil mist during commercial flights. *Proceedings of the International Congress on Occupational Health*, Conference held in Brisbane, Australia, 4–6 September 2000. ISBN 0 646 401546 (pp.196–199).

Winder, C., & Balouet, J. C. (2002). The toxicity of commercial jet oils. *Environmental Research Section A*, 89, 146–164.

14 Focal anterograde amnesia

An extraordinary case

Georgina Browne

Introduction

For the keen neuropsychologist, complex diagnostic investigation often reflects the most relished of clinical tasks. As clinicians, our ultimate goal is to deliver the most helpful of interventions to patients with neuropsychological symptoms. To this end, we must first provide a description of the disorder and an opinion on the likely aetiology. There is something exhilarating in this diagnostic process – exploring hypotheses, sifting through red herrings, assembling the crucial pieces of information, and ultimately arriving at a robust opinion on diagnosis and appropriate intervention.

Some diagnostic queries are more straightforward than others. In Cambridge, we are lucky to be presented with many rare and atypical forms of neurological and neuropsychological disorders. And so it came about that I was presented with one of my greatest diagnostic puzzles to date.

Background to the case

Mr Arthur Keller[1] was referred to our memory clinic to help determine the basis of his striking memory syndrome.

The referral came from a consultant neurology colleague and stated that two years previously Arthur had developed sudden-onset amnesia following an acute episode of disturbed speech, dizziness, and collapse (without head injury or loss of consciousness). He was taken to hospital, but initial medical and neurological investigations in A&E were apparently unremarkable and he was discharged. A CT scan undertaken a number of days later was reported as normal. Arthur had no known neurological or psychiatric history. At the time of referral, his amnesia had persisted without change and he had developed significant symptoms of anxiety. He had been seen by his local memory clinic services; however, no conclusion had been reached regarding a diagnosis to account for his amnesia. Further assessment was therefore requested in our specialist memory clinic service.

DOI: 10.4324/9781003228226-16

Memory clinic investigations

Arthur and his wife, Michelle, were seen for multidisciplinary assessment, including full neuropsychological, neurological, and psychiatric assessments, alongside various additional clinical and brain imaging investigations.

Initial assessments were consistent in documenting the following background history and episode of acute onset.

Background history and premorbid function

At the time of assessment, Arthur was a 41-year-old, right-handed gentleman, who was born and grew up in the United Kingdom. He progressed normally through school and left at the age of 16 having completed GCSEs with low-grade passes. His main occupation had been as a bus driver. He had had a difficult childhood: he had suffered sexual abuse, his father was absent, and his mother was physically abusive and neglectful.

At the time of onset, Arthur was living at home with Michelle (his partner of four years). He was functioning well at work and at home, and was undertaking evening classes (alongside Michelle) to further his education.

On a test of adult reading he scored in the average range. Alongside his educational and occupational history, his premorbid cognitive ability was estimated to fall in the average range.

Acute onset of memory problems

Arthur and Michelle had been due to undertake a history exam as part of their further educational classes. They had decided to stop at a café before sitting the exam. Arthur had good recall for events up to this moment. He described a clear and vivid recollection of being in the café and drinking tea. He recalled that he then became suddenly unable to understand what Michelle was saying to him. This was, apparently, his last episodic memory.

Correspondingly, Michelle reported that Arthur's speech had become suddenly slurred and incomprehensible. She stated that he had become pale, dizzy, and then collapsed. She described him appearing to faint, although reported no loss of consciousness. An ambulance was called and Arthur was taken to hospital, where a number of routine investigations were undertaken. However, no cause was found for his sudden collapse, he appeared well in hospital, and he was discharged home the following day.

Over the next few days, Michelle noticed that Arthur seemed unable to recall events that had occurred since his fainting episode in the café. She therefore took him back to A&E. However, further investigations including a CT head scan were reported as unremarkable and he was again discharged home. His memory difficulties nevertheless persisted. Over the following 12 months, Arthur was seen in his local memory clinic where neuropsychological assessment documented an amnesic syndrome alongside poor working memory and slowed processing speed, as determined via WAIS-III assessment. It was felt that the cognitive deficit was likely to be organic in nature; however, no firm opinion on diagnosis was reached.

At the time of his investigations with us, his memory deficit had remained stable (without deterioration, improvement, or significant fluctuation) since onset: he had formed no new episodic memory for the past two years.

Diagnostic investigations

In discussion with neurology and neuropsychology colleagues, diagnostic hypotheses and investigations of Mr Keller's symptoms were driven by our knowledge and experience of assessing and treating patients with amnesic syndromes. In considering the possible differential diagnoses, it is useful to bear in mind Parkin and Leng's (1993) taxonomy of amnesic syndromes, which sets out a classification system of organic (neurological) versus non-organic (psychogenic) features of amnesia. The authors suggest that organic amnesia may be permanent or transient and for global or selective material, whilst psychogenic amnesia is more likely to be selective for a set of events or dissociative, as seen in fugue states and multiple personality disorder. Kopelman (2002a) makes a similar distinction between global and selective amnesic syndromes. He also notes that it is difficult to fully dissociate syndromes of retrograde amnesia (i.e. memory loss for events prior to the trigger for amnesia) from anterograde amnesia (i.e. memory loss for events following the trigger for amnesia). Furthermore, whilst there are countless documented cases of focal retrograde amnesia, at the time of writing I found no cases of persistent focal anterograde amnesia.

The first aim of our investigations was therefore to determine whether Arthur's neuropsychological profile was primarily organic or psychological in origin. The second aim was to identify what specific neurological or psychological disorder could account for his difficulties.

Neuropsychological assessment

Clinical observations

Qualitatively, Arthur's presentation was striking. He was pleasant and cooperative throughout his appointments and assessments; however, he was highly anxious and constantly confused. He appeared bewildered and childlike, and was sweaty, shaky, and wide-eyed. He frequently turned to Michelle for reassurance and to answer questions put to him. He repeatedly asked where he was and who we (the clinicians) were. Though his voice trembled, his speech was fluent and there was no obvious language deficit. His conversation (for retrograde events) was full and appropriate, although repetitive, and he frequently lost his train of thought. He was able to attend to a conversation or a task for a matter of minutes but would then become distressed and ask what he was doing, and again ask where he was and who we were. He appeared unable to retain any information provided to him. In short, he seemed to have a dense and dramatic amnesic syndrome.

Arthur consistently gave the date as '*September, 2010*', as it had been at the time of his fainting episode two years previously. He was fully oriented to public and personal retrograde events. He always gave the most recent news events as those that had occurred immediately prior to his fainting episode. When discussing remote or retrograde events, his presentation changed, such that he was less anxious, with improved fluency and animation to his conversation. But when oriented to the actual date or to evidence of forgotten events, such as his wedding band, he became again distressed and confused. He never appeared able to recall or recognise new (post-onset) public or personal events. During his first appointment with me, he was unable to recall (or be cued for) the EEG or MRI scan he had undergone that same morning. When given a task to complete, he seemed able to stick to the task uninterrupted for a period of 1.5 to 2 minutes, before looking up, at a loss for what he was doing. For example, when asked to draw from memory a line drawing that he had just copied, he initially set about completing the task; however, after a minute or so he looked at me with a worried and questioning expression and asked, '*What is this? What am I drawing?*'. Despite cues and reminders, he had no apparent recollection of completing the copying task just minutes before.

Arthur was assessed and interviewed on a number of occasions and presented consistently and coherently throughout, with little to suggest poor cognitive effort. However, he was objectively anxious, was frequently distressed and confused and required constant reassurance, orientation, and repetition of questions and instructions.

Clinical interview with Arthur

After some persuasion and a note on the desk to orient Arthur to his surroundings and Michelle's whereabouts, I saw Arthur on his own. He seemed to have poor insight into his memory symptoms and endorsed little by way of cognitive symptoms generally. He thought his memory function was good. He was able to provide a detailed and full account of his life up to the point of his sudden illness in the café. He thought this incident had occurred very recently and that he had been undertaking '*usual*' work and day-to-day activities thereafter. However, he provided only generic details of post-onset '*usual*' activities and indicated no autobiographical memories of any specific events since his illness. Indeed, in the two years since onset, he had not worked and had experienced numerous significant events, including hospital appointments, brain scans, getting married, and the death of loved ones; however, upon questioning he had no recall (or recognition) for any of these events.

Arthur described a difficult childhood with his mother, but did not think that he had suffered any lasting psychological difficulties. He repeatedly noted that he was happy in his relationship with Michelle. He considered that he had been managing well at work and reported no recent (pre-onset) stressors or adverse life events.

Clinical interview with Michelle

Michelle considered that Arthur had no history of cognitive or psychological difficulties. She noted that he had been doing well at work and in their further educational courses. She gave a clear account of a sudden onset anterograde amnesia following his illness in the café. She did not endorse symptoms of any retrograde memory loss. She stated that in the days following his collapse, she had gradually become aware of Arthur's memory problems. For example, if she referred to his first hospital visit, he would look perplexed and ask what she was talking about. She stated that he behaved normally at home and went about his usual day-to-day routines. She noted, however, that he would become confused and upset if there was a change to his environment or if he became aware of an event that he had forgotten. She described symptoms of poor sustained attention. For example, she thought that whilst Arthur could engage in a task with constant prompts and stimulation (such as non-dissonant conversation), he could not sustain activities in the absence of cues and after one to two minutes would come to a halt and ask what he was doing. She thought he could watch TV and follow a film at the cinema. She did not endorse symptoms of impairment in other cognitive domains and, for example, she thought his language, way-finding, and decision making (provided he had the information in front of him and she kept him to task) were unaffected. She described no progression or significant fluctuation in his difficulties, and considered that his presentation had remained consistent over the years. She indicated that she had learnt to adapt their home environment and Arthur's activities so as to prevent any unnecessary distress. She noted, for example, that she used environmental compensatory aids, such as leaving messages on the kitchen top to alert Arthur to her whereabouts if she needed to go out.

Michelle reported that she and Arthur had married in the year following his illness, which she had organised. She stated that she could not cue Arthur's memory for this event, even with photographs, and she found it upsetting that he seemed surprised every time he noticed their wedding rings.

In terms of his psychological well-being, Michelle thought that Arthur had not had any premorbid difficulties, but had become anxious since the onset of his memory problems. She indicated that he was especially anxious with changes to his routine or day-to-day environment, and for example experienced significant distress when they were having a new bathroom fitted.

Michelle did not endorse symptoms of any gross personality or behavioural change, although noted some oddities such as Arthur trying to make a cup of coffee with a knife.

Cognitive assessment

In contrast to our usual one-stop-shop appointments, Arthur was seen on a number of occasions over a number of months and the data in Table 14.1 reflect the key findings from my cognitive assessments with him.

Overall, the assessment results reveal an amnesic profile: with marked episodic memory impairment, relative sparing of other cognitive domains, and mostly intact performance on short tests of sustained attention. However, it is worth noting his relatively poor performance on the backward digit span and N-back tasks, indicating some mildly impaired working memory function, which is not entirely typical for a pure amnesic syndrome (Hodges, 2018; Parkin & Leng, 1993), although which may reflect anxiety.

Arthur was reviewed over a period of four years. At his last appointment, his presentation and neuropsychological test results remained largely unchanged. However, there were some subtle changes. For example, his forward digit span had decreased (from F=6 to F=4) although qualitatively he appeared able to hold information in his working memory for a period of up to four minutes, reflecting an increase since his initial presentation. He reported a recurring dream and Michelle noted that he could recount his dreams upon waking. At his last assessment, he appeared generally less anxious and was aware (semantically) that he had some memory difficulties, although remained adamant that he had no episodic recollection of such symptoms.

Neurological assessment

Our neurology colleagues found that Arthur's neurological examination was entirely unremarkable. They considered that the description of his collapse may have suggested an initial vascular event; however, found no evidence of any significant neurological pathology or persistent medical illness to explain Arthur's ongoing amnesia.

Brief cognitive assessment revealed a memory dominant profile on the ACE-R, with a score of 68/100 (MMSE 21/30).

The initial neurology report stated that Arthur's amnesic syndrome most probably had an organic basis, and additional investigations were ordered, including further imaging, lumbar puncture, and blood work to investigate causes such as a lesion, tumour, autoimmune disorder, and/or epileptic disorder. The investigations, however, were all subsequently reported as normal. There was little to suggest a progressive degenerative disease.

Arthur was reviewed over the course of two years by a number of consultant neurologists. There was divided opinion as to whether Arthur's amnesia should be explained in terms of an organic and/or psychological aetiology.

Table 14.1 Neuropsychological data taken from our initial assessments

Test	Raw score	Statistical scores	Comment
Verbal memory			
BMIPB Story – immediate recall	20/60	%ile = 10th – 25th	Mild impairment.
BMIPB Story – delayed recall	0/60	%ile < 2nd	Marked impairment. (No recall of original task).
Recognition Memory Test – Words	28/50	%ile < 5th	Marked impairment.
Autobiographical Memory Interview			
Personal semantic			
First school	6/8	–	Mild impairment. Lost points on names of teachers/friends.
Secondary school	8/8	–	Unimpaired.
Recent life	2/8	–	Marked impairment. Knew current (premorbid) address only.
Autobiographical incidents			
First school	3/3	–	Unimpaired.
Secondary school	3/3	–	Unimpaired.
Recent life	0/3	–	Marked impairment.
Orientation (day, month, year)	0/3	–	Marked impairment.
Nonverbal memory			
BMIPB Figure – immediate recall	33/80	%ile < 2nd	Moderate impairment.
BMIPB Figure – delayed recall	0/80	%ile < 2nd	Marked impairment. (No recall of original task).
Recognition Memory Test – Faces	Discontinued	–	Marked impairment on completed items; Distressed.
Verbal skills			
National Adult Reading Test		Predicted premorbid 'FSIQ' = 103	Average range.
Letter Fluency – FAS	37	%ile = 20th – 30th	Unimpaired.
Category Fluency – Animals	15	%ile < 10th	Mild impairment.
Graded Naming Test	24/30	%ile = 75th – 90th	Unimpaired.

Nonverbal skills

BMIPB Figure Copy	75/80	%ile = 5th – 10th	Unimpaired copy. (Allowance made for distraction).

Attention / Working memory

WAIS–IV Digit Span	8/16 (F=6)	Scaled score = 7	Unimpaired.
	6/16 (B=3)	Scaled score = 7	Mild impairment.
WAIS–IV Coding	67	Scaled score = 9	Unimpaired.
N-back task (in-house)	3/4		Mild impairment.

Executive function

Brixton	11 errors	Sten score = 7/10 (High average)	Unimpaired.

Performance validity

Rey 15 item test	0 errors	– –	Unimpaired.
TOMM Trial 1	43/50	– –	Errors on 7 of the last 8 items.
TOMM Trial 2	43/43	–	Unimpaired. Discontinued at 43 items as became distressed.

Other

HADS Anxiety	11/21	– –	Moderate.
HADS Depression	3/21	– –	None.

At his last neurology review, his diagnosis simply read: *Unexplained amnestic syndrome.*

Psychiatric assessment

Our psychiatry colleagues reported that there was no evidence of any significant mental health history prior to the onset of Arthur's memory symptoms. They noted his difficult childhood, but considered that he had managed well from a psychological point of view premorbidly. They found no significant adverse life events or psychological stressors in the years preceding the onset of his difficulties. They found no history of alcohol misuse to suggest a Wernicke-Korsakoff's syndrome.

On brief cognitive assessment, the psychiatrists found a similar amnesic profile although noted that Arthur had also lost points on drawing a clock face and on a task of abstract thinking, which they considered as evidence against a psychogenic diagnosis.

Nevertheless, they noted some signs that could be in keeping with a psychogenic origin, including: history of childhood sexual abuse; possible secondary gain due to increased care post onset; and his prominent and consistently heightened state of anxiety.

Imaging

A CT scan undertaken a few days post onset was reported as normal. EEGs (with video) were undertaken six months post onset and repeated at two years post onset. These were both reported as normal with no epileptiform abnormalities.

An MRI scan was undertaken two years post onset and stated that the ventricles and CSF spaces appeared normal, that there were no focal abnormalities, and that the hippocampi, fornices, and mamillary bodies appeared normal. However, our neurology colleagues identified some asymmetry to the mamillary bodies (see Figure 14.1).

This scan generated much discussion and debate amongst our neurology colleagues. Most were of the opinion that the brain appeared essentially normal and that the mamillary body finding was irrelevant. Others were of the opinion that such a lesion may account for Arthur's amnesic syndrome.

Professor John Hodges, a leading authority in cognitive neurology, also reviewed Arthur's case and imaging and considered that the mamillary body finding was insufficient to account for Arthur's severe anterograde amnesia.

Interventions

Whilst no neurological illness or injury had been identified, from a functional point of view Arthur was clearly struggling to manage his confusion and was experiencing high levels of anxiety. A number of interventions were

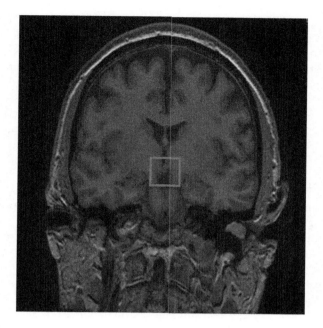

Figure 14.1 MRI brain scan reported as 'normal' with the exception of some asymmetry to the mamillary bodies (highlighted)

therefore provided with a view to reducing his anxiety and providing cognitive rehabilitation strategies to improve his day-to-day functioning.

Via the psychiatry service, he was treated with medication (including citalopram and pregabalin) and attended a number of psychological therapy sessions, which adopted an integrative approach (including elements of eye movement desensitisation and reprocessing (EMDR) therapy and cognitive analytic therapy (CAT)) to attempt to address any past trauma and current anxiety. Whilst Arthur initially attended the therapy sessions (and efforts were made by the therapist to accommodate his amnesia), he considered that he did not need therapy. Michelle considered that the therapy was a distraction and not relevant to his amnesic syndrome. In response to a therapy letter, Arthur sent an articulate (albeit somewhat frustrated) reply, raising a number of points to indicate that his anxiety related to his memory problems rather than past events. He therefore eventually disengaged with therapy and declined further input from psychological and psychiatric services.

Whilst the psychiatrists considered that his anxiety state improved with pregabalin, there was no change to Arthur's cognitive presentation either during or following his pharmacological or psychological interventions.

I provided cognitive rehabilitation support to Arthur and Michelle. This included a model for understanding cognition and the multiple factors that may contribute to poor memory function. I helped them to install external memory aids in their home and trained them to use a SenseCam, a camera that has been successful in improving autobiographical memory in other densely amnesic patients (e.g. Browne et al., 2011; Woodberry et al., 2015).

Whilst Arthur habituated to using some of the memory aids, and for example could look at an orientation screen to determine the date and upcoming activities, his amnesic syndrome remained. He found no benefit in using SenseCam, but was simply distressed to be made aware of personal events for which he had no recollection. This was at odds with our experience of using SenseCam with other amnesic patients.

Discussion of neuropsychological findings

Arthur's neuropsychological profile appeared to be largely in keeping with an organic basis for his amnesic syndrome. Indeed, in terms of his anterograde memory impairment, Arthur presented in a similar fashion to the notorious HM (Milner & Scoville, 1957). However, there remained two significant challenges to an organic explanation: (i) the absence of any significant corresponding pathology, and (ii) the absence of any retrograde amnesia.

Whilst there are reported cases of focal retrograde amnesia (e.g. Kapur, 1989; Kopelman, 2002a) and cases of transient anterograde amnesia (e.g. Anderson & Hulbert, 2021), there are no documented cases of chronic anterograde amnesia persisting in the absence of any retrograde memory impairment.

Theoretically, it is difficult to explain what process or model of memory could underpin such a persistent and focal anterograde amnesia. Anterograde amnesia usually presents with some form of temporally graded retrograde amnesia (Parkin & Leng, 1993), such that the severity of the anterograde memory deficit corresponds to the degree of the retrograde deficit. This is in keeping with the widely held 'multiple trace theory' of memory consolidation (e.g. Hodges, 2018; Nadal et al., 2000), which states that successful episodic memory function is dependent upon the age of the memory: 'traces' of a memory (for an event) may be replicated over time to enable increasingly robust memory consolidation and retrieval. What, then, could account for the abrupt onset of anterograde amnesia in a system that allows successful retrieval of all retrograde memories, including those formed just moments prior to the point of onset?

- *Perhaps we had insufficient imaging data/technology to capture a neurological injury or illness?*

This remained a plausible, although unlikely (according to the neurologists), explanation.

- *Perhaps we had failed to detect evidence of a retrograde memory impairment?*

To this end Professor Karalyn Patterson and I devised a number of further tests to look for evidence of both retrograde amnesia and of new learning.

We established a detailed list of premorbid events which had not been discussed with Arthur (by us or Michelle) previously. However, upon testing, his memory for these events was consistently intact. For a similar list of anterograde events, however, he was consistently amnesic. We revised a version of the Dead-or-Alive test (Kapur et al., 1989) for recognising public figures as having passed away or being still alive over the course of a number of years surrounding the onset of Arthur's symptoms: he showed impaired recall for post-onset deaths, but normal performance for deaths in the premorbid period, and the absence of any temporal gradient-type effect.

We devised a learning paradigm for him to complete in clinic. He was able to sustain a task and learning for a period of approximately two minutes before requiring a prompt to stick to task or becoming distressed as to what he was doing. If interrupted or following a break, he had no subsequent recall or recognition for the task.

- *Perhaps there was an initial retrograde amnesia, which had spontaneously recovered by the time Arthur came to our memory clinic?*

Michelle did not endorse such symptoms, but this remained a possibility.

- *Perhaps we had mistakenly labelled his presentation as densely amnesic for anterograde events?*

To examine this possibility, I assessed him in his home environment. He appeared less anxious; however, his confusion and amnesia remained. He was bewildered by a new (post-onset) carpet, for example, and whilst I was there he repeatedly asked about the nature of my visit and became distressed at any mention of memory problems. Nevertheless, he was calm and content when undertaking routine (and cognitively non-dissonant) activities of daily living. There was, however, some evidence of implicit procedural learning as over time he had learnt to look to his memory aids to orient himself to the date and prospective activities, and had learnt to navigate his way around a new computer game.

- *Perhaps there was an element of deliberate feigning of his symptoms, such that inconsistencies in his presentation may become apparent if observed more rigorously and more frequently?*

However, despite numerous assessments, across different environments, with multiple clinicians, and with repetition of tests and questions, his presentation remained broadly stable and consistent. On a formal test of performance validity (the TOMM), whilst his completion of the task was passable, it was somewhat unusual. On Trial 1 of the TOMM, he completed the first 42 items without error or deliberation. He then selected the incorrect answer on the following 7 of 8 items. Similarly, on Trial 2, he completed the first 43 items without difficulty, but then became disoriented and highly distressed and the test was discontinued. It is difficult to explain this sudden onset of confusion and error.

Over time, there was some subtle incongruence to his presentation. He could recall dreams; he learnt to play new computer games; he had engaged with therapy (albeit briefly) and learnt that he had memory difficulties; he could follow a film at the cinema and hold a brief discussion about it afterwards.

Differential diagnoses

Amongst neuropsychology colleagues, and with our clinical and academic colleagues in the memory clinic, Arthur's case was discussed at length as we considered possible neurological and/or psychological causes for his amnesic syndrome.

A neurological cause

Arthur was reviewed in the memory clinic over a number of years, and in that time, despite repeatedly normal investigations, his selective memory symptoms persisted (without progression or resolution). A number of clinicians felt certain that Arthur's difficulties were so circumscribed, persistent, and consistent, and with such sudden onset, that they must be explained by some neurological injury or illness. At the time of his initial assessments, this was the prevailing diagnostic opinion.

Organic causes of episodic memory impairment (as, for example, set out by Hodges, 2018) were therefore considered. Possible transient organic causes included transient global amnesia, transient epileptic amnesia, delirium, head injury, and substance misuse. Possible persistent organic causes included hippocampal damage (e.g. encephalitis, anoxia, head injury, and Alzheimer's disease), diencephalic damage (e.g. Korsakoff's syndrome, third ventricle lesion, bilateral thalamic lesion, and subarachnoid haemorrhage), and retrosplenial damage.

Arthur's amnesia appeared chronic (over a six-year period at the time of last review), thus ruling out transient organic aetiologies. There was no evidence of a head injury or of any substance or alcohol misuse. There was no evidence of a progressive disorder. In terms of other aetiologies for a persistent amnesic syndrome, it was considered that hippocampal damage, diencephalic damage, and/or retrosplenial damage should all occur with other clinical markers and/or be apparent upon imaging.

However, other than the mamillary body finding, his imaging was unremarkable. Whilst there are some cases of amnesia in patients with mamillary body lesions (cf. Vann, 2010), I could not find any reported cases of chronic anterograde amnesia as a result of selective mamillary body pathology alone. After a four-year period of review, then, the predominant (although not universal) opinion amongst our neurology colleagues was that the mamillary body finding was insufficient to account for Arthur's severe amnesia and that the absence of any other hard findings suggested a non-organic cause.

A psychological cause

It remained plausible, then, that Arthur's presentation could be entirely (or at least primarily) accounted for within the context of a psychological formulation. Kopelman (2002a; 2002b) suggests that episodes of transient or persistent amnesic syndromes can arise in response to previous significant psychological stress, to give rise to situation-specific or global (i.e. fugue state) amnesia. Arthur had retained his sense of self and personal identity, and could not be described, therefore, within the context of a global amnesia. Whilst situation-specific amnesias are usually confined to some past (retrograde) event/s, anterograde amnesia could conceivably also be described within this context. Indeed, Anderson and Hulbert (2021) describe a model of 'active forgetting' in psychogenic cases of amnesia such that the prefrontal cortex and hippocampal circuitry act to prevent the consolidation of new memories.

I considered that there were a number of factors that pointed towards such a diagnosis of psychogenic amnesia.

Firstly, there was a significant psychological history of past trauma and adverse life events. Over time, as the clinical hypotheses and assessments progressed, I became increasingly taken by the difficulties Arthur had suffered as a child at the hands of trusted adults. Approximately ten years prior to the onset of his difficulties, there had been a failed attempt to prosecute the perpetrator of his childhood sexual abuse. Arthur was living with his mother when he met Michelle, and shortly afterwards he moved out to go and live with Michelle. In the year preceding the onset of his amnesic syndrome, there had been discussion of a further court case. It is possible that this served as a trigger event for distress related to his past trauma.

Michelle and Arthur appeared to have a strong and loving relationship. In the period immediately following the onset of his memory problems, Michelle arranged his hospital visits and clinical assessments and appointments. They married in the period following the onset of Arthur's memory difficulties and Michelle eventually gave up her job to become Arthur's full-time carer.

Overall, I therefore considered that Arthur's highly unusual amnesic syndrome could be best explained within the context of a psychogenic amnesia having developed (in a dissociative fashion) to meet a set of mutually beneficial cognitive and emotional goals, which enabled survival of past trauma and ensured a future of love and care.

Indeed, cases of psychogenic amnesia frequently document some background history of psychological trauma. Whilst related cognitive symptoms tend to fluctuate over time and there are no documented cases of anterograde amnesia in the absence of retrograde amnesia, perhaps Arthur's reflects the first documented case of a persistent focal anterograde amnesia of psychogenic origin.

Perhaps his initial collapse involved some transient neurological dysfunction and accompanying memory disturbance. Perhaps thereafter, in response to the increase in care, his prefrontal cortex adapted to enable a persistent inhibition of the formation of new memories, or the active forgetting of very newly encoded information, to achieve a new and preferable cognitive and emotional state; to secure a future of unconditional care, free from harm.

Conclusions

Arthur presented with an extraordinary case of focal anterograde amnesia. No firm opinion on diagnosis was ever reached in our memory clinic. Over the years, with little change to his presentation alongside the absence of clinical findings, many of our colleagues came to the view that a psychogenic cause was the most likely explanation for Arthur's amnesic syndrome. However, a minority of others remained of the opinion that (given the initial vascular-type event, the persistence of a consistent cognitive profile, and in the absence of evidence of poor cognitive effort) his symptoms were organic in nature, but that the precise neurological diagnosis remained elusive.

In my own opinion, I considered that Arthur's neuropsychological profile reflected a non-organic, dissociative-type psychogenic amnesia, selective for anterograde events. There were a number of key findings that led to this conclusion: Arthur had a past history of significant trauma and neglect; his anxiety and bewilderment was striking; his attachment and reliance upon Michelle was a prominent feature of his presentation; Michelle was happy to become his spouse and his long-term carer post onset; his cognitive syndrome (which included the absence of retrograde amnesia and some poor working memory function) was unusual and not typical of known amnesic syndromes; he presented consistently over the years, suggesting the absence of deliberate feigning; there was an absence of sufficient pathology for a neurological diagnosis.

I would argue that when Arthur met Michelle, he found a place of love, solace, and safety. And as such, his neural circuitry adapted to sustain a memory impairment and an environment in which he could survive emotionally.

Arthur and Michelle eventually disengaged from all neuropsychology and memory clinic services. The last time I saw them they were happy at home going about their day-to-day lives.

Note

1 Demographic details have been changed to preserve anonymity. Consent was gained from the patient and his spouse for their anonymised details to be presented.

References

Anderson, M., & Hulbert, J. (2021). Active forgetting: Adaptation of memory by prefrontal control. *Annual Review of Psychology, 72*, 1–36.

Browne, G., Berry, E., Kapur, N., Hodges, S., Smyth, G., Watson, P., & Wood, K. (2011). SenseCam improves memory for recent events and quality of life in a patient with memory retrieval difficulties. *Memory, 19*, 7, 713–722.

Hodges, J. (2018). *Cognitive assessment for clinicians* (3rd ed.). Oxford University Press.

Kapur, N., Young, A., Bateman, D., & Kennedy, P. (1989). Focal retrograde amnesia: A long term clinical and neuropsychological follow-up. *Cortex, 25*, 387–402.

Kopelman, M. (2002a). Disorders of memory. *Brain, 125*, 2152–2190.

Kopelman, M. (2002b). Psychogenic amnesia. In A. Baddeley, M. Kopelman, & B. Wilson (Eds.), *Handbook of memory disorders* (2nd ed.). John Wiley & Sons.

Milner, B., & Scoville, W. (1957). Loss of recent memory after bilateral hippocampal lesions. *Journal of Neurology, Neurosurgery and Psychiatry, 20*, 11–21.

Nadal, L., Samsonovich, A., Ryan, L., & Moscovitch, M. (2000). Multiple trace theory of human memory: Computational, neuroimaging, and neuropsychological result. *Hippocampus, 10*, 352–368.

Parkin, A., & Leng, N. (1993). *Neuropsychology of the amnesic syndrome*. Lawrence Erlbaum Associates.

Vann, S. (2010). Re-evaluating the role of the mammillary bodies in memory. *Neuropsychologia, 48*, 2316–2327.

Woodberry, E., Browne, G., Hodges, S., Watson, P., Kapur, N., & Woodberry, K. (2015). The use of a wearable camera improves autobiographical memory in patients with Alzheimer's disease. *Memory, 23*, 3, 340–349.

15 'Ugly sound'

An examination of acquired receptive amusia in a skilled music critic

Sonja Soeterik

Introduction

> *Music gives a soul to the universe, wings to the mind, flight to the imagination and life to everything*
>
> (Plato)

Many of us will have a musical playlist of life, a song or piece of music that instantly transports us back to a time and place, music that connects us with a feeling and people we know. We will be able to hear a few beats of a tune and the words to the song will flood back into mind, even though it is many years since we last recalled it. We can find ourselves stuck with musical loops, that go around and around and that we can't get out of our minds and have that special tune which makes our foot tap and a desire to dance. For many, music is intimately entwined with our lives. Research suggests this relationship with music crosses all cultures (Sihvonen et al., 2017a) and begins in very early life, whilst we are in the womb. Prenatal musical exposure to rhythm and melodies has been found in fetuses, newborn babies and again at four months old (Partanen et al, 2013).

However, for some, an impairment in the perception of music, a kind of musical deafness, can occur. This is known as amusia (Kawamura & Miller, 2019) and was first reported in 1871 by Steinhals (García-Casares et al., 2013). Amusia is the loss or impairment in the ability to recognise familiar music (melodies or a particular voice), the ability to be able to distinguish between different instruments (timbre), to determine if different sounds are higher or lower (pitches), and can include the loss of the ability to read music (notation) (Sihvonen et al., 2017a; Vuvan et al., 2018; García-Casares et al., 2013). There are two primary forms of amusia described in the literature. Some people are born with a congenital form of amusia, whilst most people acquire amusia as the result of a neurological injury. It has been estimated that congenital amusia is found in up to 4% of the population, but more recent research has suggested only 1.5% (Peretz & Vuvan, 2017; Szyfter & Wigowska-Sowinska, 2022); in contrast, it is estimated that 35% to 69% of stroke survivors (Sihvonen et al., 2016) show signs of acquired amusia.

DOI: 10.4324/9781003228226-17

The processing of music within the brain involves a large cortico-subcortical network (Schmithorst, 2005; Brattico et al., 2011; Alluri et al., 2012; Burunat et al., 2014; Toiviainen et al., 2014) which is different to those networks for speech or ambient sound (Garcia-Casares et al., 2013). The right hemisphere has been described as dealing with the acoustic structure of auditory input (perception and discrimination) and the left with attributing meaning by virtue of semantic associative links (Lishman, 1988). Musical processing also differs by level of musical education and exposure (Kartsounis, 2003), and musical skill, with professional musicians using different areas of the brain (Garcia-Casares et al., 2013). Multiple brain regions have been associated with amusia, reflecting the multifactorial nature of music. Imaging studies have shown lesions in the frontal, temporal, and parietal regions can impact on acquired amusia (Sihvonen et al., 2017b). Amusia and aphasia are often comorbid (41%–65%; Sihvonen et al., 2016). More severe amusia has been noted in right-handed people who have damage to the right hemisphere following middle cerebral artery infarction (Särkämö et al., 2010). Many neuropsychological deficits may contribute to amusia including deficits in working memory and learning, semantic fluency, executive functioning, and visuospatial cognition, as well as hemisphere-specific deficits in verbal comprehension, mental flexibility, and visuospatial attention (Särkämö et al., 2009a, 2009b).

Standardised assessments of amusia have been around since the late 1930s (the Seashore Measurements of Musical Talents; Seashore, 1938, revised in 1960s by Levis and Saetveit), with the most common test cited standardised assessment of amusia in the contemporary literature being the Montreal Battery of Evaluation of Amusia (Sihvonen et al., 2017b).

Case presentation

Jacob (a pseudonym) was a writer, intellectual, and music critic[1] for large national and international newspapers. His family reported that he was a very intelligent and able man, for whom music played a central and significant role in his life. He was often asked to write reviews for the sleeves of compact disc recordings of classical music collections. He had a number of close friends who were musicians and composers. Whilst his favourite composer was Mozart, he had a particular interest in modern classical music and had given a number of public lectures on this genre. A review of a sample of his writings evidenced his great expertise and depth of musical knowledge, identifying individual instruments within the orchestra, the pitch and tone of sections of the orchestra, and the subtlety of how the overall qualities of the music evoked emotional connotations.

When Jacob was in his early fifties he had a myocardial infarction ('heart attack'), which required angioplasty and stenting. He was noted to have hypercholesterolaemia. Some five years later, in his mid-fifties, he sustained a series of cerebrovascular accidents (known as CVAs or 'strokes') leading to multiple bilateral intracerebral haemorrhages and a predominately right hemiparesis. Subsequent to his CVAs, Jacob developed epilepsy and had two periods of status epilepticus.

Reason for referral

Jacob was in a Level 1 hyperacute stroke service who had considered that he was potentially refusing support, or was too apathetic, or too cognitively impaired to benefit from further neuro rehabilitation. The team recommended he was transferred directly to a long-term residential nursing care placement. Jacob's family appealed this decision and requested a specialist assessment. Jacob was therefore referred to a Level 1 specialist inpatient neurobehavioural rehabilitation service. The intake assessment suggested a differential diagnosis between an initiation impairment and/or clinical depression, noting apparent dysphasic and dyspraxic concerns on bedside screening. The intake assessment showed that having rapport, controlling the environmental distractions, using simple language supported with gesture, and providing physical prompts led to increased participation levels. His participation levels appeared influenced by his sensory, language, and cognitive abilities rather than a deliberate desire to refuse sessions and his mood did not appear to be optimal. He was therefore accepted for further inpatient neurobehavioural rehabilitation.

Jacob was assessed as lacking the mental capacity to consent to the admission and his care plan. All assessments and care were conducted in line with the Mental Capacity Act (2005) Best Interests decision-making processes. On admission, around one year after his CVAs, Jacob was completely dependent on two healthcare assistants for all washing and dressing on his bed as well as all his grooming activities (such as shaving, combing hair, and brushing teeth). He was doubly incontinent. Jacob was unable to eat or drink orally at all, and was completely reliant on clinically assisted nutrition and hydration (via a percutaneous endoscopic gastrostomy 'PEG'). He spent most of the day wearing noise cancelling headphones and listening to music selected by the staff from his personal items in bed. Once a specialist wheelchair was prescribed, Jacob was often positioned near the radio in the communal day areas on the ward.

Jacob was reviewed by the consultant neuropsychiatrist who considered that although aphasiac, there may be an elective component to his mutism and prescribed a combined anti-depressant medication approach that creates noradrenergic and serotonergic effects (a combination of two anti-depressant medications: mirtazapine and venlafaxine) known as 'California Rocket Fuel' (Silva et al., 2016). However, Jacob was unable to tolerate this and suffered from nausea and vomiting. Instead, mirtazapine was trialled and gradually increased to 45mg per day. Other medication changes were made to his anti-epileptic medications (from phenytoin to lamotrigine) following a prolonged generalised seizure which required a temporary transfer back to acute care.

During his admission Jacob became more medically well and was able to eat some food orally for pleasure (about 50% of his daily needs) and gain some weight. This appeared to coincide with higher levels of arousal and initiation of conversation.

Brief neuropsychological assessment summary

Formal standardised neuropsychological assessment was challenging. Jacob's educational and occupational background suggested his premorbid general cognitive abilities would have been at least average to above average relative to others of a comparable age.

Jacob demonstrated severe oral and verbal dyspraxia and alongside this he appeared to have a likely moderate to severe dysphasia. He showed severe word finding problems, a total inability to generate the names of people he knew well with the exception of a sibling, and semantic and phonemic paraphasias. He used circumlocution in his language. His volitional speech was very infrequent, typically only for automatic social phrases (such as 'excuse me' when sneezing or when word finding 'I know that word but can't say it'). Occasional instances of jargon were evident. He had an unreliable yes/no response dependent on the complexity of the question. He was unable to write. He was able to read and comprehend single written words in context but not written phrases. He showed some intact pragmatic communication skills for greeting people, but appeared to have difficulties understanding when people were ending conversations and trying to leave.

Initial behavioural observations suggested Jacob had some sensory changes (likely double vision), severe difficulty with motor initiation and praxis on his less affected side, perseveration, pattern recognition and sequencing, and severe memory impairments in new learning, confabulation and disorientation.

As the admission progressed, in general conversation he displayed some intellectual awareness of his physical changes (for example that he was sat in a wheelchair and needed hoist transfers). But he showed difficulty with abstract concepts and extensive confabulation in his attempts to maintain a conversation and to account for his extreme disorientation (oftentimes believing the hospital was his office) and demonstrated difficulties with 'time tagging' of his memories, recalling times from long ago and fitting them into the present day (for example 'Mummy and Daddy have been looking after me here') and severe deficits in his ability to encode new memories.

A chance observation

The service's neuropsychologist noticed Jacob was in the unit day area positioned by the radio in his wheelchair with the radio playing pop music – the Spice Girls. Following an apology for the generic music, Jacob stated it was 'ugly sound'. The radio station was changed to a station more in keeping with his documented pre-injury preferences, Classic FM. However, Jacob continued to say 'ugly sound'. This statement was hypothesised to be a form of perseveration. Jacob was supported to be pushed around the wider ward area, drawing his attention to people and things in the environment. The other part of the neurobehavioural ward had a number of very agitated clients who were shouting and screaming loudly. He did not make any response to the loud noises in this part of the unit. On return to near the radio playing the Classic FM station, he promptly again said 'ugly sound'. The radio was then turned off and discussion moved to talk about visual things in the environment, with the neuropsychologist slowly raising the volume on the radio, without his awareness. As soon as sound became audible to him, he again stated 'ugly sound'. Finally, he was moved to his own bedroom and after looking at his own CD collection and discussing his preferred music, composers, arrangements, and conductors, a CD of his choice was played and again he agitatedly exclaimed it to be 'ugly sound'. This chance observation and 'bedside' experimentation indicated more detailed understanding of how a previously beloved activity, listening to music, was apparently now so aversive.

Whilst standardised tools to assess amusia existed, it was clear the combination of his cognitive deficits coupled with his communication impairments and dyspraxia would not allow these to be administered in a standardised way and therefore drawing off the normative information would not be useful as he was likely to perform at floor on the test. It was decided it was necessary to personalise the assessment using the multidisciplinary team in order to obtain the most useful information about his current abilities. Due to the complexity of his presentation, opinions and advice were sought from the specialist speech and language therapist as to how to optimise his receptive and expressive language skills, and the neurological occupational therapist to navigate his praxis issues, and a joint assessment with the music therapist was conducted.

Given the initial chance observation had shown increased agitation to the volume of music, Jacob was observed in order to determine the volume at which he began to attend to the sound and what his responses were. He consistently remarked on the sound when it was louder than talking volume and described it only in negative terms 'noise', 'awful noise', and 'ugly sound'. Jacob displayed a reduction in agitation when music was stopped. He was occasionally observed to be moving his head or finger like he was conducting and listening to music when there was no audible sound.

Jacob was invited to talk about each CD in his personal collection (who was the composer, who performed this, and the era) and he was able to recognise factual details about composers and their music such that he could participate in conversation about composers and be accurate in his knowledge of their compositions on a surface level. He had a scrapbook of many of the detailed and pointed articles he had written and enjoyed hearing these read to him, appearing to agree with some of his points.

A number of bespoke materials were collaboratively designed by the team to support the assessment. To circumvent his word-finding difficulties, it was planned to have all the key words presented visually in front of him accompanied by the relevant image. The visual array needed to be small – only 3–5 items at a time. This meant he could freely say the word, or he could point to the relevant word on the sheet or point to the image on the sheet or be asked closed forced choice questions (such as yes/no or x or y style questions) supported by the sheet. This was tested with a variety of high frequency words (such as cup, plate) and then done for a variety of musical instruments (for example, a picture of a harp was next to the word HARP) and for composers (for example, a picture of Mozart was next to his name) and musical genres (for example Orchestral and Choir).

To determine whether Jacob could recognise different musical characteristics (such as Orchestral, Choir, Jazz, Gospel, Pop) Jacob was provided with a visual prompt sheet but could not correctly do this even for music that he had spent his career listening to and writing about.

To assess whether he could recognise familiar melodies that were recorded, selected recorded classical music from his personal collection was used. This was initially played at different volumes to observe his response; then, to assess whether he could recognise the music and then select the corresponding composer. To determine whether he could recognise what was making the sound (the timbre) he was asked to identify the instruments. Jacob was asked to do this freely; then, using the provided visual prompt sheets, and finally from a forced choice of two. Even when he was asked to select instruments that he could hear on the music track from a forced choice of two provided verbally and visually (for example is this a string instrument like a violin or a brass instrument like a trumpet?) he was unable to do this.

To assess whether he was able to recognise familiar melodies that he heard live, Jacob was invited to listen to familiar tunes and asked to identify when you would hear them. The music therapist played these familiar tunes which would be recognisable to British nationals (such as Happy Birthday and God Save the Queen). The music therapist played these pieces on a keyboard, live in his bedroom. He was not able to use the music to prompt the production of any of the lyrics (for example Happy Birthday to …?). Jacob was quick to become agitated and expressed this as 'awful noise' and 'ugly sound'. He was unable to freely recognise the melody and did not agree when he was told what the tune was (stating only 'if you say so'). However, in conversation he could intellectually confirm the British National Anthem is God Save the Queen and that it is played at international sporting events. Jacob could not discriminate between two tones of different pitches (for example, if the sound was higher or lower than the last sound), describing all musical sounds played live to him as 'noise'.

Intervention

The brief, bedside, structured behavioural observation assessment suggested that Jacob had acquired receptive amusia as the result of his CVAs and was experiencing hearing music as aversive. There are no known treatments for this condition. The assessment allowed the formation of several hypotheses to guide disability management-based interventions. Firstly, that Jacob was still able to use his pre-injury semantic and declarative memory to draw from in conversations about music, when these conversations were heavily supported by props (his scrapbook of reports, his CD collection, visual prompts) and the conversation partner. He appeared to enjoy and derive pleasure from talking about how much music meant to him and mattered to him. He appeared to draw pleasure from seeing his extensive collection of CDs, concert programmes, musical reviews, and ticket stubs from concerts he had attended. This indicated that the network of people in his life, many of whom were musicians and appreciated similar music greatly could best engage with Jacob to talk together about music rather than listening together to music. Guidelines were created for family and friends and the staff who supported him by the music therapist. Many of his friends could not believe this could be right as music was so integral to who Jacob was and their own relationships together. They considered the MDT opinion may be incorrect and in reality the findings were just a factor of the poor quality of the unit sound system or the portable one he had in his bedroom. They grouped together to buy him a better quality sound system, but unfortunately this did not alter his experience of being played recorded music. His friends and family also thought that it could be explained by listening to music in the unit rather than being in a concert venue. He was taken to concerts in the Royal Albert Hall and other venues, but typically left mid-way through as he seemed to them to be agitated. The neuropsychologist supported the family and friends through psychoeducation and development of a shared formulation about amusia so that they could begin to think about how to best transform their shared passion to make use of his existing knowledge and interest in music, without listening to it.

Secondly, this assessment indicated that environmental and ecological strategies were going to be needed on discharge as many residential care homes provide group-based music activities and someone with his history was likely to be individually set up by staff to listen to music daily. These strategies and ideas for alternatives were made clear to the current inpatient unit staff and the discharge care home.

Conclusion

Although formal standardised neuropsychological assessment was challenging as a result of the complexity of Jacob's presentation, structured behavioural-based assessment did provide information to try to understand more about his cognition. This assessment information was combined with the speech and language therapist findings and advice from the neurological occupational therapist, to guide the development of how to best approach the bespoke and personalised assessment of possible amusia in the context of being unable to administer the standardised amusia assessments due to Jacob's significant neuro-disability. Working jointly with the music therapist, in as much as we were able to ascertain, Jacob demonstrated both receptive amusia (failure to discriminate between melodic patterns, timbre and pitch and experience sounds as aversive) and musical amnesia (failure to identify familiar melodies). He seemed to hear jumbled sounds which he perceived as 'ugly' and could not recognise as being music; nor could he recognise the much cherished music he enjoyed pre-injury ('if you say so'). As professionals the ability to optimally assess using standardised tools needs to be part of our skill set, but also we need to develop our abilities to design single case experiments with complex client presentations to investigate their skills using our knowledge of the condition, paradigms of assessment, and underlying neuropsychology – we should not be scared away by what may seem 'unassessable' at first glance. We may not be able to get a complete answer to questions about a person's skill, but it is possible to obtain some important and useful information nonetheless. This case also raises the issue of how our profession is being reduced to commenting only on the core components of cognition, formed through neuropsychological assessments across a desk, as a feature of the time pressures on busy clinicians, yet we too have skills in making key observations of cognition in function and in day to day life.

This case illustrates the challenges common for family, friends (and indeed professionals) to try to honour the pre-injury person and interests by reverting to known wishes and values of the person in designing neurorehabilitation and care on their behalf. Playing music for a person after an injury is a common thing friends, family, and professionals like to do. Whilst that strategy had naturally been employed, as new (albeit imperfect) behavioural-based assessment data evolved, so too did the management plans. It became clear that it was important not to rely on Jacob's premorbid interests and use music indiscriminately. By using the aspects of musical knowledge that were preserved for Jacob, conversations reflecting on his life-long love of music and deep understanding of it could still be shared with those who cared for him. This potentially helped connect and maintain his identity, provide space for his expertise to be heard and admired, and ensured his interests and passions were maintained in a new way.

Note

1 The Oxford Companion to Music defines music criticism as 'the intellectual activity of formulating judgments on the value and degree of excellence of individual works of music, or whole groups or genres'.

References

Alluri, V., Toiviainen, P., Jääskeläinen, I. P., Glerean, E., Sams, M., & Brattico, E. (2012). Large-scale brain networks emerge from dynamic processing of musical timbre, key and rhythm. *Neuroimage, 59*, 3677–3689.

Brattico, E., Alluri, V., Bogert, B., Jacobsen, T., Vartiainen, N., Nieminen, S., & Tervaniemi, N. (2011). A functional MRI study of happy and sad emotions in music with and without lyrics. *Frontiers in Psychology, 2*, 308.

Burunat, I., Alluri, V., Toiviainen, P., Numminen, J., & Brattico, E. (2014). *Dynamics of brain activity underlying working memory for music in a naturalistic condition. Cortex*, 57, 254–269.

García-Casares, N., Berthier Torres, M. L., Froudist Walsh, S., & González-Santos, P. (2013). Model of music cognition and amusia. *Neurología*, 28, 3, 179–186.

Kartsounis, L. D. (2003). Assessment of perceptual disorders. In P. W. Halligan, U. Kischka, & J. C. Marshall (Eds.), *Handbook of clinical neuropsychology* (pp. 108–124). Oxford University Press.

Kawamura, M., & Miller, M. W. (2019). History of amusia. *Frontiers of Neurology and Neuroscience*, 44, 83–88.

Latham, A. (2002). *The Oxford companion to music*. Oxford University Press.

Lishman, W. A. (1988). *Organic psychiatry: The psychological consequences of cerebral disorder* (3rd ed.). Blackwell Science.

Partanen, E., Kujala, T., Tervaniemi, M., & Huotilainen, M. (2013). Prenatal music exposure induces long-term neural effects. *PLoS ONE*, 8, 10.

Peretz, I., & Vuvan, D. T. (2017). Prevalence of congenital amusia. *European Journal of Human Genetics*, 25, 5, 625–630.

Särkämö, T., Tervaniemi, M., Soinila, S., Autti, T., Silvennoinen, H. M., Laine, M. & Hietanen, M. (2009a). Amusia and cognitive deficits after stroke: Is there a relationship? *Annals of the New York Academy of Sciences*, 1169, 441–445.

Särkämö, T., Tervaniemi, M., Soinila, S., Autti, T., Silvennoinen, H. M., Laine, M., & Hietanen, M. (2009b). Cognitive deficits associated with acquired amusia after stroke: A neuropsychological follow-up study. *Neuropsychologia*, 47, 12, 2642–2651.

Särkämö, T., Tervaniemi, M., Soinila, S., Autti, T., Silvennoinen, H.M., Laine, M., Hietanen, M., & Pihko, E. (2010). Auditory and cognitive deficits associated with acquired amusia after stroke: A magnetoencephalography and neuropsychological follow-up study. *PLoS One*, 5(12). https://doi.org/10.1371/journal.pone.0015157

Schmithorst, V. J. (2005). Separate cortical networks involved in music perception: Preliminary functional MRI evidence for modularity of music processing. *Neuroimage*, 25, 444–451.

Sihvonen, A. J., Ripollés, P., Leo, V., Rodríguez-Fornells, A., Soinila, S., & Särkämö, T. (2016). Neural Basis of Acquired Amusia and Its Recovery after Stroke. *The Journal of Neuroscience*, 36, 34, 8872–8881.

Sihvonen, A. J., Särkämö, T., Ripollés, P., Leo, V., Saunavaara, J., Parkkola, R., Rodríguez-Fornells, A., & Soinila, S. (2017a). Functional neural changes associated with acquired amusia across different stages of recovery after stroke. *Scientific Reports*, 7, 11390.

Sihvonen, A. J., Ripollés, P., Rodríguez-Fornells, A., Soinila, S., & Särkämö, T. (2017b). Revisiting the neural basis of acquired amusia: Lesion patterns and structural changes underlying amusia recovery. *Frontiers in Neuroscience*, 11, 426.

Silva J., Mota, J., & Azevedo, P. (2016). California rocket fuel: And what about being a first line treatment?. *European Psychiatry*, 33, S1, S551.

Szyfter, K., & Wigowska-Sowińska, J. (2022). Congenital amusia—pathology of musical disorder. *Journal of Applied Genetics*, 63, 127–131.

Toiviainen, P., Alluri, V., Brattico, E., Wallentin, M., & Vuust, P. (2014). Capturing the musical brain with Lasso: Dynamic decoding of musical features from fMRI data. *Neuroimage*, 88, 170–180.

Vuvan, D. T., Paquette, S., Mignault Goulet, G., Royal, I., Felezeu, M., & Peretz, I. (2018). The Montreal protocol for the identification of amusia. *Behaviour Research*, 50, 662–672.

16 Variability and validity

Challenges to meaningful neuropsychological assessment in mental health settings

Victoria Teggart

Introduction: clinical neuropsychology in mental health

The application of clinical neuropsychological assessment and intervention within adult mental health services has received limited attention in academic literature and service development guidance. Whilst there has been longstanding academic interest in the neuropsychological features of conditions commonly seen within mental health services (O'Carroll, 2010), these are not generally recognised in commissioning guidance documents[1] (The Community Mental Health Framework for Adults and Older Adults, Joint Commissioning Panel for Mental Health, 2019).

The description of the work of clinical neuropsychologists on the website of the British Psychological Society (BPS) does not include mental health conditions in the list of key areas of work.

> Neuropsychologists work with people of all ages dealing with patients who have had traumatic brain injury, strokes, toxic and metabolic disorders, tumours and neurodegenerative diseases.
>
> (https://careers.bps.org.uk/area/neuro)

The subsequent text recognises that clinical neuropsychologists 'require knowledge of the range of mental health problems'; however, there is no recognition that this may be the primary area of work for some people, with the focus remaining squarely on work within neurology and neurorehabilitation settings.

> Neuropsychologists most commonly work in acute settings, usually in regional neuroscience centres where their main focus is on the early effects of trauma, neurosurgery and neurological diseases. They also work in rehabilitation centres providing post-acute assessment, training and support for people who have sustained brain injury, or who have other neurological problems.
>
> (https://careers.bps.org.uk/area/neuro/
> where-do-neuropsychologists-work)

DOI: 10.4324/9781003228226-18

Similarly, guidance documents to promote the development of more robust and equitable clinical neuropsychology across the United Kingdom do not list mental health services as an area for investment, noting that the guidance is relevant to those commissioning services in the following areas:

- Care for long-term neurological conditions such as stroke, epilepsy, dementia, multiple sclerosis, Parkinson's disease, neurodisability and motor neurone disease.
- Care for patients following traumatic or acquired brain injury.
- Inpatient neurosurgery, neurology and neurological rehabilitation.
- Neuro-oncology.
- Outpatient neurological rehabilitation.
- Care for functional neurological disorders such as non-epileptic attack disorder.

(The British Psychological Society, 2015)

For the minority of clinical neuropsychologists who specialise in this area and work primarily for Mental Health Trusts, the limited recognition is associated with a number of difficulties:

- Lack of high quality evidence base to guide and shape practice.
- Few examples of good outcomes and no recognised 'gold standard' service models to present to commissioners to drive investment.
- Limited opportunity for professional networking and peer support.

The lack of interest and developments in clinical neuropsychology within mental health is all the more surprising, given the longstanding recognition that:

- Many psychiatric conditions have concomitant cognitive effects (e.g. Heinrichs & Zachzanis, 1998; Pavuluri et al., 2009; Bourne et al., 2013).
- Populations often served by mental health services, such as those with alcohol and drug addictions, are at high risk of developing brain injuries (Svanberg, 2015).
- People seen by mental health services have high levels of physical health comorbidity, often with neurological complications (Daré et al., 2019).

Given the complex needs of the mental health population, it is unlikely that a clinical neuropsychologist would ever be the sole professional working with an individual. However, there are many opportunities for a neuropsychological perspective to add to the understanding of an individual's presentation, to support teams in care planning, decision making and tailoring appropriate treatments, and to avoid potential errors that may arise from a misunderstanding of a person's neuropsychological needs. These ideas are not new; a quarter of a century ago, Keefe (1995) published an article titled 'The Contribution of Neuropsychology to Psychiatry' and highlighted that,

> neuropsychological data serve as a window into the everyday mental processes of the psychiatric patent.
>
> (p. 7)

> the greatest contribution of the neuropsychological evaluation of patients with psychiatric disorders may be that it provides important, objective data about mental deficiencies that shape patients' lives.
>
> (p. 11)

> neuropsychological assessment can improve the quality of individualized therapeutic management.
>
> (p. 12)

This description highlights the core principles of neuropsychological practice, to identify the cognitive abilities and areas of difficulty of an individual in order to understand their everyday function and make adaptations as needed. It is encouraging that it moves away from the focus on diagnostic questions that often dominate (in the experience of the author) the referrals from within Mental Health Services. Requests such as, 'Does this person have alcohol related brain damage?' or, 'Can you test for IQ please?' have some validity in terms of access to specialist services but limit the scope and potential impact of a comprehensive neuropsychological assessment.

Alongside direct assessment, clinical neuropsychology has the potential to contribute to mental health practice through providing supervision and consultation to other colleagues, providing neuropsychological expertise and ensuring that cognitive assessments are used correctly and to their full potential. The use of free-to-access cognitive screening measures, such as the Addenbrooke's Cognitive Examination (ACE-III; Hsieh et al., 2013) and the Montreal Cognitive Assessment (MoCA; Nasreddine et al., 2005) is widespread within mental health services and these may be administered by clinicians who have had limited access to training regarding the administration and interpretations of psychometric measures. It is recognised that these tools should be used mindfully and ethically, with recommendations for training (e.g. www.mvls.gla.ac.uk/aceiiitrainer/; www.mocatest.org/training-certification/) and ongoing supervision, as well as keeping up with developments in these tools. Clinical neuropsychologists are well placed to offer training and consultation to other professionals in the use of these tools to avoid potential mistakes.

Whilst clinical neuropsychologists within the mental health workforce are a rarity, clinical psychologists are better represented, and often have a presence within community mental health teams (CMHTs) and inpatient mental health wards. The BPS Accreditation Standards (2019) for Clinical

Psychologists in training emphasise the need for some foundational training in neuropsychological approaches, including:

- Acquired knowledge and understanding of psychological testing.
- 'Knowledge of neuropsychological processes across the lifespan'.
- 'Competence in performance based psychometric measures'.
- Knowledge of 'neurological presentations'.
- 'Psychometric theory and approaches to understanding assessment findings including statistical and clinical significance'.
- Experience of administering certain cognitive assessments.

Therefore clinical psychologists can offer aspects of neuropsychological assessment where this fits within the expectations of their role. However, it would be necessary for them to be able to access appropriate expert supervision from someone who has expertise in clinical neuropsychology specifically. This is particularly important within the mental health population where co-morbidities are common, neuropsychological presentations are often complex and multifactorial, and there are multiple non-neurological factors that may influence cognitive test performance.

The case study presented here demonstrates the different ways in which a clinical neuropsychologist may be involved in a patient's care across multiple time points. It highlights some of the difficulties in providing high quality neuropsychological input from poorly resourced services and the importance of having data from behavioral observations to aid the interpretation of test scores. It also highlights the complexities of assessment in cases where there are multiple diagnoses or existing problems.

Case presentation

Service context

Our neuropsychology service sits within a mental health trust. We accept referrals from a subset of secondary care services (i.e. CMHTs and inpatient mental health wards) within the Trust and offer a consultation and assessment service. It is a very limited provision in terms of resources (approximately 0.6 whole-time equivalent) and covers a population of more than 500,000 people. Consequently, links with referring services are poor and there is little opportunity for upskilling teams in the benefits and limitations of neuropsychological assessments within this setting through the provision of training or wide-scale case consultation. We are not resourced to provide intervention or follow-up.

The following case presents neuropsychological assessment at three different time points in the patient's contact with mental health services.

Assessment 1: April 2012

Reason for referral

The referral was received from a consultant psychiatrist on an inpatient mental health ward, where Mr A had been a patient since October 2011. Initially there had been concerns about disinhibited behaviour towards females. There had been a deterioration in the weeks following his admission including staff reports of attention and memory problems, and reduced engagement in activities of daily living. The referral requested further assessment to consider the possibility of Korsakoff's syndrome or other alcohol-related cognitive impairment, given the patient's history of alcohol use.

Social background

Mr A is a white British male born in 1983. There were no indications of developmental difficulties or childhood illnesses. He completed an NVQ level qualification and worked as a financial advisor with a bank. He had not been in employment since 2011 due to his mental health difficulties and substance misuse.

Psychiatric history and current presentation

Mr A was first admitted to an inpatient mental health unit in 2004, where he was diagnosed with and treated for psychotic depression. He was discharged to the community. He remained well until October 2008, when he began to state that household items were going missing and that his family were in imminent danger.

His alcohol intake increased, and Mr A reported that he was drinking more to help him cope with the symptoms of his mental health condition. It also became apparent that he had stopped taking his medications. He received support from the CMHT and, following the reinstatement of a medication regime, he was discharged to the care of his GP in May 2010.

He stopped taking his prescribed medication again from around June 2010, and this marked the beginning of a gradual deterioration in his mental health. By May 2011 his family was reporting concerns about Mr A's drinking, and increased aggression and irritability. A pattern of heavy drinking and attendance at A&E continued until September 2011 when Mr A presented to the emergency department. He was subsequently reviewed by psychiatry and was admitted to a mental health unit initially under Section 2 of the Mental Health Act (MHA).

During this admission his diagnosis was updated to bipolar affective disorder with psychotic features. He was prescribed regular quetiapine and haloperidol as needed, which was given frequently.

Disinhibited behaviour towards females was reported early during this admission. From around November 2011 a notable deterioration in functioning was reported. Mr A needed frequent prompts to engage in personal care tasks, appeared to be disorientated and distressed, was generally uncommunicative, had poor concentration and attention, and was struggling to remember information presented to him on a regular basis, for example, staff members' names.

Medical history

No significant head injuries or neurological illnesses were reported. Following his admission to the mental health ward, Mr A showed mild symptoms of alcohol withdrawal and was treated with a Librium regime.

Possible neurological complications from substance misuse were considered as contributory factors to his presentation. In October 2011 a CT scan revealed:

> There is no evidence of a space occupying lesion identified. The ventricles are normal in size. Mild cortical atrophy is noted, this is slightly more than you would expect in a patient of this age.

However a subsequent MRI scan in February 2012 reported no abnormalities, and a review by a consultant neurologist in March 2012 indicated that there was no clear neurological reason for his presentation.

Substance misuse

It was documented in the mental health records that Mr A began binge drinking (around 7 or 8 cans of lager each day at the weekend) in approximately 2004. Around 2010 he was drinking more heavily and frequently around one litre of vodka and two cans of strong lager per day for about five days of the week. An inpatient detox was arranged for September 2011 but Mr A only stayed for a few hours before absconding.

It was reported that Mr A had accessed alcohol during a leave period from the Mental Health Unit. It was unclear how many times this had occurred, or how much alcohol he had consumed on these occasions.

Brief summary of relevant literature

Research findings suggest there are higher levels of cognitive impairment among individuals with psychotic affective disorders compared with non-psychotic affective disorders (Schatzberg et al., 2000; Glahn et al., 2007). The profile of difficulties is described as similar in nature to those seen in schizophrenia, but with less severity (Hill et al., 2004). Deficits have been observed in the domains of sustained attention (Nelson et al., 1998), processing speed and working memory (Hill et al., 2004), response inhibition (Scatzberg et al.,

2000), reasoning and flexibility (Pavuluri et al., 2009), and verbal memory (Gomez et al., 2006), although the latter is generally attributed to attentional and encoding difficulties. It has been proposed that the cognitive abilities usually impacted by affective disorders with psychosis are those mediated by the prefrontal cortex and hippocampus (Fleming et al., 2004). Cognitive abilities can be negatively affected by fluctuations in mental health symptoms, with greater deficits observed when the individual is experiencing acute psychosis (Mulligan et al., 2017).

Drinking to harmful levels can result in damage to the brain and subsequent cognitive and behavioural changes (Beaunieux et al., 2015). The mechanisms underlying alcohol related brain damage (ARBD) are complex and include the neurotoxic effects of alcohol, thiamine deficiency, withdrawal syndromes, and medical complications associated with alcohol use including hepatic encephalopathy and cerebrovascular disease (Savage, 2015). This can result in both grey and white matter changes that affect multiple brain networks. Deficits are commonly reported in executive functioning (Oscar-Berman & Marinković, 2007), episodic memory (Noël et al., 2012), impulse control or inhibition, and decision making (Le Berre at al., 2014). It is recognised that presentations in ARBD are heterogenous. In the early stages, cognitive impairment may be subtle (Svanberg et al., 2015). Wernicke Korsakoff's syndrome is a particular type of ARBD resulting from thiamine deficiency and leads to significant anterograde and retrograde amnesia (Scalzo et al., 2015), as well as executive functioning difficulties.

Alongside underlying psychiatric and neurological causes, the potential impacts of medication also need to be considered in this population. Antipsychotic medications such as quetiapine have been shown to have negative effects on cognitive functioning when used to treat bipolar disorder (Arts et al., 2013) and haloperidol can impact on cognitive functioning at high doses (Woodward et al., 2007). The cognitive effects of medication are often transient (Stoner et al., 2020), and therefore may result in variability in cognitive functioning on a daily basis.

Finally, the issue of motivation to engage in the assessment process is particularly relevant in inpatient mental health settings, where concerns regarding cognition are usually raised by the clinical team rather than the patient themselves and assessments may be requested without full discussion. Reduced engagement with standardised assessments, often referred to as 'poor effort', significantly impacts on the validity of the assessment process, referred to as 'performance validity', and limits the conclusions that can be drawn from test performance. Studies have shown high levels of failure on tests of performance validity within psychiatric populations (McWhirter et al., 2020).

Neuropsychological assessment

Mr A was seen in the inpatient unit on four occasions. At the first three appointments he was able to engage in conversation but was too tired or fatigued to attempt any standardised assessment. On one occasion he refused to get out of bed for the session. He showed very limited understanding of the reason for the assessment. Following changes in his medication, including a reduction in quetiapine and haloperidol, his fatigue improved and standardised cognitive assessment was undertaken in session four. The Repeatable Battery for the Assessment of Neuropsychological Status (RBANS; Randolph, 1998) was selected as an initial broad screen and to provide information regarding effort via embedded measures.

Mr A appeared anxious about his performance, often requiring reassurance in order to continue. At times, he appeared to lose concentration and stated that he was not listening to instructions or test items.

Mr A was oriented to time, person, and place. He showed good recall for events earlier in the day such as the outcome of ward round discussions. His performance on tests suggested mild to moderate deficits in a range of cognitive domains including processing speed, attention, verbal learning and memory, visual memory, naming, and fluency.

The embedded performance validity calculation of Silverberg et al. (2007) did not indicate an invalid response pattern. However, observations of his approach to testing, notably being frequently distracted from the task, raised some concern about effort being consistently applied throughout the assessment.

It was concluded that the results may indicate a degree of cognitive deficit, but caution was required in the interpretation. In addition, it was highlighted that there were multiple static and dynamic risk factors for cognitive impairment and that it would not be possible to draw conclusions about aetiology at this stage. Brain damage resulting from alcohol use was considered a possible contributory factor; however, the assessment had not highlighted the severe episodic memory impairments often seen in Korsakoff's syndrome. It was highlighted that Mr A's presentation appeared to fluctuate, based on the observations of ward staff, which would suggest that his mental health condition and/or medications were impacting on his cognitive abilities.

Although the broad screen had not covered the important area of executive functioning, the presence of possible reduced effort, along with ongoing medication changes and fluctuating mental health led to the decision that further assessment was unlikely to be beneficial at that time. It was recommended that a more comprehensive assessment be undertaken following a period of stability in his mental health and medication regime, ideally following his discharge from hospital. Unfortunately, Mr A was lost to follow up and this assessment was not completed.

Assessment 2: May 2018

A further referral was received when Mr A was again an inpatient under Section 3 of the MHA. He was reported to be confused, disoriented, and repetitive in conversation. He was described as anxious, preoccupied, and distractible, but there were no active symptoms of psychosis. He was also noted to be socially inappropriate towards female staff. There were indications of self-neglect in terms of personal hygiene and lack of ability to manage finances. The referring psychiatrist did not consider his presentation to fit with his psychiatric diagnoses and wanted to explore a neuropsychological or neurological explanation.

Updated psychiatric information

Mr A had a long inpatient mental health admission between December 2013 and January 2015, which was preceded by the death of his mother. Following a period of relative stability, he was reported to be drinking heavily again in late 2016 and there were concerns about self-neglect. At some stage, Mr A's psychiatric diagnosis had been changed to schizophrenia, which might be associated with more severe cognitive impairments.

Prior to the inpatient admission in February 2018, Mr A was described as drinking heavily and anxious in presentation. He was not observed to present with active symptoms of schizophrenia, nor did he appear low in mood. He was deemed to be vulnerable to physical violence and financial exploitation.

On the mental health ward, he was reported to appear anxious and preoccupied, with self-reported anxiety and reduced motivation. He was observed to occasionally mutter or appear distractible, but did not appear to be responding to unseen or unheard stimuli for the majority of the time. He denied experiencing auditory or visual hallucinations. He was described as appearing confused on the ward, and was at times intrusive, socially inappropriate and sexually disinhibited, particularly to female members of staff.

At the time of the assessment his prescribed medications were quetiapine, amisulpride, depakote, and melatonin.

Updated medical information

In 2016, Mr A was diagnosed with pulmonary embolism and was placed on anticoagulant medication.

Assessment

Mr A was seen on two occasions on the ward. During both sessions he appeared inappropriate in manner, requesting 'fist bumps' from the clinician, and on one occasion he asked to leave the room to attend the bathroom, and returned with a pair of underwear, which he invited the clinician to smell. This behaviour was socially inappropriate but did not seem to be disinhibited, as there appeared to be a degree of preplanning and intent behind the behaviour, rather than being impulsive.

He paused for long periods of time prior to answering questions and provided information unrelated to the question asked on a number of occasions. He struggled to provide concrete examples when asked about his life and prior experiences and presented conflicting information regarding past events. At times he held prolonged eye contact.

Mr A's verbal comprehension and expression appeared well preserved. Despite the long pauses, his speech was fluent. He was able to leave the session for a cigarette and remembered to return five minutes later without prompting.

Cognitive assessment was attempted using the RBANS. A standalone performance validity test (PVT) was also included. Reduced effort was apparent on both the embedded (RBANS performance validity index) and explicit measures. His pattern of responses was highly suggestive of deliberate underperformance as he scored below the chance level and there was significant variability in his responses across trials.

It was concluded that, whilst a degree of cognitive impairment could not be ruled out given the known history, it was unlikely that this would account entirely for Mr A's current presentation, and primarily the role of his mental health condition should be considered in understanding his behaviour. It was recommended that it would be beneficial to take a functional analysis approach to his behaviour in order to understand his presentation in more detail. Furthermore it was highlighted that additional cognitive assessment was unlikely to be beneficial due to questionable engagement with the process.

Consultation to medical staff

A few weeks later a member of the psychiatry team from the ward requested a consultation to discuss the results of an ACE-III assessment that they had completed with Mr A due to his ongoing confusion. They felt that this indicated that he had significant cognitive impairment, and that this was much worse than in previous assessments. On discussion, they considered that Mr A had put forth sufficient effort during this assessment based on their clinical opinion and experience of having administered the measure many times before.

I agreed to review the ACE-III. I highlighted my concerns regarding judgements of effort based on observation alone, as research has indicated that this is generally fallible and inaccurate (e.g. Garb, 1998).

The ACE-III scores were: attention 13/18, memory 18/26, fluency 1/14, language 21/26, and visuospatial 16/16. My review of the ACE assessment suggested that the difficulties highlighted were mild in nature and consistent with those found on the previous assessment in 2012, and there was no clear indication of deterioration over time and possibly indication of an improvement. I noted that he had refused to complete one half of the verbal fluency test and this had been included as '0' in the final scoring, thus skewing the results toward a more severe level of impairment. The refusal also led me to question his level of engagement in the assessment process. I reiterated the benefits of focusing on functional and behavioural assessments rather than cognitive tests.

At the time, there were discussions that Mr A should be discharged to a nursing home due to the severity of his cognitive impairments. These circumstances meant it was vital that assessments of cognitive functioning were reliable and valid, given the potential consequences of misinterpretation of test performance.

Assessment 3: July 2019

By this time, Mr A had moved to an inpatient psychiatric rehabilitation unit, where the focus of treatment was more on skills development than stabilizing mental health. The clinical psychologist who worked on the unit wanted to complete cognitive assessment with Mr A, as he continued to present with a number of difficulties in function. Mr A was reported to struggle to organise himself, neglect his self-care if not prompted, and needed reminders for appointments. There was evidence of making in-the-moment decisions that were at odds with his expressed intentions, particularly in relation to making food choices in keeping with his dietary needs. An occupational therapy (OT) assessment had been completed, which demonstrated functional deficits.

The clinical psychologist reported that Mr A's mental health was currently stable. They had developed a good working rapport with Mr A and therefore wanted to complete the assessment themselves; however they recognised the complexity of the case and the need to consider effort, given the outcome of the earlier assessment, and therefore requested supervision.

Standardised assessment was completed using the RBANS, Similarities and Block Design subtests from the Weschler Abbreviated Scale of Intelligence 2nd Edition (WASI-II; Wechsler, 2011) and the Key Search and Zoo Map subtests of the Behavioural Assessment of the Dysexecutive Syndrome (BADS; Wilson et al., 1996).

Effort was assessed via the embedded measures in the RBANS and there was no indication of invalid responding. Whilst it would have been preferable to include a standalone PVT, none was available within the rehabilitation service.

The assessment indicated impairments in processing speed and attention (<1st percentile), which impacted upon verbal learning and memory (1st percentile). Learning was enhanced by repetition of new information and delayed memory was supported by the provision of cues in the recognition memory task. Visual memory was found to be a relative strength (37th percentile), as was verbal abstract reasoning (37th percentile). Difficulties in executive functioning were observed with problem solving and planning, with both described as impaired. Observation of Mr A's approach to tasks suggested difficulties with flexibility and perseverance on tasks that he found challenging.

These results of the assessment were used to develop the team's understanding of Mr A's behaviour in certain situations. It was suggested that his difficulty with sticking to stated intentions related more to difficulties with problem solving and flexibility in unfamiliar situations rather than being a sign of impulsive behaviour or non-compliance with pre-agreed plans. It was highlighted that clear guidelines and instructions, along with ongoing prompts and cues would be helpful to support decision making. The use of compensatory strategies such as a diary or notebook was recommended.

Discussion

This case highlights the need for access to clinical neuropsychological expertise in mental health services for cases where there are concerns regarding cognitive functioning on a background of comorbid psychiatric and potential neurological conditions. The contribution of clinical neuropsychology within these settings spans direct assessment, consultation and supervision to ensure the accurate and proper use of measures of cognitive functioning, and that potential confounding variables are considered in interpretation.

The difficulties with providing a comprehensive neuropsychological formulation in this case reinforces the need for a broad approach to assessment, especially in complex cases. Neuropsychology assessment should be multidimensional and include, where possible, observations of client behaviour in a range of structured and unstructured settings, along with collateral history from a range of sources. Due to limited resources and the service structure, our input in this case was restricted to clinical interviews and cognitive assessments. We were unable to undertake behavioural observations or work alongside occupational therapy colleagues to review Mr A's abilities in functional activities. Attendance at multidisciplinary case discussions was also not possible, which limited our ability to feed into the formulation of his presentation and stay updated with fluctuations in his presentation. The limited resources and stand-alone nature of the service also meant we were not able to actively pursue further assessment following his discharge in 2012 and we did not get updates regarding his progress following the final assessment in 2019. This latter point makes it difficult to evaluate the impact of neuropsychological input in such cases, data that is essential to make the case for additional resources. Research into the benefits of neuropsychological assessment and consultation in mental health settings is much needed to inform service developments.

In addition, the case demonstrates a number of important points regarding the provision of neuropsychological assessments with a mental health population:

- Timing of assessments is important: undertaking assessments when mental health is unstable, medications are being changed, or the individual is not fully engaged with the assessment process means that results of standardised tests may be invalid and the assessment findings are unlikely to add to the understanding of the person's presentation.
- Rapport is important: the third assessment was undertaken within the context of an established therapeutic relationship, rather than by a clinician unfamiliar to the person. It is possible that this led to greater willingness to engage with the process.

- Effort is important: given the impact on validity of assessment findings, it is vital to consider effort at any time that cognitive tests are undertaken, even if there is no obvious secondary gain.
- Neuropsychological formulation, rather than diagnosis, is important: the third assessment was undertaken to enhance the understanding of Mr A's behaviour in certain situations and was supported by robust observations undertaken by staff. This led to recommendations for adapted treatment plans that were useful despite the ongoing lack of clarity around the underlying cause of these impairments.

Neuropsychological perspectives have the potential to contribute to the understanding of cognitive and behavioural presentations in people with psychiatric conditions. Given the complexity of such cases, clinical neuropsychology services within mental health settings need to be sufficiently resourced to build relationships with referring teams, provide training and supervision, and respond flexibly to requests for assessments.

Note

1 Adult mental health services in the context of this chapter refers to adults of working age. It is acknowledged that neuropsychological difficulties such as those associated with dementia are addressed within mental health services for older adults.

References

Arts, B., Simons, C. J., Drukker, M., & van Os, J. (2013). Antipsychotic medications and cognitive functioning in bipolar disorder: Moderating effects of COMT Val108/158Met genotype. *BMC Psychiatry, 13*(1), 1–8.

Beaunieux, H., Eustache, F., & Pitel, A-L. (2015). The relation of alcohol-induced brain changes to cognitive function. In J. Svanberg, A. Withall, B. Draper & S. Bowden (Eds.), *Alcohol and the adult brain*. Psychology Press.

Bourne, C., Aydemir, Ö., Balanzá-Martínez, V., Bora, E., Brissos, S., Cavanagh, J. T. O., ... & Goodwin, G. M. (2013). Neuropsychological testing of cognitive impairment in euthymic bipolar disorder: An individual patient data meta-analysis. *Acta Psychiatrica Scandinavica, 128*(3), 149–162.

Daré, L. O., Bruand, P. E., Gérard, D., Marin, B., Lameyre, V., Boumédiène, F., & Preux, P. M. (2019). Co-morbidities of mental disorders and chronic physical diseases in developing and emerging countries: A meta-analysis. *BMC Public Health, 19*(1), 1–12.

Fleming, S. K., Blasey, C., & Schatzberg, A. F. (2004). Neuropsychological correlates of psychotic features in major depressive disorders: A review and meta-analysis. *Journal of Psychiatric Research, 38*(1), 27–35.

Garb, H. N. (1998). *Studying the clinician: Judgment research and psychological assessment*. American Psychological Association.

Glahn, D. C., Bearden, C. E., Barguil, M., Barrett, J., Reichenberg, A., Bowden, C. L., ... & Velligan, D. I. (2007). The neurocognitive signature of psychotic bipolar disorder. *Biological psychiatry, 62*(8), 910–916.

Gomez, R. G., Fleming, S. H., Keller, J., Flores, B., Kenna, H., DeBattista, C.,... & Schatzberg, A. F. (2006). The neuropsychological profile of psychotic major depression and its relation to cortisol. *Biological Psychiatry, 60*(5), 472–478.

Heinrichs, R. W., & Zakzanis, K. K. (1998). Neurocognitive deficit in schizophrenia: A quantitative review of the evidence. *Neuropsychology, 12*(3), 426.

Hill, S. K., Keshavan, M. S., Thase, M. E., & Sweeney, J. A. (2004). Neuropsychological dysfunction in antipsychotic-naive first-episode unipolar psychotic depression. *American Journal of Psychiatry, 161*(6), 996–1003.

Hsieh, S., Schubert, S., Hoon, C., Mioshi, E., & Hodges, J. R. (2013). Validation of the Addenbrooke's Cognitive Examination III in frontotemporal dementia and Alzheimer's disease. *Dementia And Geriatric Cognitive Disorders, 36*(3–4), 242–250.

Joint Commissioning Panel for Mental Health (2019). The Community Mental Health Framework for Adults and Older Adults.

Keefe, R. S. (1995). The contribution of neuropsychology to psychiatry. *The American Journal of Psychiatry, 152*(1), 6–15.

Le Berre, A. P., Rauchs, G., La Joie, R., Mezenge, F., Boudehent, C., Vabret, F., ... & Beaunieux, H. (2014). Impaired decision-making and brain shrinkage in alcoholism. *European Psychiatry, 29*(3), 125–133.

McWhirter, L., Ritchie, C. W., Stone, J., & Carson, A. (2020). Performance validity test failure in clinical populations: A systematic review. *Journal of Neurology, Neurosurgery & Psychiatry, 91*(9), 945–952.

Mulligan, O., Tan, W. T., Lowry, G., & Adamis, D. (2017). Cognitive dysfunction in acute psychosis. *European Psychiatry, 41*(S1), S745–S745.

Nasreddine, Z. S., Phillips, N. A., Bédirian, V., Charbonneau, S., Whitehead, V., Collin, I., ... & Chertkow, H. (2005). The Montreal Cognitive Assessment, MoCA: a brief screening tool for mild cognitive impairment. *Journal of the American Geriatrics Society, 53*(4), 695–699.

Nelson, E. B., Sax, K. W., & Strakowski, S. M. (1998). Attentional performance in patients with psychotic and nonpsychotic major depression and schizophrenia. *American Journal of Psychiatry, 155*(1), 137–139.

Noël, X., Van der Linden, M., Brevers, D., Campanella, S., Hanak, C., Kornreich, C., & Verbanck, P. (2012). The contribution of executive functions deficits to impaired episodic memory in individuals with alcoholism. *Psychiatry Research, 198*(1), 116–122.

O'Carroll, R. (2010). Clinical presentation of neuropsychiatric disorders. In J. Gurd, & U. Kischka (Eds.), *The handbook of clinical neuropsychology.* Oxford Academic.

Oscar-Berman, M., & Marinković, K. (2007). Alcohol: Effects on neurobehavioral functions and the brain. *Neuropsychology Review, 17*(3), 239–257.

Pavuluri, M. N., West, A., Hill, S. K., Jindal, K., & Sweeney, J. A. (2009). Neurocognitive function in pediatric bipolar disorder: 3-year follow-up shows cognitive development lagging behind healthy youths. *Journal of the American Academy of Child & Adolescent Psychiatry, 48*(3), 299–307.

Randolph, C. (1998). *The Repeatable Battery for the Assessment of Neuropsychological Status.* Pearson.

Savage, L. (2015) Alcohol-related brain damage and neuropathology. In J. Svanberg, A. Withall, B. Draper & S. Bowden (Eds.), *Alcohol and the adult brain.* Psychology Press.

Schatzberg, A. F., Posener, J. A., DeBattista, C., Kalehzan, B. M., Rothschild, A. J., & Shear, P. K. (2000). Neuropsychological deficits in psychotic versus nonpsychotic major depression and no mental illness. *American Journal of Psychiatry*, *157*(7), 1095–1100.

Silverberg, N. D., Wertheimer, J. C., & Fichtenberg, N. L. (2007). An effort index for the Repeatable Battery for the Assessment of Neuropsychological Status (RBANS). *The Clinical Neuropsychologist*, *21*(5), 841–854.

Stoner, C. R., Knapp, M., Luyten, J., Kung, C., Richards, M., Long, R., & Rossor, M. (2020). The cognitive footprint of medication: A review of cognitive assessments in clinical trials. *Journal of Clinical Pharmacy and Therapeutics*, *45*(4), 874–880.

The British Psychological Society (2015). *Clinical Neuropsychology Services: Delivering value for the NHS*. A briefing paper for NHS commissioners and policy makers. BPS.

Scalzo, S., Bowden, S., & Hillbom, M. (2015). Wernicke-Korsakoff syndrome. In J. Svanberg, A. Withall, B. Draper & S. Bowden (Eds.), *Alcohol and the adult brain*. Psychology Press.

Svanberg, J. (2015). *Introduction*. In J. Svanberg, A. Withall, B. Draper & S. Bowden (Eds.), *Alcohol and the adult brain*. Psychology Press.

Svanberg J., Morrison, F., & Cullen, B. (2015). *Neuropsychological assessment of alcohol-related cognitive impairment*. In J. Svanberg, A. Withall, B. Draper & S. Bowden (Eds.). *Alcohol and the adult brain*. Psychology Press.

Wechsler, D. (2011). *Wechsler Abbreviated Scale of Intelligence (WASI-II)* (2nd ed.). Pearson.

Wilson, B. A., Alderman, N., Burgess, P. W., Emslie, H., & Evans, J. J. (1996). *The Behavioural Assessment of the Dysexecutive Syndrome (BADS)*. Pearson.

Woodward, N. D., Purdon, S. E., Meltzer, H. Y., & Zald, D. H. (2007). A meta-analysis of cognitive change with haloperidol in clinical trials of atypical antipsychotics: Dose effects and comparison to practice effects. *Schizophrenia Research*, *89*(1–3), 211–224.

17 Recognising autism in adult neuropsychology services

Sally Finnie

Introduction

Autism is characterised by persistent deficits in social communication and social interaction across multiple contexts, as well as restricted, repetitive patterns of behaviour, interests, or activities and sensory sensitives (American Psychiatric Association, 2013). In the UK, the estimated prevalence is about 1% (National Autistic Society, 2018).

Autism was not recognised in the *Diagnostic and Statistical Manual of Mental Disorders* (DSM) until 1980. Asperger's syndrome (an outdated but still popular term to describe autistic individuals with normal intellectual functioning and no history of speech and language delay) was added in 1994. As a result, many adults grew up in a time when parents, educators, and healthcare providers were not aware of the symptoms of Autism, particularly in children without intellectual impairment. These individuals will usually have attended mainstream school, may have worked, had relationships, and lived independently. They may have been viewed as *quirky*, *odd*, or *painfully shy* without anyone recognising their behaviours as symptoms of Autism.

The pathway to an Autism assessment can be long and laborious. Geurts and Jansen (2011) found that prior to the Autism assessment, clients had first contacted mental health clinics with social problems, feelings of anxiety, and mood disturbances on average 15 years earlier. The most common earlier diagnoses were anxiety and mood disorders or psychosis-related disorders.

Autistic adults are more likely to experience mental health conditions such as depression (Cassidy et al., 2014), eating disorders (Westwood & Tchanturia, 2017) and obsessive-compulsive disorder (Wikramanayake et al., 2018). Autistic people are at significantly increased risk of experiencing suicidal thoughts and behaviours and death by suicide (Cassidy et al., 2021) compared to non-autistic people. Autistic people who have experienced delay in autism diagnosis until adulthood show the highest estimates of lifetime suicidal thoughts (66%) and suicide attempt(s) (35–36%) (Cassidy et al., 2014).

As a result of late diagnosis, autistic adults (and often females, see Rynkiewicz et al., 2019) may have learnt to mask or camouflage their differences. This term has been coined to describe the considerable efforts autistic people

DOI: 10.4324/9781003228226-19

may go to to hide their difficulties in order to fit in. Autistic adults describe learning tricks such as appearing to make eye contact, the use of social scripts as well as exhausting efforts to suppress stereotypical stimming behaviours (e.g., sensory seeking or avoiding behaviours). Masking is thought to contribute to the high levels of mental health difficulties in this population.

Autism increases the likelihood of other neurodevelopmental conditions. Attention deficit hyperactivity disorder (ADHD) is the most common comorbidity in autistic children with comorbidity rates in the 40–70% range (Antshel et al., 2016; Johnston et al., 2013). ADHD is characterised by inattention, impulsiveness, and/or hyperactivity that remain relatively persistent over time and result in impairment across multiple domains of life activities. Furthermore, 11% of children with dyslexia (Brimo et al., 2021) and 3% of children with dyscalculia (Morsanyi et al., 2018) are autistic. In one of the few adult studies in this area, Cassidy and colleagues (2016) found that autistic adults were significantly more likely to report a diagnosis of dyspraxia (6.9%) than those without Autism (0.8%).

Finally, autistic adults are more likely to have other neurological conditions such as epilepsy, macrocephaly, hydrocephalus, cerebral palsy, migraine/ headache, and congenital abnormalities of the nervous system (Pan et al., 2020), Tourette's disorder (Darrow et al., 2017), and epilepsy (Tuchman & Rapin, 2002). Given the prevalence, range of symptoms, and co-occurring conditions, it is inevitable that clients, with or without a formal diagnosis of autism, will cross the desks of neuropsychologists.

Neuropsychological profile of Autism

The idea that autism is part of the *brain wiring* is popular amongst clinicians and autistic advocates. These theories tend to focus on brain connectivity. It is well documented that there is increased brain growth and altered synaptic pruning in the first four years leading to some areas of the brain being over-connected and others under-connected. MRI studies have identified a smaller corpus callosum and cerebellum (linked with social cognition as well as more traditionally with motor coordination), possibly explaining why an autistic individual may be socially and physically clumsy (Powell, 2021). Misra (2014) has suggested that various neural systems involved in social and emotional tasks are less connected in autistic people. These regions, termed the '*Social Brain Network*' include the fusiform face area (perception of personal identity), inferior frontal gyrus (facial expression imitation), posterior superior temporal sulcus (perception of facial expressions and eye gaze tasks), superior frontal gyrus (theory of mind, i.e., taking another person's perspective), and the amygdala (emotion processing).

Extensive research has defined impairments across domains associated with Autism such as emotion perception and regulation, perspective-taking, pragmatic language, language comprehension, concept formation, cognitive flexibility, face perception, self-regulation, and motor praxis, and these results have been widely replicated (for a review see Gallagher & Varga, 2015). However, neuropsychological differences in the domains more commonly assessed by neuropsychologists are also apparent.

Autistic adults, compared with neurotypical controls, have been shown to present with a constellation of neuropsychological strengths and weaknesses. It is not usual for autistic adults to perform in the superior range on some tasks and impaired range on others. This spikey profile can also be seen in real world examples: an autistic person could be a leading expert on nuclear physics but unable to remember to brush their teeth or clean their clothes.

When tested with Wechsler intelligence scales, autistic individuals usually produce deficits in verbal comprehension tasks and strengths on the nonverbal Block Design task. These peaks have been classified as *islets of ability* and contributed to the theory of *weak central coherence* (Frith & Happé, 1994; Happé & Frith, 2006). This theory suggests that autistic people have a processing bias for detailed and local information, and relative failure to extract gist or *see the big picture* in everyday life. This hypothesis can account for some unusual attentional features seen in autism; for example, fascination/preoccupation with unusual objects or unusual aspects of objects and insistence on sameness. This theory has led to a huge amount of research and has been well accepted by the autistic community whose autobiographical accounts often included descriptions of specialist interests requiring attention to detail. There is also evidence that autistic brains have an excess of relatively short neural fibres producing local over-connectivity and limited range of connectivity. This idea has been used to explain why autistic people can be detail oriented and in contrast struggle to integrate complex ideas which may be seen as requiring whole brain thinking. It also helps explain sensory sensitivities in autism: imagine one auditory cortical neuron being over-connected to lots of others – any stimulus would be amplified (Powell, 2021). The idea of islets of ability has also directed research into savant syndrome (neurodiverse people with remarkable talent in one or more domains (e.g., music, memory; see Hughes et al., 2018 for a review).

Slow processing speed has been suggested as a potential mechanism that underlies the diverse profile of neuropsychological deficits observed in Autism. Haigh et al. (2018) found that, compared to matched controls, autistic adults without intellectual impairments performed slower on all standardised measures of processing speed. Furthermore, they found lower processing speed was associated with poorer communication and reciprocal interaction skills. However, these tasks measure motor speed as well as components of executive functioning, which have also been found to be impaired in autistic adults. There is also suggestion that autistic people are better at processing tasks that require singular, systematic processing, but struggle on tasks of parallel processing. Nason (2014) explains,

> When your brain cannot simultaneously integrate information, it has to sort through the information sequentially ... this sequential reasoning slows down the processing, leaving the individual missing much of the

rapidly changing information … this is very draining and often leaves people on the spectrum struggling to keep up.

(Nason, 2014, p. 39)

Autistic people have been shown to have average or above average skills in sustained and selective attention; however, they have challenges switching or dividing attention (Johnston et al., 2013). Indeed, the autistic brain can achieve hyper focus for activities of interest and importance. This can be a strength and disadvantage as clients have reported forgetting to eat, sleep, or engage in essential tasks when engaged in a special interest leading to failure to complete the more mundane activities of daily living. King et al. (2018) may have found a reason for difficulties shifting attention. They used functional MRI to measure sustained connectivity, i.e. how long connectivity persists between brain regions or networks after a task is completed. They found increased sustained connectivity in autistic adolescents and adults that was related to severity in autism symptoms. The idea that sustained connections between different regions of the brain are slower to fade out when there is a required shift was likened to a phone that won't hang up.

Impairments in executive functioning are widely cited in Autism (see Wallace et al. 2016 for review) and overlap with a core Autism symptom: cognitive inflexibility. Johnston et al. (2019) compared autistic clients with no intellectual impairments or co-occurring ADHD and found the autistic group to have lower scores relative to controls on tasks of planning, generativity, and flexibility. A significant greater proportion of the Autism group had scores below the fifth percentile on tasks of generativity (35%) and response initiation (24%). The Autism group also took significantly longer to complete executive tasks, consistent with previous reports of a slow and accurate response style (Johnston et al., 2019). The Autism group also reported high levels of dysexecutive difficulties on a standardised questionnaire. However, one-third of the Autism group were not in the clinically impaired range on any of the tasks, suggesting a subset of people with Autism who do not have difficulties in this area. These findings have been replicated and added to by Xie et al. (2020). She also found executive dysfunction in the domains of inhibition, working memory, as well as flexibility, planning, and fluency in adults with high functioning autism as compared to typically developing adults. Importantly Wallace et al. (2018) found that executive dysfunction occurs outside of the neuropsychological assessment in a cohort of autistic adults with high average IQ. Informant reports using the BRIEF-A showed weaknesses in flexibility and planning that were associated with adaptive functioning deficits and comorbid symptoms of anxiety and depression. Increasingly research implicates a broader influence of executive dysfunction in Autism, including impacts on mental health, and the ability to perform activities of daily living needed for independent function such as dressing, shopping, and cooking (Demetriou et al. 2018). Those autistic individuals affected by executive functioning deficits have significantly lower quality of life (De Vries et al., 2015; Johnston et al., 2019).

Case: Mr H

Mr H, a 36-year-old, right-handed, self-employed cleaner, was referred to the neuropsychological outpatient department by Children's Services. His son had been referred to social care due to alleged domestic abuse perpetrated by Mr H to his partner. The professionals working with Mr H believed that he lacked understanding about the consequences of his actions and was difficult to work with. He had written incomprehensible emails in which he repeated the same statement or question several times. He could not work flexibly with children's services and could not tolerate small changes from what was expected, for example if he did not receive a phone call at a set time. The social worker hoped a better understanding of Mr H's cognitive profile would support her work with him.

Presentation and presenting difficulties

Mr H attended the appointment alone. He was neatly presented in casual clothes. He avoided eye contact and his affect was flat. He was able to explain to me the reason for his referral. He expressed a desire to be involved with his son and was hoping this assessment would help him to access appropriate support. He agreed that he struggled to engage with services but expressed that he generally found communication baffling and was unclear what was expected of him. He felt his communication difficulties were life long and that the current stressors were exacerbating these difficulties. He did not report concerns with his attention, memory, or other aspects of his thinking.

Relevant background

Mr H is the eldest of three siblings. He described a good relationship with his parents and there was no evidence of childhood trauma. His birth was described as 'difficult' but there was no indication he required oxygen or specialist care. He met his milestones within the expected time frame and had not experienced any significant illness or neurological conditions. There are no diagnoses of Autism or ADHD in the family. Both he and his younger sister have a diagnosis of dyslexia.

As a child, he recalled teachers reporting difficulties with his concentration and that he was often 'in his own world'. He reported bullying throughout school and believes that this was about his communication and speech. He recalled that his pronunciation was unusual, and he often did not understand the games being played in the playground. He felt that other children seemed to be more advanced and understand what they were supposed to do when playing, whereas it seemed to be a 'complete mystery to me [him]'.

He was diagnosed with dyslexia and received one to one support in primary and secondary school. There was talk of holding him back a year, but this did not come to fruition, and he left school with Ds, Es, and Fs in his GCSEs. He completed a GNVQ in Business Studies and Leisure and Tourism which he found very challenging because he received less structure and support with his learning than he had at school.

As a young adult, his parents separated, and he felt that this may have precipitated an episode of depression. He was prescribed antidepressants. Unfortunately, his mood deteriorated and he attempted suicide. His sister found him, and he did not require hospitalisation. His antidepressant medication was changed; however, he did not access any further mental health support. He reported very limited contact with health professionals, including the GP and dentist, due to social avoidance.

Since this time, he has not had any further episodes of suicidal ideation or self-harm and has not taken antidepressants. However, he reported 'brain fog' where he experiences 'feeling like a zombie'. He said this is different from fatigue or tiredness as he feels that his 'head is just not in the right place' and he lacks motivation. He struggles with day-to-day activities, for example getting up, dressed, and washed. He estimated that he spends at least one day a fortnight in bed due to this difficulty. He denied alcohol or drug use.

Mr H has worked in numerous minimal wage jobs, such as stacking shelves. He has left jobs when asked to do something unexpected or challenging. A few years ago, he set up a cleaning business with his partner. He said he enjoyed cleaning due to the repetitive nature of the work and has been able to maintain some repeat customers due to the high quality of his work. He reported that he struggled with the communication and administration side of work; for example, he struggles with small talk when meeting new potential customers and has learnt scripts to manage this. His business had been impacted by the COVID-19 pandemic and the loss of his partner who tended to manage the administrative side. He reported considerable financial difficulties.

Mr H has had one long-term relationship with his ex-partner, which lasted for 16 years. Mr H was surprised when the relationship ended and had not been able to explain his role in this. They have a three-year-old son. It was interesting to note that his son's language development was delayed, though he was not currently on a pathway for assessment.

Neuropsychological formulation

Mr H has been referred for neuropsychological assessment due to difficulties with communication and flexible thinking/executive functioning. However, his presentation (poor eye contact, limited facial expressions, and need for direct questions) and features of his background (dyslexia, poor attention at school, bullying, difficulties with social interaction, preference for routines, and difficulty with change) raised concern that a potential cause of his difficulties may be undiagnosed Autism.

Assessment

Due to the nature of the original referral, I proceeded with a brief neuropsychological assessment. Results showed borderline-impaired verbal comprehension skills (WAIS-IV Similarities scaled score 5, Vocabulary scaled score 6), average visual constructional skills (WAIS-IV Block Design scaled score 8), and impaired processing speed (WAIS-IV Coding scaled score 2) where he showed a preference for working slowly and accurately. Mr H hence presented with a variable cognitive profile, consistent with my provisional formulation of ASD. When I explained this formulation to Mr H he consented to further assessment for ASD. I switched hats and pulled out my autism assessment kit.

The Autism Diagnostic Observation Schedule (ADOS-II; Gotham et al., 2007) is recognised by National Institute for Health and Care Excellence (2021) to be part of a gold standard assessment of ASD. It uses various activities to assess social communication, emotional literacy, social insight, and rigid/repetitive behaviours.

Mr H's score on the ADOS-II was above the cut-off indicative of Autism. He showed difficulties with social initiation and response; for example, he did not offer personal information unless asked very directly nor did he ask questions to extend a conversation. He reported that he gets frustrated with communication, does 'not like talking', and often misunderstands intention. There was evidence of difficulties with relationships and emotional understanding: he described himself as 'not a people person' and does not enjoy social occasions. He described being overwhelmed by people. When asked to interpret a story (a task deigned to illicit social and emotional understanding as well as obtain communication sample) there was a lack of reference to characters relationships or emotional states.

With reference to nonverbal communication behaviour, Mr H struggled to use eye contact to initiate or maintain social interaction and reported that he struggles to interpret facial expressions and body language in others. In exploring his use of language, his speech was observed to be repetitive and rigid, he struggles to understand humour, to read between the lines, and has a literal interpretation of language. He described stereotypical behaviours as a child, such as head banging, and reported a preference for sameness (wears the same clothes daily, goes to the same places via the same routes) and difficulties with change, which had resulted in problems in the workplace. He reported sensory sensitivities related to smell, hearing, and touch.

As Autism is a neurodevelopmental condition with childhood onset, I spoke to his mother by phone to collect further developmental history. She described him as a 'handful' when he was young, 'hyperactive with frequent tantrums'. He was not a talkative child and would take things literally. He would talk quickly and slur his words. He would lose the listener because he was not explaining what he was talking about. He struggled to play imaginatively or socially. He fell in with a small group of close-knit friends whom he maintained through school. Outside of this group he found social interaction very difficult and was bullied.

Based on the above information, Mr H demonstrated persistent deficits in social communication and social interaction across contexts, including deficits in social–emotional reciprocity, deficits in nonverbal communicative behaviours, and deficits in developing and maintaining relationships. There was evidence of restricted, repetitive patterns of behaviour, including stereotyped speech and movements, resistance to change, and sensory differences. He did not demonstrate any highly restricted or fixated interests – an important but not essential feature of ASD. These symptoms were present in early childhood but did not become fully manifest until social demands exceeded limited capacities and were considered to limit and impair everyday functioning within school, employment, and with mental health. This case was discussed with a multidisciplinary team, and it was deemed that he met the diagnosis of Autism Spectrum Disorder without intellectual impairment as per the DSM-V criteria 299.00. This would well explain his difficulties engaging with Children's Services.

Care planning and recommendations

Mr H expressed satisfaction with the outcome of this assessment. As he had not been initially referred for an autism assessment, he was somewhat surprised, but as we explored how difficulties he had experienced across his life span could be explained by autism, he expressed relief.

Autistic adults are covered by The Equality Act 2010 and therefore entitled to reasonable adjustments to access appropriate education, employment, housing, goods and services, and legal systems. Examples of appropriate reasonable adjustments for healthcare professionals and children services when engaging with Mr H would be use of direct language, breaking down expectations and tasks, prior warning of changes to events, agreed times to contact, making every effort not to change staff members involved in his case, support from a familiar person, written information provided before and after meetings, access to a quiet space for appointments free of sensory stimulation, and regular breaks to reduce social fatigue.

Following the diagnosis, Mr H reported that his interactions with children's services had improved. He has found it helpful to have information broken down in a way that he can understand and to have a family member present to support him and provide responses on his behalf. His nonverbal communication and rigidity have been understood as a symptom of autism rather than an indication of lack of interest or motivation to parent his son or engage with children's services. His insistence on routine has also been understood as part of his condition as opposed to awkward or difficult behaviour.

Autistic adults can experience alexithymia (difficulty feeling, recognising, or having words to express emotions). During the assessment it was apparent that Mr H struggled to identify and speak about emotions. He was able to report 'brain fog' that prevented him from getting out of bed on occasion but was not the same as tiredness. Mr H was encouraged to access talking therapies to help him identify and develop strategies to support low mood. Talking therapies can be successful for autistic clients, particularly when modifications are made (NICE, 2021), and helpful guidance on making mental health talking therapies more accessible for autistic people has recently been published (National Autistic Society & Mind, 2021).

Discussion

Mr H posed a conundrum to Children's Services. A working man, capable of engaging in a long-term relationship but with poor communication and whose insistence on routines made him appear cantankerous and difficult to engage. Many autistic adults remain undiagnosed, given the lack of understanding of symptoms in adulthood and limited adult autism diagnostic services. Given the prevalence, range of symptoms, and co-occurring conditions it is inevitable that clients, with or without a formal diagnosis of autism, will cross the desks of neuropsychologists.

Mr H showed many features of Autism such as poor eye contact, difficulty expressing and understanding emotions, as well as having some core features in his history − bullying, dyslexia, depression with suicidality, and social difficulties, and he expressed some elements of masking. Neuropsychological assessment, albeit brief, revealed a strength in perceptual tasks over verbal tasks, and poor processing speed consistent with the autism literature.

Competency frameworks ensure all neuropsychologists have a good knowledge of neurodevelopmental conditions such as autism. However, as these conditions are usually diagnosed by specialist multidisciplinary services and by professionals with specific training in autism it remains likely that these conditions at times remain undiagnosed after input from neuropsychology or that clients require onward referral to specialist services with lengthy delays. To reduce the instance of missed diagnosis we recommend the following:

- Neuropsychologists must listen carefully to neurodevelopmental histories and consider the possibility of neurodiversity in their clients (see Table 17.1 for a list of indicators to be aware of).
- Neuropsychologists should have knowledge of onward referral options, for example the local autism assessment service.
- Where Autism is suspected, a screening tool such as the freely available Autism Quotient-10 (Allison et al., 2012) may be useful.
- Interested healthcare professionals may seek training in the ADOS-II (provided by Pearson and Kings College London as well as others); however, they should be aware that NICE guidelines (2021) recommend multidisciplinary assessments, which may not be possible in all services.

Table 17.1 Suggested circumstances in which autism assessment may be indicated

- The referral includes information about social communication difficulties and rigid thinking styles or behaviors.
- When there does not seem to have been an event or trigger of change, indicating the symptoms are lifelong.
- When the client reports a long history of social interaction difficulties such as social isolation, bullying, or impaired friendships or feelings of difference/ isolation.
- When there is a family history of Autism, ADHD, or other neurodiverse conditions e.g., dyslexia.
- When the client has underachieved despite intact intellectual ability.
- When the client presents with nonverbal communication difficulties such as poor eye contact, neutral facial expressions, or incongruent verbal and nonverbal behaviour, e.g., smiling when discussing poor mental health.
- When the cognitive profile is variable (spikey), indicating extremes of strength and weakness, or when there are executive functioning or attentional difficulties that cannot otherwise be explained.
- The presence of unusual behaviours during the neuropsychological assessment such as repetitive language, counting, or sensory-seeking behaviours. There is a useful checklist of behaviours associated with Autism that can present during an assessment (Meem, 2015).
- AQ-10 screening measures scores >6.

References

Allison, C., Auyeung, B., & Baron-Cohen, S. (2012). Toward brief 'red flags' for autism screening: The short autism spectrum quotient and the short quantitative checklist in 1,000 cases and 3,000 controls. *Journal of American Academy Child and Adolescent Psychiatry, 51*, 202–212.

American Psychiatric Association. (2013). *Diagnostic and statistical manual of mental disorders* (5th ed.). APA.

Antshel, K. M., Zhang-James, Y., Wagner, K., Ledesma, L., & Faraone, S. V. (2016). An update on the comorbidity of ASD and ADHD: A focus on clinical management. *Expert Review of Neurotherapeutics.* https://doi.org/10.1586/14737175.2016.1 146591

Brimo, K., Dinkler, L., Gillberg, C., Lichtenstein, P., Lundström, S., & Åsberg Johnels, J. (2021). The co-occurrence of neurodevelopmental problems in dyslexia. *Dyslexia, 27*, 277–293.

Cassidy, S., Bradley, P., Robinson J., & Allison, C. (2014). Suicidal ideation and suicide plans or attempts in adults with Asperger's syndrome attending a specialist diagnostic clinic: A clinical cohort study. *Lancet Psychiatry, 1*, 142–147.

Cassidy, S., Hannant, P., Tavassoli, T., Allison, C., Smith P., & Baron-Cohen, S. (2016). Dyspraxia and autistic traits in adults with and without autism spectrum conditions. *Molecular Autism, 7*, 48.

Cassidy, S. A., Bradley, L., Cogger-Ward, H., Cassidy, S. A., Bradley, L., Cogger-Ward, H., & Rodgers, J. (2021). Development and validation of the suicidal behaviours questionnaire: Autism spectrum conditions in a community sample of autistic, possibly autistic and non-autistic adults. *Molecular Autism, 12*, 46.

Darrow, S. M., Grados, M., & Sandor, P. (2017). Autism spectrum symptoms in a Tourette's disorder sample. *Journal of American Academy Child and Adolescent Psychiatry, 56* (7), 610–617.

Demetriou, E. A., Lampit, A., Quintana, D. S., Naismith, S. L., Song, Y. J. C., Pye, J. E., & Guastella, A. J. (2018). Autism spectrum disorders: A meta-analysis of executive function. *Molecular Psychiatry, 23*(5), 1198–1204.

De Vries, M., & Geurts, H. (2015). Influence of autism traits and executive functioning on quality of life in children with an autism spectrum disorder. *Journal of Autism and Developmental Disorders, 9*, 2734–2743.

Frith, U., & Happé, F. (1994). Autism: Beyond 'theory of mind'. *Cognition, 50*(1–3), 115–132.

Gallagher, S., & Varga, S. (2015). Conceptual issues in autism spectrum disorders. *Current Opinion in Psychiatry, 28*(2), 127–132.

Geurts, H. M., & Jansen, M. D. (2011). A retrospective chart study: The pathway to a diagnosis for adults referred for ASD assessment. *Autism, 16*(3), 299–305.

Gotham, K., Risi, S., Pickles, A., & Lord, C. (2007). The Autism Diagnostic Observation Schedule: Revised algorithms for improved diagnostic validity. *Journal of Autism and Developmental Disorders, 37*(4), 613–627.

Haigh, S. M., Walsh, J. A., Mazefsky, C. A., Minshew, N. J., & Eack, S. M. (2018). Processing speed is impaired in adults with autism spectrum disorder, and relates to social communication abilities. *Journal of Autism and Developmental Disorders, 48*(8), 2653–2662.

Happé, F., & Frith, U. (2006). The weak coherence account: Detail-focused cognitive style in autism spectrum disorders. *Journal of Autism and Developmental Disorders, 36*(1), 5–25.

Hughes, J. E. A., Ward, J., & Gruffydd, E. (2018). Savant syndrome has a distinct psychological profile in autism. *Molecular Autism, 9*, 53.

Johnston, K., Dittner, A., Bramham, J., Murphy, C., Knight, A., & Russell, A. (2013). Attention deficit hyperactivity disorder symptoms in adults with autism spectrum disorders. *Autism Research, 6*(4), 225–236.

Johnston, K., Murray, K., Spain, D., Walker, I., Russell, A. (2019). Executive function: Cognition and behaviour in adults with autism spectrum disorders. *Journal of Autism and Developmental Disorders, 49*(10), 4181–4192.

King, J. B., Prigge, M. B., King, C., Morgan, J., Dean, D., Freeman, A., Alfonso, J., Villaruz, M., Kane, K. L., Bigler, E. D., Alexander, A. L., Lange, N., Zielinski, B. A., Lainhart, J. E., & Anderson, J. A. (2018). Evaluation of differences in temporal synchrony between brain regions in individuals with autism and typical development. *JAMA Network Open, 1*(7), e184777. https://doi.org/10.1001/jamanetworkopen.2018.4777

Meem, L. (2015). Cognitive Assessment Behaviour Checklist: 89 behaviours worth noting when writing reports and referring on (paper presented at the Asia Pacific Autism Conference, September 9, 2015). Brisbane, Australia.

Misra, V. (2014). The social brain network and autism. *Annals of Neurosciences, 21*(2), 69–73.

Morsanyi, K., van Bers, B. M., McCormak, T., & McGourty, J. (2018). The prevalence of specific learning disorder in mathematics and comorbidity with other developmental disorders in primary school-age children. *British Journal of Psychology, 109*, 917–940.

Nason, B. (2014). *The autism discussion page on stress, anxiety, shutdowns and meltdowns.* Jessica Kingsley Publishers.

National Autistic Society. (2018). *Autism facts and history.* National Autistic Society. www.autism.org.uk

National Autistic Society & Mind. (2021). *Good practice guide for professionals delivering talking therapies for autistic adults and children.* www.mind.org.uk/media/11912/nas-good-practice-guide-a4.pdf

National Institute for Health and Care Excellence. (2021). Autism spectrum disorder in adults: Diagnosis and management (NICE Guideline No. 142]. www.nice.org.uk/guidance/cg142

Pan, P. Y., Bolte, S., & Kaur, P. (2020). Neurological disorders in autism: A systematic review and meta-analysis. *Autism, 25*(3), 812–830.

Powell, T. (2021) *Recognising autism and Asperger's syndrome: A practical guide to adult diagnosis and beyon* (2nd ed.). Routledge, ISBN 9780367427610.

Rynkiewicz, A., Janas-Kozik, M., & Słopień, A. (2019). Girls and women with autism. *Psychiatria Polska, 53*(4), 737–752.

Tuchman, R., & Rapin, I. (2002). Epilepsy in autism. *The Lancet Neurology, 1*(6), 352–358.

Wallace, G. L., Kenworthy, L., & Pugliese, C. E. (2016). Real-world executive functions in adults with autism spectrum disorder: Profiles of impairment and associations with adaptive functioning and co-morbid anxiety and depression. *Journal of Autism and Developmental Disorders, 46*, 1071–1083.

Westwood, H., & Tchanturia, K. (2017). Autism spectrum disorder in anorexia nervosa: An updated literature review. *Current Psychiatry Reports, 19*(7), 41.

Wikramanayake, W. N. M, Mandy, W., Shahper, S., Kaur, S., Kolli, S., & Osman, S. (2018). Autism spectrum disorders in adult outpatients with obsessive compulsive disorder in the UK. *International Journal of Psychiatry in Clinical Practice, 22*, 54–62.

Xie, R., Sun, X., Yang, L., & Guo, Y. (2020) Characteristic executive dysfunction for high-functioning autism sustained to adulthood. *Autism Research, 13*(12), 2102–2121.

18 What's in the diagnosis of 'ASD' in the context of Paediatric ABI?

Jenny Jim, Laura Carroll, Enrique Childress, Louise Owen, Elizabeth Roberts, Isabelle Sharples, and Valeria Lowing

Introduction

I've been fully diagnosed as autistic, which was very expected and good as it has given me a lot of closure.

(Annabel, 16 yrs, who welcomed a diagnosis of ASD in the context of developmental trauma and ABI)

When meeting people for the first time it's easier to mention X has autism, a label which more people understand these days, rather than try to explain the intricate details of an unfamiliar diagnosis such as hemiconvulsive hemiplegic epilepsy.

(Parents of Zenah, 9 yrs, whose intractable epilepsy and ASD symptoms appeared concurrently, very early in development)

Someone finally understood what they had been trying to say for years.

(Parents of Carlo, 13 yrs, who successfully challenged the legitimacy of a post-brain injury ASD diagnosis given when he was 10 yrs)

Autism spectrum disorder (ASD) is characterised by a dyad of core symptomatology encompassing social communication and restricted and repetitive behaviours, including sensory symptoms (DSM-V, APA, 2013a). As a neurodevelopmental disorder, ASD symptoms must be present in early childhood, even if these are not recognised at the time (APA, 2013b). ASD aetiology is complex. Myriad environmental factors are potentially associated, including pollution, extreme prematurity, and birth complications (Crump et al., 2021; Curran et al., 2015; Maramara et al., 2014) but effect sizes are small. Genetically, there is 50% heritability (Sandin et al., 2014) and a number of rare genetic disorders are associated with ASD, such as Angelman syndrome, tuberous sclerosis, and Phelan-McDermid syndrome (Persico & Napolioni, 2013). Although effect sizes are large for these syndromes, a child does not *always* develop ASD in these cases and no single gene variation process has

DOI: 10.4324/9781003228226-20

yet been identified (Pinto et al., 2010). Crucially, by its very definition as a neurodevelopmental disorder, there is no concept of ASD as an acquired disorder. The average age of diagnosis in the UK is around 5.5 years (Howlin & Asgharian, 1999), suggesting that symptoms should be apparent at least from this age, if not prior. A very recent research focus is to identify early signs and early intervention effectiveness, almost from infancy (such as the British Autism Study of Infant Siblings network, www.basisnetwork.org/) and indeed diagnostic stability in children identified before the age of three is remarkably high (Ozonoff et al., 2015).

However, it is erroneous to assume that ASD was either not present, or conversely always present in a child's early development, waiting to be discovered or refuted. As clinicians, we are aware of the controversies in early markers when delving into a child's developmental history to assess whether an individual was at risk of developing ASD. Very early markers, such as attenuated gaze shifts at 6–9 months (Elsabbagh et al., 2013), or reduced sensitivity to social auditory stimuli over the superior temporal sulcus at five months (Lloyd-Fox et al., 2013) are currently represented at group level in research, and are inaccessible to assess for most clinicians working with the family some years later. Even behavioural markers, such as atypical eye contact, or reduced joint attention in the first few years of life (Woolfenden et al., 2012) rely on accurate parent report and are not necessarily specific to ASD.

These so called 'early signs' *could* lead to ASD, but can also be associated with later ADHD, or indeed global, or even no overall impairment (Johnson et al., 2015). During developmental history taking we may uncover behaviours that lead us to hypothesise ASD might have been present, but crucially, these early markers also do not always reflect later deficits (Gliga et al., 2014). We are also aware that differences between high- versus low-risk ASD groups could be equally well explained by genetic correlates or familial environment (Gliga et al., 2014), and identifying ASD in the context of an acquired brain injury (ABI) is therefore particularly challenging.

As neuropsychologists, we also reflect on recent theories of brain development. These posit an activity-dependent process which is bi-directional between environment and genetics, set against a backdrop of probabilistic epigenesis (Johnson & de Haan, 2015). The causal pathway to ASD symptomatology is therefore likely to be probabilistic, rather than deterministic. Perhaps a child was at risk of developing ASD and an ABI has compounded that risk. Perhaps the child would not have developed ASD without the ABI. The underlying developmental mechanisms leading to ASD are likely to implicate both atypical cortical development (including disruptions to development, such as prematurity, or ABI) and resulting adaptations alongside environmental factors. It is therefore paramount to consider the causal pathway of the individual child's development and hypothesise in which ways the ABI has potentially interacted with this path. Part of our role is also to assess whether the ASD diagnostic pathway makes sense for an individual on a neuroanatomical, functional, and psychosocial level and whether this can lead to life improvement for that individual.

Our practice is guided by the core question, 'What is likely to lead to positive change for the CYPF we work with?' and in reality, this outcome is co-constructed with the children, young people, and families (CYPF). It changes and is influenced by many factors including access to resources, the systems around them and biases in terms of knowledges that we have or do not have, the information that is elicited and said, and the information that is not asked about and therefore not said. We accept that by taking this position we do not seek an ultimate and objective truth but construct together a narrative with our interpretations of multiple sources of evidence that 'fits' at the time. What we are advocating for is a reflexive process that allows us to keep the CYPF in the centre and highlights that labels are a form of language that constructs realities that can unwittingly serve to close off multiplicity in our hypotheses, lose engagement, and at worst, result in inappropriate intervention and compromise recovery and add to secondary unnecessary impairment. Diagnosis may alienate key agents of change: caregivers, professionals, and crucially the CYP themselves. However, at best, we see that diagnosis can serve to reinforce an ego-syntonic sense of self at a time when validation of identity is crucial to progress and recovery.

Our stance is one of holistic formulation. We have developed specific models such as 'SPECS' (taking into account social, physical, emotional, cognitive, spiritual/identity strengths and needs; see Jim & Liddiard, 2019) and NIF-TY (Neuropsychological Integrated Formulation model; see Jim & Liddiard, 2019) based on comprehensive assessment (Watson & Gracey, 2020), essentially, using our expertise that covers risk and resiliency factors across the lifespan within a biopsychosocial model shaped by our professional backgrounds as clinical and educational psychologists. With this in mind, we present Annabella, Zenah, and Carlo, three CYP and their families for whom the question of ASD was paired with life-changing implications. Through these stories we hope to illustrate the diverse and complex nature of ASD within ABI and suggest a framework/reflections for practice that helps hold each CYP and their family's unique circumstances in mind.

Annabella

Annabella is a 14-year-old with a background of developmental trauma and pre-existing mental health difficulties. Difficulties with social communication are evident from Annabella's own formulation of her needs, as well as her early history. Annabella had unusual special interests, a lack of imaginative play, and difficulty initiating or maintaining social interactions at around four years. There was a paternal family history of neurodevelopmental disorders, including ASD. Annabella also experienced significant developmental trauma. Her mother reported she suffered post-natal depression following Annabella's birth. Annabella herself reported a history of traumatic experiences including being homeless as a young child, witnessing frequent conflict between her parents, being bullied, and she also experienced verbal abuse within the home. Annabella also described how she had difficulty with introspection, leaving her feeling she had no mastery over her internal state. She felt disconnected, unsafe, and mistrusting of the adults in her life. Annabella very expertly hid her feelings and emotions for fear of seeming weak and vulnerable. Her mental health was affected as a result. This culminated in suicidal ideation and multiple suicide attempts. The most serious of these occurred when she was fourteen. On this occasion, she jumped from the fourth floor of a multi-storey car park, leading her to sustain a severe brain injury including a haemorrhage in the frontal region of her brain, as well as diffuse axonal injury. As a result of her acquired needs, Annabella was offered an eight-week placement for residential neurorehabilitation. Her neurorehabilitation placement was used to further explore this formulation, given that social communication difficulties and childhood trauma are associated with later mental health difficulties, including suicidal ideation and attempt (Yong-Chun et al., 2017; Barbosa et al., 2014).

ASD diagnosis

As part of her neurorehabilitation placement, holistic assessment was completed with Annabella and her family. Although the assessment covered many facets, including systemic factors, neuropsychological skills, emotional well-being, trauma, risk, and social communication, the focus in this chapter is the formulation of Annabella's social communication skills (Figure 18.1).

The formulation illustrates that Annabella had several needs that fit the criteria for ASD. She has a history of difficulty initiating and maintaining social relationships, alongside difficulties with introspection. She shows rigidity in her thinking, seeking perfection, having 'black and white' thinking patterns and having difficulty seeing situations from the perspectives of others. She has a tendency to mask her true feelings, a common trait amongst high functioning girls with ASD (Tubío-Fungueiriño et al., 2021). She also has diagnoses of anxiety and depression, which are often observed co-morbidly with ASD, particularly within those that mask (Soloman et al., 2012).

Outcome

Whilst Annabella certainly meets a great deal of the diagnostic criteria, there are potential differential diagnoses to consider (e.g., developmental trauma, brain injury, mood disorder). As such, there needs to be caution and consideration before making a diagnosis of ASD. Whilst Annabella has familial risk factors and reported atypical social communication development, her brain injury might underpin some of her current presentation. Frontal lobe brain injuries are known to affect social skills and understanding (Rosema et al., 2012) and may well be a root cause of Annabella's current needs. In addition,

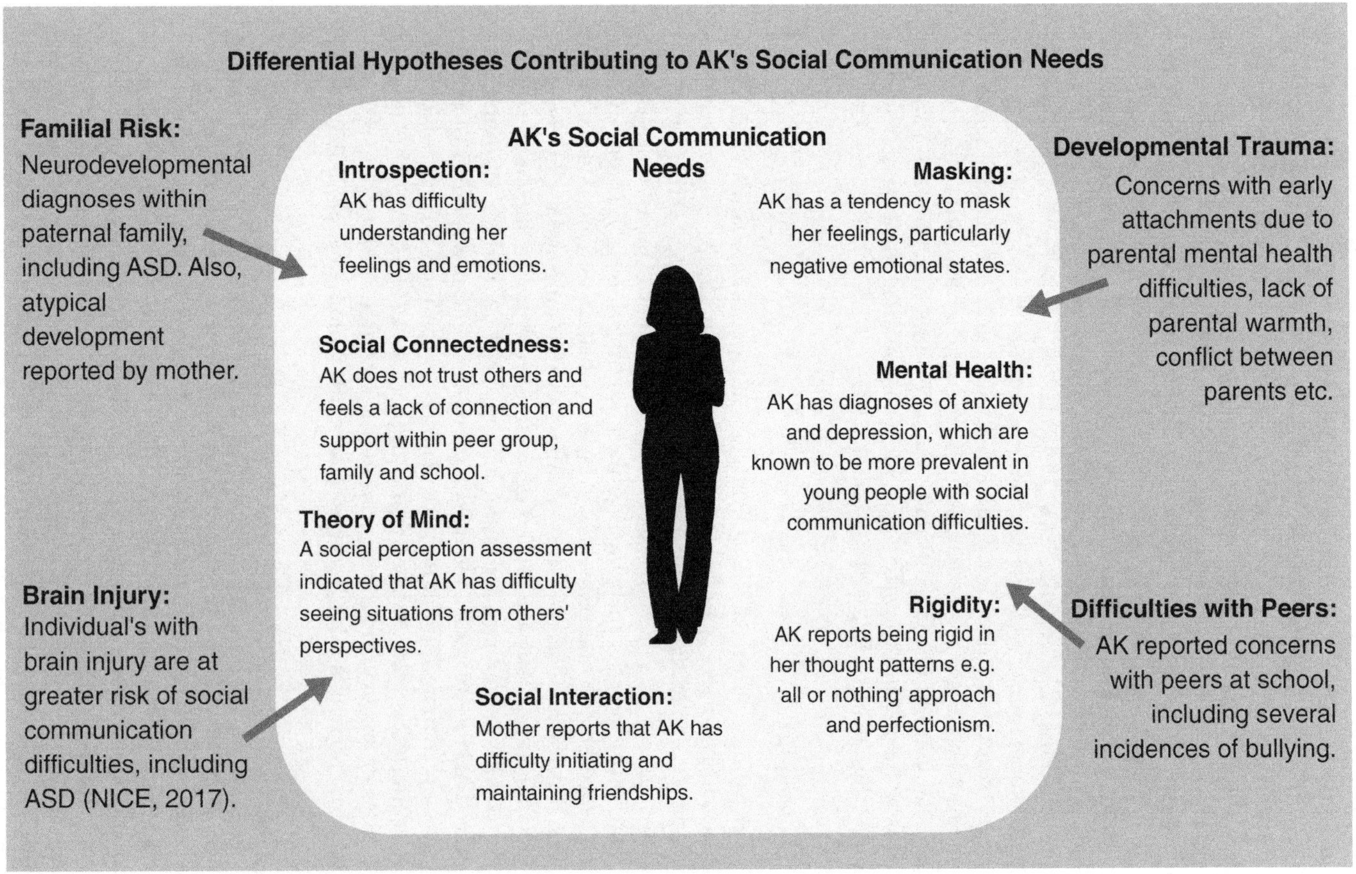

Differential Hypotheses Contributing to AK's Social Communication Needs

Familial Risk:
Neurodevelopmental diagnoses within paternal family, including ASD. Also, atypical development reported by mother.

Brain Injury:
Individual's with brain injury are at greater risk of social communication difficulties, including ASD (NICE, 2017).

Developmental Trauma:
Concerns with early attachments due to parental mental health difficulties, lack of parental warmth, conflict between parents etc.

Difficulties with Peers:
AK reported concerns with peers at school, including several incidences of bullying.

AK's Social Communication Needs

Introspection:
AK has difficulty understanding her feelings and emotions.

Social Connectedness:
AK does not trust others and feels a lack of connection and support within peer group, family and school.

Theory of Mind:
A social perception assessment indicated that AK has difficulty seeing situations from others' perspectives.

Social Interaction:
Mother reports that AK has difficulty initiating and maintaining friendships.

Masking:
AK has a tendency to mask her feelings, particularly negative emotional states.

Mental Health:
AK has diagnoses of anxiety and depression, which are known to be more prevalent in young people with social communication difficulties.

Rigidity:
AK reports being rigid in her thought patterns e.g. 'all or nothing' approach and perfectionism.

Figure 18.1 Annabella's formulation

she has experienced developmental trauma as the result of a number of adverse family circumstances. Such experiences are also known to affect social communication development (Moran, 2010), but are not always indicators of ASD. Despite the complexities with differential diagnosis, Annabella received a diagnosis of ASD. This was a multidisciplinary team decision, which took place over several weeks of Anabella's placement, involving Annabella, her mother, her neurorehabilitation team, and a visiting neuropsychiatrist.

The formulation and diagnosis was shared with Annabella to explore her views about this. Annabella shared that she found the label of ASD useful, as it helped her to understand some of her ways of thinking and interacting in a way that she had not made sense of them before. She also felt that it would provide a way for those around her to have more of an understanding of her needs, as well as connecting her with wider options for support.

We can never be really sure whether Annabella 'truly has' the neurodevelopmental disorder of ASD; or whether her impaired social communication skills are a result of a more complex interaction of social, environmental, and ABI factors. However, it is also important to ask whether this distinction is meaningful, or helpful. In the end, Annabella's diagnosis of ASD was the most appropriate description of her needs and the key reason this was advocated for was because Annabella said that she felt it would be helpful to her.

Zenah

Zenah was a typically developing child at age two when she first experienced a prolonged convulsive seizure following a febrile illness. She was hospitalised and needed intubation and ventilation and her seizures continued. Zenah was diagnosed with intractable epilepsy and explosive onset of right focal seizures evolving to focal status epilepticus. She acquired a right hemiplegia with dystonia and a regression in developmental skills and language. Zenah was admitted to intensive paediatric neurorehabilitation, making significant gains in her dystonia and communication skills, but her seizures continued once weaned off medication. During this time her parents noted a significant regression in developmental skills, including speech and language. When Zenah started preschool aged four, her parents noticed she was delayed in her social skills compared to her peers. They raised their concerns to the local community team but it was concluded that Zenah's difficulties were largely due to her brain injury and no further assessment was needed.

ASD diagnosis

Zenah was assessed several times following her initial onset of seizures. Most noteworthy was when she was assessed prior to left-hemispherectomy aged seven. Her behaviour was described as nervous, apprehensive, self-directed, and challenging, and it was noted that she struggled to connect with the adults around her. This aligned with her parents' concerns, who also highlighted her challenging behaviours and difficulties interacting with peers, together with difficulties with eye contact, and repetitive and sensory seeking behaviours. Difficulties with both receptive and expressive language were also noted, despite good single word vocabulary. At this age, Zenah experienced significant difficulties with behaviour, daily skills, social communication, and emotional well-being. Her behaviour during the assessment was self-directed and repetitive, with little understanding of the world of others. It was during the pre-surgery neuropsychological assessment that Zenah was diagnosed with ASD, as well as mild/moderate intellectual disability.

Zenah came for a period of rehabilitation, following a left hemispherectomy when she was eight. She now had hemianopia which impacted her performance on vision-based tests but she was able to access further assessments. The results of these assessments were broadly in line with her pre-surgery formulation and indicated Zenah had moderate executive functioning difficulties, as well as mild memory difficulties. She experienced significant attention difficulties and these may have been exacerbated by sensory difficulties. However, as Zenah remained seizure free, a significant difference in her social skills began to emerge. She became more interested in building social relationships with the people around her and she was more engaged in her neuro-rehab sessions. She also started seeking out support from those around her and connected well to her therapy team.

The complexity of Zenah's ASD diagnosis is exacerbated by the early onset of her seizures. Although her early development was similar to her twin sister, Zenah was very young for early ASD symptoms to have been particularly apparent. Zenah's parents noted significant skill regression after the onset of her seizures, in particular in speech, language, and social domains. ASD and epilepsy often co-occur (Besag & Vasey, 2021; Sunderlin et al., 2016) and, unsurprisingly, skill regression often coincides with seizure onset (Velíšková et al., 2018). Recent research suggests a common aetiology for co-occurring ASD/epilepsy is likely although, controversially, no causal mechanism has been elucidated (Besag & Vasey, 2021; Velíšková et al., 2018). Nevertheless, the hypothesis that Zenah's presentation at age seven is predominantly a result of brain injury cannot be excluded and continued monitoring and assessment will be key to identify whether, in the absence of seizures, continued improvements are seen in her social communication.

Outcome

Zenah's parents felt the ASD label remained useful as it provided a shortcut to the description of her needs without the need for them to describe the complexities of an ABI. The challenge as clinicians was to evaluate the utility of the diagnostic label alongside the impact of ABI in a comprehensive formulation within a holistic framework. We were able to provide brain injury education to Zenah's school and community which enabled the systems around her to consider a dynamic approach to meeting her needs. She continues to make progress both in her learning and in her social interactions and has access to ASD services which support her appropriately. Perhaps in the future, Zenah will be given the opportunity to reflect on her ASD diagnosis and whether she finds this a helpful framework to explain her strengths and needs.

Carlo

When Carlo was seven he experienced a vacant episode, headaches, vomiting, double vision and sixth nerve palsy, following sinusitis. After numerous visits to the GP, Carlo eventually had a scan which revealed a right frontal lobe abscess. The abscess was large enough to cause a midline shift and mass effect. A few months after the abscess was removed, Carlo's parents noticed gradual changes in his mood and behaviour. He had a 'different personality': sleep disturbances and bouts of acute anger, aggression, and depression accompanied by wild mood swings. Sadly, 'at times he would threaten us, attack us physically, and talk about wanting to die, and even tied a scarf around his neck saying he would kill himself'.

ASD diagnosis

Carlo underwent many assessments during the following years. Much time was spent on waiting lists. Nine months after his injury he underwent a neuropsychological assessment and when he was eight, he was diagnosed with specific needle phobia and separation anxiety with generalised anxiety disorder. Following this, at age ten Carlo had a neurodevelopmental assessment diagnosing historical (pre-ABI) autism spectrum disorder (ASD) of Asperger's phenotype. From this point forward, Carlo received intervention focusing predominantly on specific phobias and ASD within his school and local community. None of which were effective in meeting his needs or helping him function. Crucially, professional input was disjointed, addressing specific issues in isolation.

Carlo and his parents disagreed with his ASD diagnosis, maintaining that marked changes in Carlo's behaviour arose six months post-brain injury and were not present through his early development. They felt professionals considered behavioural responses separately and were 'not joining up the dots'. Carlo and his family lived with the ASD diagnosis for three years before it was finally removed following a multidisciplinary assessment, referred by the GP. Carlo, now aged 13, had a deep lack of trust in professionals as continued ineffective provision was put in place which never did support him. Unfortunately, despite the removal of the ASD diagnosis, this still dominated Carlo's narrative in the school system. Relationships at school were deteriorating and Carlo had regular emotional outbursts. He became disengaged, caught in a vicious cycle of escalating behaviour and punitive behaviour management.

Challenging the ASD diagnosis

At the time we met Carlo, aged 13, he understandably expressed a dislike of psychologists. The ASD-dominant narrative had impacted Carlo's self-esteem, mental health, and academic progress. To challenge the power of this narrative, an ABI-based re-formulation of Carlo's needs was collaboratively constructed (Figure 18.2). It was subsequently used alongside information gathered from Carlo, his parents, and school staff to identify their priorities for specialised support.

Using neuropsychological knowledge within a subsequent holistic multidisciplinary team (MDT) assessment, Carlo's frontal lobe injury was re-formulated to be a causative factor for both emotional/mood regulation challenges *and* severe executive dysfunction affecting cognition and learning. The behavioural presentation of difficulties with transition, adjusting to change, peer relationships, and a limited range of interests could now be accounted for by executive dysfunction, cognitive difficulties with planning and sequencing, social anxiety, and cognitive rigidity, which were in keeping with right frontal lobe injury.

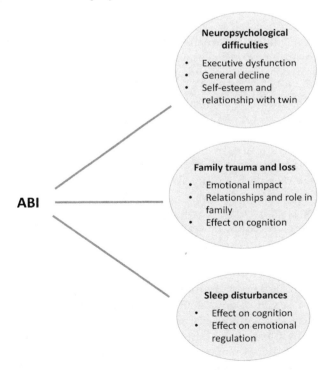

Figure 18.2 re-formulation of difficulties in context of ABI

Outcome

The re-formulation became a core component of the intervention. It was strengthened by ABI psychoeducation for Carlo, his family, and the school system. By constructing a shared family narrative (siblings were included) of what brain injury is and how it has impacted Carlo, the family felt that 'someone finally understood what they had been trying to say for years'. Psychoeducation for school staff were key to dismantling the ASD narrative. Sharing images of Carlo's brain scans from the time of his abscess demonstrated tangible differences and thereby proved a tangible learning tool. This helped the school differentiate Carlo's support from other pupils with ASD. The session promoted empathy and understanding, paving the way for new and more bespoke behavioural and cognitive planning with the school staff based on an ABI framework. Cognitive and learning support was tailored to a shared agreement that others provide role-modelling and 'be his frontal lobes'.

Further interventions provided support on different levels. At an individual level, Carlo and his siblings took part in a cognitive behavioural therapy (CBT) based intervention exploring links between thoughts, feelings, and behaviour. School-level consultation with staff supported implementation of cognitive rehabilitation and reviewing of emotional support and behavioural plans. Parent-level support was provided to implement sleep routines and strategies. Carlo's behavioural incidents at the school significantly reduced, and the family experienced greater family positivity and empowerment. Carlo felt able to engage with further psychological intervention. When Carlo moved to a new school his re-formulation was shared with staff, alongside a psycho-education session, and this lay foundations for a successful transition.

Discussion

From working with young people and their families in our rehabilitation service we have learnt that an ASD diagnosis in the context of ABI has powerful consequences and is never straightforward. For Annabel the diagnosis was an integral component of her story, and for Zenah's family it was a useful shortcut to explaining her needs to others without having to delve into painful recollections of the ABI. Conversely, in Carlo's case the ASD diagnosis was detrimental to the formulation of his needs. It was a source of frustration for Carlo and his family and led community services and the school to misunderstand him, misinterpret his behaviours, and therefore provide inappropriate intervention. Three key themes emerge from our case studies and reflections follow below. Firstly, we consider ASD symptoms in early development in the context of ABI. Secondly, we evaluate the concept of acquired ASD and why this may not be appropriate. Thirdly, and perhaps most importantly, we outline the ways in which ABI and ASD differ with regard to impact on a young person's identity and narrative.

ASD symptoms in early development: the importance of a developmental history

The current definition of ASD states that characteristics including aspects of social communication and restricted, repetitive behaviours must be present early in development (APA, 2013b). This was certainly the case for Annabel, supporting her diagnosis. Carlo's case is somewhat different. Initially, his diagnostic report mentions early ASD 'symptoms' but his diagnosis was later removed since his parents strongly refuted this claim, explaining that his 'symptoms' only appeared after the age of seven, the time at which Carlo had his ABI. So, in fact, Carlo never really had any ASD symptoms, and his presenting characteristics should always have been formulated within an ABI framework. These two cases illustrate the importance of obtaining an accurate developmental history in order to support or refute a diagnostic pathway to ASD.

Zenah's case, however, shows it is not always possible to untangle ABI from ASD behaviours, since her ABI was acquired at such a young age. Her developmental history alone would have been insufficient to support a route to diagnosis and other factors would need to be considered. There is a 20–30% overlap of ASD and epilepsy (Besag, 2015; Seidenberg et al., 2009; Tuchman & Rapin, 2002), which is more common in girls (Tuchman et al., 2010). Although common underlying mechanisms for this phenomenon are currently elusive, it may be that one or the other nudged Zenah's neurodevelopment onto a pathway that led her towards an ASD outcome. It will not be possible to ascertain whether Zenah's autism pre-dated her intractable epilepsy, whether the epilepsy and ASD shared aetiologies, or whether the ASD behavioural features were an outcome of the brain injury. However, the crux is that, for Zenah's family, the diagnosis provided not only meaningful understanding, but also access to resources.

ASD symptoms post ABI: the risks of considering acquired ASD

The question of whether one can 'acquire' ASD is provocative. Currently, the definition does not allow for this, nor perhaps should it. On the one hand, the term acquired, secondary or atypical ASD, could be a way of packaging a presentation into a familiar label that others can understand and will take seriously. Access to resources and intervention is likely to be enabled. And, indeed, many of the interventions will focus on characteristics for which a young person may need support. For example, children with ASD can often have difficulties with emotional regulation and/or executive functioning (Mazefsky et al., 2013; Woodcock et al., 2020) and many interventions are already up and running in community settings, especially in schools (Robinson et al., 2018). A child with ABI and a diagnosis of 'secondary ASD' could readily access a world of support and intervention, perhaps much like Zenah is currently thriving on. On the other hand, ABI is complex and heterogenous and acquired/secondary ASD risks an over-simplification and misinterpretation of a young person's presentation. This, as we saw in Carlo's case, can have catastrophic long-term consequences.

The acquired/secondary ASD contention is particularly salient depending on the nature of the brain injury. Carlo's injury was the result of an abscess, and this can be associated with high rates of neurological impairment (Gelabert-González et al., 2008). However, there is a paucity of research and in the study referenced, only seven children (out of 28) with a brain abscess had neurological sequelae and none was identified with social communication difficulties (Gelabert-González et al., 2008). Perhaps injury location is a more useful consideration, where frontal lobe injury may mirror some difficulties associated with ASD. Theoretically, it is reasonable to assume a frontal lobe abscess may lead to frontal lobe associated difficulties such as executive dysfunction, which is also a common area of need for children with ASD (Geurts et al., 2014). Children with bilateral orbitofrontal damage and children with ASD have similar deficits in Theory of Mind tests (Stone & Gerrans, 2006). Frontal lobe injury can be associated with resisting interference from salient alternative responses (Stuss et al., 2001) which could be argued is an overlapping characteristic with ASD. It is therefore particularly important to be alert to a false ASD narrative within the context of a frontal lobe injury, such as Carlo's.

ASD and ABI: identity formed, identity changed

Even when similarities are drawn between ASD and types of ABI, and behavioural symptoms and characteristics appear similar, there is often a crucial difference to one component of a young person's neurorehabilitation: identity. The unique experience of ABI contrasts a neurodevelopmental ASD profile. When a child or young person acquires a brain injury, they often have a memory of being able to do things that are now difficult. They may have an awareness of being changed, or different. Not only is their sense of self affected on a personal level, but their families and friends may have a sense of loss and even grieve for what the person could previously do or how they previously presented. With ABI there is unpredictability and a longing for improvement. As clinicians in neurorehabilitation we work within a framework of reasonable hope and an expectation that things may change. Identity within the context of a neurodevelopmental disorder will be different. The process is likely to be more gradual, often without a single traumatic event that changed everything, as with ABI. The impact of an ASD diagnosis after ABI will have its own challenges for identity. It needs to be carefully woven into identity work together with the young person and their families to help them construct meaningful and adaptive narrative of their unique situation.

Implications for practice

We face complex issues when working with severely brain injured children and young people and their families, especially when their injured child displays 'symptoms' that appear to relate to a diagnosis of ASD. This complexity is not only linked to whether the CYP's needs fit a diagnosis, but also whether a diagnosis will resonate with the CYP and whether it will continue to be helpful throughout their lifetime. A diagnosis can lead to helpful and rapid access to resources and intervention. But in the longer term, there is a real risk of a CYP's ABI needs being overshadowed by the ASD label. Community teams are often less familiar with the fluctuation in presentation of a CYP with ABI. They may assume that since the ABI happened long ago, it may not be linked to new emerging difficulties. Continuous assessment and re-formulation, alongside brain injury education, is important to help equip the CYPF to advocate for their ABI needs when these change or become more apparent.

There is learning that we as clinicians can take from our experiences which mediates our thinking when a child or young person presents with ASD symptoms, or an ASD diagnosis.

(i) *Comprehensive assessment within a biopsychosocial model*

The practice examples of Annabel, Zenah, and Carlo demonstrate the importance of assessment incorporating a thorough understanding of environmental, family, cognitive, social, emotional, and behavioural characteristics from birth through to current age. These are integrated into a biopsychosocial model using frameworks for practice such as SPECS, NIF-TY, and SNAP (Systematic Neuropsychological Assessment Profile, see Jim & Liddiard, 2019), which enable us to create formulations that can be shared with the family and young person. This enables us to gain their views, check our understanding, and ensure the route to intervention is helpful and relevant.

(ii) *Identity rehabilitation is key*

Whilst developmental, neuropsychological, and psychiatric assessments are important parts of a formulation, understanding the identity factors for the CYP is also paramount. We find it useful to consider a concept of rehabilitation as needing to look beyond the loss of skills to the young person's 'sense of self' (Perkins, 2020). This involves paying attention to the young person's identity, and the resilience of their identity.

(iii) *Interdisciplinary communication and active participation*

In order to ascertain a thorough developmental picture of a CYP, communication between professionals is crucial. This includes sharing assessment information and ensuring an ongoing dialogue. It is important that formulations are reviewed regularly and updated based on new information and evidence from ongoing assessments.

Alongside co-constructing a formulation between professionals, the views of CYPF should be central to all discussions. As clinicians, we are well versed in ascertaining the views of CYPF. We also find that many more professionals are beginning to ask CYP for their views. Whilst we commend this first step, our experience in a paediatric neurorehabilitation service suggests that, in order to be effective, eliciting views should lead to further work to include the CYP in their own plans. CYPF need to be active participants in discussions and formulation. This can lead to a shared understanding and agreed ways forward in how best to meet a CYP's needs with a focus on strengths. This joint approach of shared formulation, careful planning and active participation has led to improved tangible outcomes for Annabel, Zenah, and Carlo, as well as other young people and their families who have come for neurorehabilitation.

Acknowledgements

With thanks to Gemma Costello, Amanda Davies, and Susan Lawton at The Children's Trust.

References

American Psychiatric Association (2013a). *Diagnostic and statistical manual of mental disorders: DSM-5* (5th ed.). American Psychiatric Publishing.

American Psychiatric Association, (2013b). file:///media/fuse/drivefs-6f480b-77c7e9461180a471a8da7812c0/root/Book%20Chapter/APA_DSM-5-Autism-Spectrum-Disorder.pdf; accessed 29th September 2021.

Barbosa, L. P., Quevedo, L., da Silva, G. D. G., Jansen, K., Pinheiro, R. T., Branco, J., ... & da Silva, R. A. (2014). Childhood trauma and suicide risk in a sample of young individuals aged 14–35 years in southern Brazil. *Child Abuse & Neglect*, *38*(7), 1191–1196.

Besag F. M. (2015). Current controversies in the relationships between autism and epilepsy. *Epilepsy & Behavior: E&B*, *47*, 143–146.

Besag, F., & Vasey, M. J. (2021). Seizures and epilepsy in autism spectrum disorder. *The Psychiatric Clinics of North America*, *44*(1), 51–68.

Crump, C., Sundquist, J., & Sundquist, K., (2021). Preterm or early term birth and risk of autism. *Pediatrics*. *148*(3), e2020032300. https://doi.org/10.1542/peds.2020-032300

Curran, E. A., O'Neill, S. M., Cryan, J. F., Kenny, L. C., Dinan, T. G., Khashan, A. S., & Kearney, P. M. (2015). Research review: Birth by caesarean section and development of autism spectrum disorder and attention-deficit/hyperactivity disorder: A systematic review and meta-analysis. *Journal of Child Psychology and Psychiatry*, *56*(5), 500–508.

Elsabbagh, M., Fernandes, J., Webb, S. J., Dawson, G., Charman, T., Johnson, M. H., & British Autism Study of Infant Siblings Team. (2013). Disengagement of visual attention in infancy is associated with emerging autism in toddlerhood. *Biological Psychiatry*, *74*(3), 189–194. https://doi.org/10.1016/j.biopsych.2012.11.030

Gelabert-González, M., Serramito-García, R., García-Allut, A., & Cutrín-Prieto, J. (2008). Management of brain abscess in children. *Journal of Paediatrics and Child Health*, *44*(12), 731–735.

Geurts, H. M., de Vries, M., & van den Bergh, S. F. (2014). Executive functioning theory and autism. In *Handbook of executive functioning* (pp. 121–141). Springer.

Gliga, T., Jones, E. J., Bedford, R., Charman, T., & Johnson, M. H. (2014). From early markers to neuro-developmental mechanisms of autism. *Developmental Review, 34*(3), 189–207.

Howlin, P., & Asgharian, A. (1999). The diagnosis of autism and Asperger syndrome: findings from a survey of 770 families. *Developmental Medicine and Child Neurology, 41*(12), 834–839. https://doi.org/10.1017/S0012162299001656

Jim, J., & Liddard, H. (2019). Using biopsychosocial formulations in paediatric neurorehabilitation. In J. Jim, & E. Cole (Eds.), *Psychological therapy for paediatric acquired brain injury: Innovations for children, young people and families* (pp. 70–89). Routledge.

Johnson, M., & de Haan, M. (2015). *Developmental cognitive neuroscience: An introduction*, (4th ed.). Wiley Blackwell, ISBN: 978-1-118-93808-9

Johnson, M. H., Gliga, T., Jones, E., & Charman, T. (2015). Annual Research Review: Infant development, autism, and ADHD – early pathways to emerging disorders. *Journal of Child Psychology and Psychiatry, 56*(3), 228–247.

Lloyd-Fox, S., Blasi, A., Elwell, C. E., Charman, T., Murphy, D., & Johnson, M. H. (2013). Reduced neural sensitivity to social stimuli in infants at risk for autism. *Proceedings of the Royal Society B: Biological Sciences, 280*(1758), 20123026. https://doi.org/10.1098/rspb.2012.3026

Maramara, L. A., He, W., & Ming, X. (2014). Pre-and perinatal risk factors for autism spectrum disorder in a New Jersey cohort. *Journal of Child Neurology, 29*(12), 1645–1651. https://doi.org/10.1177/0883073813512899

Mazefsky, C. A., Herrington, J., Siegel, M., Scarpa, A., Maddox, B. B., Scahill, L., & White, S. W. (2013). The role of emotion regulation in autism spectrum disorder. *Journal of the American Academy of Child & Adolescent Psychiatry, 52*(7), 679–688.

Moran, H. J. (2010). Clinical observations of the differences between children in the autism spectrum and those with attachment problems: The Coventry Grid. Good Autism Practice, 11(2), 46–59.

Ozonoff, S., Young, G. S., Landa, R. J., Brian, J., Bryson, S., Charman, T., Chawarska, K., Macari, S. L., Messinger, D., Stone, W. L., Zwaigenbaum, L., & Iosif, A. M. (2015). Diagnostic stability in young children at risk for autism spectrum disorder: A Baby Siblings Research Consortium study. *Journal of Child Psychology and Psychiatry, 56*(9), 988–998. https://doi.org/10.1111/jcpp.12421

Perkins, A. (2020), Psychological support using narrative psychotherapy for children with brain injury. *Neuropsychological Rehabilitation of Childhood Brain Injury, 18*, 215–234. https://doi.org/10.1057/9781137388223_11

Persico, A. M., & Napolioni, V. (2013). Autism genetics. *Behavioural Brain Research, 251*, 95–112. https://doi.org/10.1016/j.bbr.2013.06.012

Pinto, D., Pagnamenta, A. T., Klei, L., Anney, R., Merico, D., Regan, R., … & Yaspan, B. L. (2010). Functional impact of global rare copy number variation in autism spectrum disorders. *Nature, 466*(7304), 368–372.

Robinson, L., Bond, C., & Oldfield, J. (2018). A UK and Ireland survey of educational psychologists' intervention practices for students with autism spectrum disorder. *Educational Psychology in Practice, 34*(1), 58–72. https://doi.org/10.1080/02667363.2017.1391066

Rosema, S., Crowe, L., & Anderson, V. (2012). Social function in children and adolescents after traumatic brain injury: A systematic review 1989–2011. *Journal of Neurotrauma, 29*(7), 1277–1291.

Sandin, S., Lichtenstein, P., Kuja-Halkola, R., Larsson, H., Hultman, C. M., & Reichenberg, A. (2014). The familial risk of autism. *Jama, 311*(17), 1770–1777. https://doi.org/10.1001/jama.2014.4144

Seidenberg, M., Pulsipher, D. T., & Hermann, B. (2009). Association of epilepsy and comorbid conditions. *Future Neurology*, *4*(5), 663–668.

Soloman, M., Miller, M., Taylor, S. L., Hinshaw, S. P., & Carter, C. S. (2012). Autism symptoms and internalizing psychopathology in girls and boys with autism spectrum disorders. *Journal of Autism and Developmental Disorders*, *42*, 48–59.

Stone, V. E., & Gerrans, P. (2006). What's domain-specific about theory of mind?. *Social Neuroscience*, *1*(3–4), 309–319. https://doi.org/10.1080/17470910601029221

Stuss, D. T., Gallup Jr, G. G., & Alexander, M. P. (2001). The frontal lobes are necessary for theory of mind. *Brain*, *124*(2), 279–286. https://doi.org/10.1093/brain/124.2.279

Sundelin, H. E., Larsson, H., Lichtenstein, P., Almqvist, C., Hultman, C. M., Tomson, T., & Ludvigsson, J. F. (2016). Autism and epilepsy: A population-based nationwide cohort study. *Neurology*, *87*(2), 192–197.

Tubío-Fungueiriño, M., Cruz, S., Sampaio, A., Carracedo, A., & Fernández-Prieto, M. (2020). Social camouflaging in females with autism spectrum disorder: A systematic review. *Journal of Autism and Developmental Disorders*, *51*, 1–10. https://doi.org/10.1007/s10803-020-04695-x

Tuchman, R., Cuccaro, M., & Alessandri, M. (2010). Autism and epilepsy: Historical perspective. *Brain and Development*, *32*(9), 709–718.

Tuchman, R., & Rapin, I. (2002). Epilepsy in autism. *The Lancet Neurology*, *1*(6), 352–358.

Velíšková, J., Silverman, J. L., Benson, M., & Lenck-Santini, P. P. (2018). Autistic traits in epilepsy models: Why, when and how?. *Epilepsy research*, *144*, 62–70.

Watson, S., & Gracey, F. (2020). Assessment in paediatric acquired brain injury. In J. Jim & E. Cole (Eds.), *Psychological therapy for paediatric acquired brain injury: Innovations for children, young people and families* (pp. 43–69). Routledge/Taylor & Francis Group. https://doi.org/10.4324/9780429296932-4

Woodcock, K. A., Cheung, C., Marx, D. G., & Mandy, W. (2020). Social decision making in autistic adolescents: The role of theory of mind, executive functioning and emotion regulation. *Journal of Autism and Developmental Disorders*, *50*(7), 2501–2512.

Woolfenden, S., Sarkozy, V., Ridley, G., & Williams, K. (2012). A systematic review of the diagnostic stability of autism spectrum disorder. *Research in Autism Spectrum Disorders*, *6*(1), 345–354.

Yong-Chun, B., Seon-Kyeong, J., Kee-Hong, C., & Seung-Hwan, L. (2017). The relationship between childhood trauma and suicidal ideation: Role of maltreatment and potential mediators. *Psychiatry Investigation*, *14*(1), 37.

Part 3

Controversial issues and conditions

19 The dilemmas surrounding the decision to reject or accept a postgraduate research student with known cognitive difficulties and a history of an arteriovenous malformation several years prior

Rudi Coetzer

Introduction

Clinical neuropsychology folklore has it that the late Kevin Walsh during the 1990s famously (or perhaps infamously!) suggested, maybe even *insisted*, that 'Neuropsychology is a contact sport'. Considering the neuropsychology *zeitgeist* of that era, his statement (if true) was most likely made during a period of clinical practice when the 'bread and butter' work of most clinical neuropsychologists involved predominately cognitive testing, often for diagnostic purposes. *Patients* referred were 'seen' for neuropsychological testing, often during a single, very long session. Practitioners administered objective standardised tests and observed their patients' performance to come to some conclusion. Daily practice was mainly concerned with diagnostics and anatomical localisation. However, clinical neuropsychology as a profession has of course significantly changed and developed over the past three to four decades. Now rehabilitation has as important a role as assessment, if not even more significant, at least to those to whom it matters most – our clients. However, it would be unfair to say the one is more crucial than the other. Each informs the other in modern-day practice. Neuropsychological assessment informs which cognitive areas should be targeted during rehabilitation. However, neuropsychological rehabilitation often requires more than cognitive rehabilitation.

Generally speaking, neuropsychological rehabilitation often requires sustained hands–on involvement with clients. There can often be less immediate outcomes, and the clinician continually has to keep in mind the whole picture of the person, their difficulties, and the systems around them, to inform the ongoing, complex decision-making process underpinning modern rehabilitation. In contrast, assessment is immediate, cross-sectional, and short term, whereas rehabilitation tends to be long term, longitudinal, and ongoing. Furthermore, broadly speaking, today neuropsychological rehabilitation consists

DOI: 10.4324/9781003228226-22

of more than assessment (testing) and cognitive rehabilitation. Wilson and colleagues (2017) provide an excellent overview and perspective on the historical development of neuropsychological rehabilitation, theories, practice, and contemporary issues in the field. In essence, they make the point that given the complexity of each individual client's difficulties in the areas of cognition, behaviour, and emotion, it is unlikely that one theory or approach can cover 'all bases'. Indeed, it would most likely be considered poor clinical practice to be too closely aligned to only one theoretical model or approach to neuropsychological rehabilitation.

Let us now return to consider Walsh's historical metaphor in the context of current day clinical neuropsychology practice. Perhaps then it would be reasonable to suggest that if neuropsychological assessment is (was) thought to be a 'contact sport', by default neuropsychological rehabilitation should not automatically be assumed to be the opposite, a 'spectator sport'. Viewed completely dispassionately, neuropsychological rehabilitation is so much more than observation and measurement. To further develop the metaphor, good rehabilitation professionals, rather than spectators, are perhaps more like experienced coaches who do not just watch a specific match to figure out what is happening in the moment, but take care of a forever changing *season*, full of small successes and heart-breaking setbacks, trying to see things through to the goals mutually agreed with the team. In many respects brain injury rehabilitation is defined by ups and downs, unpredictability, ethical dilemmas, and the constant question of what is best for this client, now. For example, what exactly constitutes 'rehabilitation', who is it for, and how long is 'long term'? In this chapter a case of unusual neuropsychological rehabilitation is presented to illustrate some of these complexities and decision making integral to providing longer-term neuropsychological rehabilitation that is meaningful to the person for whom it matters most: the 'patient'.

Case presentation (part 1)

In this chapter, the 'patient' was Ms N, a right-handed female aged 37 (at the time of writing), who had a complex acute diagnostic presentation. Ms N was 17 at the time she first presented with seizures. At that time, she worked part time in a pub, and had a history of migraine. Initially the cause of the seizures could not be determined, but later during a hospital admission it transpired that she most likely had some form of space occupying lesion. Fortunately, Ms N was then rapidly transferred to a regional neuro-surgery unit for emergency management. Neuroimaging revealed that she had a right parietal arteriovenous malformation (AVM), which required immediate neurosurgery. After her acute and sub-acute medical care, Ms N was eventually discharged home. At age 24 Ms N was referred to a regional community brain injury rehabilitation service by her general practitioner. She was then seen by various members of the multidisciplinary team where the author was based, including neurology, clinical neuropsychology, and physiotherapy. Neurological examination was completed and reported migraine, an inferior quadrantanopia, a Riddoch effect, and possible difficulties with cognition. As part of her initial multidisciplinary assessments to inform further community-based rehabilitation, Ms N completed a baseline neuropsychological assessment.

Neuropsychological testing was completed during 2008, with a view to inform Ms N's post-acute community rehabilitation. The main challenge with interpreting the findings from the testing was that her performance was adversely affected by impaired vision, or visual processing, secondary to her brain injury, and accordingly her scores were clearly artificially reduced. However, besides the unsurprising problems with visual–spatial perception and processing (given the right parietal lobe location of the lesion in a right-hander), which made interpretation of the rest of the test results problematic, there were potentially some difficulties with memory (retention and recall), mild social disinhibition, and executive function as well. The remainder of neuropsychology input included helping Ms N with compensatory strategies for some of the cognitive difficulties, most notably for possible problems with memory (new learning). These were mainly delivered by an assistant psychologist under the supervision of the consultant neuropsychologist (the author). However, Ms N also reported non-cognitive difficulties, most notably anxiety. This was further explored with Ms N, and it transpired that her anxiety was specific to walking around in unfamiliar towns. Psychological therapy aimed to develop a formulation to help understand Ms N's anxiety. The formulation incorporated the following factors: loss of confidence; fear of getting lost (potentially related to a difficulty with spatial memory); and a fear of falling on cobbled, uneven road surfaces (possibly related to Ms N's visual spatial perceptual impairments).

A further development during Ms N's neuropsychology intervention concerned the changes in her level of self-awareness. Initially Ms N presented with some, and steadily increasing, intellectual awareness. To some extent this was to be expected, as a function of her engagement in rehabilitation and willingness to use compensatory strategies – which in themselves provide 'feedback' that there is a 'problem' to work around. With time Ms N's self-awareness further progressed, perhaps as a function of more non-cognitive (affect) issues such as anxiety, and 'being different', which were being discussed in psychological therapy. As time went on, Ms N also increasingly devoted herself to learning everything she could about her own neurological diagnosis and acquired brain injury more generally. To some extent the evolution of Ms N's self-awareness, from limited, to an intellectual understanding, and then to a more predictive, affect-informed awareness of potential difficulties mirrored some of the well-described models of self-awareness after acquired brain injury, for example that of Crosson et al. (1989) and also Toglia and Kirk (2000). Regular neuropsychology input ended at this point. Four years later, a routine neurological review took place at the service and an EEG was requested due to concerns about possible seizures. The EEG was subsequently reported as being mildly abnormal, thought to be consistent with Ms N's structural lesion, but that there were no epileptic features on the protocol. It was now four years after Ms N's formal community-based rehabilitation had ended. Or had it? What is neuropsychological rehabilitation, who is it for, and when does it 'end'?

Case presentation (part 2)

A decade later, when least expected, Ms N appeared on my radar again – but not as a re-referral or self-referral in one of my outpatient clinics .... As already highlighted above, during the time of her community rehabilitation, Ms N developed a desire to develop an in-depth understanding of the nature of her acquired brain injury, perhaps as a function of increasing self-awareness. Unbeknown to me, as part of this personal endeavour, Ms N continued to further her progress and rehabilitation in a way that was ecologically valid (to her) by completing a BSc Psychology degree at a local university. This was the very same university where I was now seconded part time from my NHS post at the time. I had not seen Ms N in my NHS role during the previous ten years for further neuropsychology input or review. And then, one day her name came up during an informal discussion about applications for one of our MSc degree programmes with other academic colleagues. The specific situation was that Ms N desperately wanted to enrol for our MSc Neuropsychology programme at the university – a programme I was now involved in as a lecturer and research supervisor. Clearly, quite a few coincidences had occurred. However, much more importantly, during the conversation I became aware that there was some reticence about Ms N's application. It then transpired that the apprehension was related to her undergraduate academic results. Let us now return to the above question: *What* is neuropsychological rehabilitation, *who* is it for, and *when* does it end?

When confronted with questions as complex as these, we face what one might want to term 'the selection phenomenon'. In the United Kingdom, the majority of clinical neuropsychologists complete clinical psychology training first, as an entry requirement. However, selection for clinical psychology training is by far the hardest part of the journey. We know that the odds are stacked against the vast majority of applicants, however good their academic grades are. And there may be a (potentially one of several) very good, possibly universally true, reason why selection is so incredibly hard. The truth is that almost anyone could, in theory at least, *at their own pace*, complete the individual academic and practical components of clinical training, or for that matter any highly selected profession, vocation, sport, or other elite role. No setbacks, no multiple demands to face, no emotional and physical exhaustion, no failures – just a little bit every day, week, or month. To use a metaphor, we can all achieve the record time for a 500 metre elevation climb for a specific sector in the mountains, provided we were allowed to break it up into many smaller sections to be completed when we felt like it .... Selection for clinical psychology training attempts to identify, over and above academic ability, those personal characteristics (of which there are several, including for example compassion, sensitivity, warmth, and empathy) that are crucial to being a practising clinical psychologist. And one of these is making highly complex clinical decisions under pressure, and where there is unlikely to be a 'right answer'. The ability to be reasonably comfortable with ambiguity and uncertainty is important.

So, what were the complexities surrounding the seemingly simple question of Ms N's application to do an MSc degree? One of the ethical complexities seemed to cut to the heart of neuropsychological assessment: awareness, to some degree, relies on cognition. And Ms N had quite significant cognitive impairment. Or did she? Did the 'contact sport' neuropsychological testing suffer a hiccup? Was most of the variance explained not by percentiles and Z scores, but perhaps simply by her visual perceptual and mathematical difficulties? Was there a mind well suited to advanced study underneath these 'cognitive impairments'? Thinking back about the clinical interpretation of her assessment, I thought so. But I was also aware that Ms N, who was after all one of our service's (and my) ex-clients, was now keen on doing an MSc degree and did not actually have the grades thought necessary to successfully complete such a programme of study. There was a much bigger problem though. It became increasingly clear that Ms N had more pronounced difficulties than her undergraduate grades. The main challenge, given her grades and the common knowledge that she had a brain injury (Ms N was very open about this in the university environment), was going to be finding an academic member of staff to be her research supervisor. I wasn't sure others would take her on. Should I consider volunteering to take on Ms N and act as her project (research) supervisor? This was the question facing me, and all the ethical complexities integral to it.

The first, and obvious aspect of the ethics to consider in this case, was about the supervisory relationship. Would this constitute a dual relationship? On reflection this seemed highly unlikely. I had not seen Ms N for ten years, and most of her hands–on neuropsychology input was in fact delivered by the assistant psychologist, whom I supervised. Furthermore, Ms N was *asking* me to *help* her with what was clearly a long–term aspiration and goal close to her heart. The principle of *primum non nocere* (do no harm) underpins most ethical codes. If Ms N were unable to find a supervisor, she was very likely to experience harm as she would not be able to continue her studies, and in the process potentially increase her chances of gainful employment. Which raises another question. Whose goals are the most important during rehabilitation – those of the clinician, and clinical team? Or those of the patient? Hence, considering this, there is an important further ethical issue to think about: autonomy. We should facilitate autonomous decision making of those who come to us for our rehabilitation, care, support, or advice. And ultimately, from an ethics perspective, it is of course very much also about respect, and preserving a person's dignity.

Let us now turn to another ethical aspect identified above: who is it (rehabilitation, care) for? Do we see only one or two clients, and 'give them our everything', but neglect the many more who may need our care? Furthermore, do we rather invest the vast majority of our time not seeing clients directly, but supervising, supporting, training, and skilling-up others to do that? No other clinical profession does .... Is it even (theoretically speaking) possible that if it is so hard to get selected, training is so long and complex, and lengthy, that we can simply 'show others how to do neuropsychology' in a very short period of time? Or do we, the same as every other clinical profession, aspire to care for as many as we can, *and* skill up colleagues in other professions? It is a complex, and potentially uncomfortable ethical question. An interesting thought experiment to perform here might be to reflect on hypothetically how much *direct* client input the *same* neuropsychologist performs, who is employed in *different* settings: for example, an NHS hospital; their own private practice; an independent provider; a higher education institution; and so forth. I have worked in all these settings – state-funded hospitals, including the NHS; private practice; independent healthcare provider; higher education institutions – and my own take is that our care is always for *everyone* who needs it wherever we work, not only a select few. Hawley et al. (2019) provide an interesting discussion of the ethical factors relevant to long-term brain injury rehabilitation. Considering all these complexities, in the situation thus far described in this chapter, was Ms N still my responsibility?

Clinicians often dwell on the negative and can ruminate for days over complex decisions such as those illustrated in this chapter. I speak from personal experience! Taking a few steps back though, perhaps it is more important that we realise we have to consider not only potential harm, but also possible *benefits* that might come from our decisions and actions as practising clinicians. Reconstructed and expanded from the universal ethics perspective of doing no harm, 'in the first instance do no harm, and if possible, do good'. With this in mind, on reflection I thought that I had some insight into Ms N's difficulties and could almost certainly provide the academic support, and maybe even cognitive strategies, to increase the chances of success for Ms N during her studies – which had in essence become her 'rehab'. It may be possible *to do good*. To return to Walsh's metaphor, I could have been a 'spectator' to Ms N's application, considering the apprehension around accepting her, and crucially, decided that finding a supervisor for her was not a 'contact sport', and hence 'not my problem'. After careful consideration of the above complexities, I put myself forward as a supervisor. A supervisor with hopefully enough understanding to inconspicuously fuse the roles of academic supervisor and putting in place some supportive mechanisms to optimise her learning and as a result (hopefully) the chances of success in a highly motivated student. So, yes, Ms N was still my responsibility. And that was that, I forgot about it all in the whirlpool of academic and clinical demands of the next few months.

The new academic year, and intake, was upon us much sooner than it felt it would be at the time, a few months earlier, when we were considering Ms N's application. Those who teach at universities, know that October usually flashes by in a blur with the new intake of students. But lectures went well, Ms N's attendance and participation was impeccable. Ms N was very well engaged, and highly motivated for her coursework. Towards the winter, we started to meet with our research project students. The project Ms N chose was going to look at social isolation after acquired brain injury. Ms N was very enthusiastic about the topic and collecting data. She had an excellent strategy (plus boundless energy and enthusiasm!) for recruiting participants through a local group of Headway, which she also chaired. The only potential problems were that recruitment and data collection of course relies heavily on researchers' organisational skills, memory, and, unfortunately, mathematical/statistical ability. Keeping in mind the site of Ms N's lesion, the latter could possibly have posed some big hurdles for her .... Was trying to do good by accepting Ms N as a postgrad, going to end badly in failure, and doing harm?

As part of compensatory strategies for her cognitive difficulties, Ms N had to make use of technology to aid her with her studies. This she had long ago spontaneously recognised herself. However, one of the challenges here was to together identify the most suitable apps/software for her to use during her MSc studies. Bower et al. (2021) provide an overview of factors that influence clinicians' choice of software platforms to use in rehabilitation. Whilst Ms N was very proficient in the use of mainstream social media, the challenge was to find apps that could be used as part of compensatory tools in cognitive remediation. Although there are literally thousands, and more, options, in contrast to the most popular social media apps, the vast majority of these other apps and software were unsuitable due to their poor stability, being overly complex to use, having regular disruptive 'updates', and containing too much redundancy in the form of pointless additional 'features'. In the end, three tech strategies were identified and put in place for Ms N. The first was a simple calendar app to prevent memory lapses, for example for attending supervision appointments. The second was the use of a Word document platform that could easily track changes and prevent 'version confusion' concerning Ms N's written work, which she had to regularly submit to me for review. The third was a map and location share function to overcome getting lost on campus and elsewhere, or for directing others to where she was at a given time. Using these was considered the best way forward. Thinking about Ms N's case, on reflection, there is perhaps some truth in the late Steve Jobs' saying that 'Simplicity is the ultimate complexity' when it comes to apps and software to be used in compensatory strategies as part of the cognitive rehabilitation of persons with acquired brain injury.

One of Ms N's main cognitive difficulties, which was not directly amenable to tech-supported compensatory strategies, soon revealed itself during our weekly supervision sessions. Ms N had difficulties with sustained attention, or more specifically, being highly distractible. As a result of this problem, Ms N often in the moment rather quickly strayed quite far off task (the research project). This took the form of extensive talking about a particular off-topic point in the narrative which suddenly caught her attention. These 'stimuli' within a narrative appeared to usually have an emotional valence, and hence quite powerfully drew her (sustained) attention away from the discussion directly pertaining to the research project. Discussion and feedback of my observation of her distractibility slowing down her progress, and indeed Ms N's own awareness of this difficulty, led to us together thinking about a strategy to support her. Much has been written about goal setting *with* clients, rather than *for* them, as well as the role of the therapeutic relationship in doing this successfully. Especially during the post-acute, longer-term phases of follow-up, about which in fact very little has been written, our clients' goals are not necessarily the same as those of their treating clinicians (Hawley et al., 2019). In this case, working collaboratively, Ms N and I together found a *simple* answer (remember student and supervisor learned from our forays in the world of bloated apps what to avoid!). We came up with the simplest of simple strategies. A memorable (for Ms N specifically) mantra in the form of the word 'Focus', was used to 'distract' Ms N back from her distraction, to the task at hand during supervision. Initially I would very regularly during meetings 'disrupt her distraction', by saying out aloud: 'Focus'. After some time this generalised to internal monitoring, and Ms N would spontaneously after going *off piste* and becoming aware of it, say: 'Yes, I know, focus!' This strategy was very similar to the principles to manage problems of attention already described many years earlier by Robertson and colleagues (1995). In Ms N's case, the generalisation of an external compensatory strategy to the use of internal self-monitoring was a good outcome, with benefits beyond the university environment, as will later be pointed out.

During the final stages of her studies, Ms N continued to provide truly remarkable input to her local Headway branch. Ms N was also very active within the university community, and very effectively used social media to more generally advocate for persons with acquired brain injury. Whilst nearing the end of studying for her post-graduate degree, Ms N (appropriately so) started applying for many posts. Some of her experiences illustrated the not to be underestimated difficulties our clients face out there in the real world, many years post-injury. For many applications, Ms N secured an interview, but then never secured the job, after being told 'You did so well, but on this occasion there was this one person who was a stronger candidate than you', or words to that effect. Understandably these 'failures' in the real world, despite having worked so hard at her rehabilitation, often had a negative effect on Ms N's mood. At times we reflected on these during her supervision sessions, and I was able to provide her with some support regarding her disappointment.

It was very important for Ms N to have a sense of purpose and meaning in her life. One pragmatic area where this was possible to sustain concerned her links as a student with the university, where her contribution was genuinely valued. Accordingly, we remained in contact in my academic capacity, as Ms N's contribution through her project work was very significant, and made a substantial contribution to the research beyond her own project. And then at the start of 2020 the Covid-19 pandemic engulfed everybody's lives. I got caught up and overwhelmed by a whirlpool of non-stop direct work with sometimes very unwell patients in NHS inpatient or isolation wards and clients in their own homes. Almost everything beyond patient care under unimaginable conditions stopped. Meanwhile Ms N did her best to support her Headway members during this terrible time. Our paths temporarily separated. Seventeen months into the pandemic I left the NHS, but remained at the university in an honorary capacity, and (virtually) in touch with Ms N. The height of the pandemic brought a whole new set of very complex ethical questions and decisions on how to best support those we care for and ensure that they receive the best rehabilitation under circumstances that were 'not covered in our clinical training', while sometimes ourselves being very near being broken.

At the time (end of 2021) of writing this chapter, I approached Ms N to obtain her final consent (she had already consented when I contacted her prior to the commencement of its writing) after she had an opportunity to read and approve the chapter. After reading over this chapter, and consenting, Ms N spontaneously asked if she could provide me with an update on how things had worked out. She reported that she was now settled in a job she enjoyed, and was doing well in. Reflecting on some factors that could possibly be contributing to her successful return to employment, Ms N spontaneously reported that she felt the following had been important. The first was that she found the strategies we used to counteract her distractibility very helpful in her work to remain focused on the tasks at hand. And not only that, but she also used the same strategies to focus the people she was assisting through her work. Finally, Ms N also commented that prior to her brain injury, she did not have a lot of empathy, but that now felt she could truly empathise and identify with the difficulties others might be experiencing. This she felt was particularly beneficial in her job. It had been a very long journey, but it sounded as if after many years there had finally been some good outcomes, of real significance to her.

All decisions about rehabilitation interventions in the final analysis are intended to culminate in desirable outcomes for our clients, including recreation, relationships, and employment (Prigatano, 1989). But in the complex situation described in this chapter, Ms N was clearly not a client, but primarily a student out there in the real world, who happened to have an acquired brain injury, with a supervisor who was aware of her clinical history. Are outcomes as important (beyond the generic desired outcomes of academic institutions – that students pass and have a positive learning experience) in this situation? I would reason that they are as, if not *more*, important. Outcomes in the worlds where our clients live their lives long after more formal, clinic-based, structured clinical input has ceased, can potentially have profound positive (and negative) effects on their well-being. Speaking of outcomes, one obvious, glaring question remains to be answered in this case report. What happened to Ms N? Ms N proved to be an excellent, hard-working student. On reflection, I could not have hoped for a better project student. Through her involvement with Headway, she turned out to be by far the most successful recruiter of participants for the dissertation project (one of my research projects) Ms N was assigned to. She was by far the most conscientious Masters degree student I have ever supervised to date. But most readers of this chapter would by now probably suspect that the elephant in the room of whether Ms N actually passed her degree is being avoided ... Did Ms N pass her degree?

Yes, she did. With merit.

Conclusion

Reflecting on the time I spent supervising Ms N, I did ask myself many questions, some explored in greater depth above. Was Ms N really 'a complex case'? No, she was not. Rather, in this chapter a case of complex diagnostics, assessment, and 'rehabilitation' beyond the traditional period of active intervention was described, as a platform for us to consider some of the universal ethical and philosophical factors underpinning the overall process of when situations don't neatly fit those we were trained for. Are the skills underpinning clinical neuropsychology really so complex? Maybe it is not complexity in isolation, but time, that explains most of the answer to this question. Selection for training is a long, anxiety-provoking process. Training (if we are lucky enough to secure a place), is long and demanding on all levels; gaining experience, on the other hand, is akin to the generalisation and gradual cementing down over time of what we have learnt. Perhaps then the main learning points from this chapter are that the journey to becoming a clinician is never quick, not for everyone, and littered with very ambiguous crossroads testing our ability to make the decisions and provide the input that has the potential to effect change that is meaningful to our clients and the complex world where they live long after formal rehabilitation has ended. And that to make this happen, entails numbers, and more numbers.

References

Bower, K. J., Verdonck, M., Hamilton, A., Williams, G., Tan, D., & Clark, R. A. (2021). What factors influence clinicians' use of technology in neurorehabilitation? A multisite qualitative study. *Physical Therapy*, *101*(5), 1–9.

Crosson, B., Barco, P. P., Velozo, C. A., Bolesta, M. M., Cooper P. V., Werts, D., & Brobeck, T. C. (1989). Awareness and compensation in postacute head injury rehabilitation. *Journal of Head Trauma Rehabilitation*, *4*, 46–54.

Hawley, L., Hammond F. M., Cogan, A. M., Juengst, S., Mumbower, R., Pappadis, M. R., Waldman, W., & Dams-O'Connor, K. (2019). Ethical considerations in chronic brain injury. *Journal of Head Trauma Rehabilitation*, *34*(6), 433–436.

Prigatano, G. P. (1989). Work, love, and play after brain injury. *Bulletin of the Menninger Clinic*, *53*(5), 414–431.

Robertson, I. H., Tegnér, R., Tham, K., Lo, A., & Nimmo-Smith, I. (1995). Sustained attention training for unilateral neglect: Theoretical and rehabilitation implications. *Journal of Clinical and Experimental Neuropsychology*, *17*(3), 416–430.

Toglia, J., & Kirk, U. (2000). Understanding awareness deficits following brain injury. *NeuroRehabilitation*, *15*, 57–70.

Wilson, B. A., Winegardner, J., Van Heugten, C. M., & Ownsworth, T. (2017). *Neuropsychological rehabilitation. The international handbook.* Routledge.

20 Mild traumatic brain injury

Diagnostic difficulties and legal controversies

Karen Addy

Introduction

Within the literature there has been a growing shift away from referring to the mildest form of traumatic brain injury (TBI) as 'concussion'. Whilst this term has been previously used and is common in lay language, the term concussion is steadily being replaced with mild traumatic brain injury (mTBI) as clinicians and researchers argue that concussion as a construct lacks diagnostic precision and does not refer to the underlying pathological neurological processes that unpin the symptomatology of mTBI (Smith & Stewart, 2020). As technological advances in scanning and diagnostic assessment of mTBI have demonstrated, this condition occurs as a result of mechanical forces (following a blow to the head) affecting brain tissue (Wagner et al., 2000). Rapid rotational velocity/acceleration (inertial loading) is thought to be a key component of mTBI injury (Smith et al., 2000). Although referred to as 'mild', individuals can still experience a variety of physical, emotional, and cognitive problems, including attentional and memory impairments, sleep disturbance, increased anxiety, and depression (Dewan et al., 2018.)

Diagnosing TBI severity is usually based on four indices: (1) initial Glasgow Coma Scale scores (GCS), (2) loss of consciousness (length of), (3) length of post-traumatic amnesia (PTA), and (4) neuroradiological evidence of brain damage. Estimates of severity based on any one single index may be of limited prognostic value due to confounding variables. For example, retrospective estimates of the duration of post-traumatic amnesia may be invalid when a patient has been given certain medications or has undergone procedures, which can interfere with memory function. A number of classification systems have therefore been developed to combine these indices to give an overall indicator of the severity of a traumatic brain injury (see Table 20.1).

However, mTBI remains a heterogeneous category, and as such there is often variation in the neuropathology and survivors can experience varying symptoms (Smith & Stewart, 2020), making accurate clinical diagnosis difficult. Despite extensive research into novel imaging biomarkers of mTBI (for review see Shenton et al., 2012), such methods are not ready for use in general diagnostic practice. Therefore, the presence of visible lesions on computed

DOI: 10.4324/9781003228226-23

Table 20.1 Comparison of classification systems for determining the severity of head injury

	GCS[*]	Loss of consciousness	Length of post traumatic amnesia	Abnormal structural imaging
Severe TBI	3–8[3,7]	>24 hours[1,2,4,7] >30 minutes[3]	>24 hours[1,2,3] >7 days[4]	Present[1,2,3] Present or not present[4,7]
Moderate TBI	9–12[3,7]	30 minutes to 24 hours[1,4,7] >30 minutes[3]	30 minutes to 24 hours <24 hours[3] >1 and < 7 days[4]	Not present[1,3] Present or not present[4,7]
Complicated mild TBI	13–15	<30 minutes[6]	<30 minutes[5]	Present[6] (on enhanced MRI)
mild TBI	13–15[2,3,4,7] 15 13–15 after 30 minutes[5]	<30 minutes[1,2,3,4,5,7] Up to 24 hours[7][**]	<30 minutes[1] or <24 hours[2,3,4,5]	Not Present[1,2,3,4,7]
No brain injury	15	None	None	Not present

[*]without subsequent deterioration
[**]alteration of mental state
1 Annegers et al. (1998)
2 Christensen et al. (2009)
3 Malec et al. (2007)
4 ICD-10 (WHO, 1993)
5 American Congress of Rehabilitation Medicine (1993)
6 Iverson et al. (2012)
7 Frieden & Collins (2013)

tomography (CT) and clinical magnetic resonance imaging (MRI) reported by neuroradiologists is still the standard option for severity classification in clinical practice. However, these methods are unreliable, with the reported frequency of traumatic lesions on CT and MRI in mTBI varying enormously across studies (Shenton et al., 2012).

The cognitive and emotional changes associated with mTBI are due to microscopic injury to white matter fibres and diffuse axonal injury (DAI) (for review see Biagianti et al., 2020). Diffuse axonal injury is defined as the presence of small foci of brain injury with maximum diameter <15 mm, located in loci minoris resistentiae of the brain, such as the grey-white matter junction and the midline structures (Scheid et al., 2006). Microscopic injury to white matter fibres in mTBI cannot, however, be identified on standard CT or 1.5T MRI available to clinicians in acute care. Several MRI sequences have been proposed to increase the sensitivity of the MRI techniques to identify DAI (Rutgers et al., 2008). With studies using advanced diffusion tensor imaging (DTI) (for review see Asken et al., 2018) and enhanced 3T MRI scanning (Jolly et al., 2021). As the sensitivity of MRI increases roughly linearly with field strength, high-field MRI is more sensitive than low-field

MRI and studies have shown that 3T MRI is almost twice as sensitive as 1.5T MRI in identifying DAI. This highlights that, in diagnostic decision making, low magnetic field MRI scanning data can be unreliable as an indicator of neurological damage.

With advances in diagnostic accuracy and the use of enhance scanning data to identify the clinical signs of mTBI, improvements are being made. However, as the literature highlights, for many patients the standard clinical care pathway is CT scan or 1.5T MRI, both of which cannot identify microbleeds, which may indicate DAI associated with mTBI. This can lead to significant problems in terms of accurate clinical diagnosis and the misattribution of symptoms.

mTBI is now recognised as a major public health concern as clinicians and researchers are becoming more aware of the dangers and potential long-term consequences (Ponsford et al., 2013). Whilst most mTBI survivors can recover and return to their pre-morbid self, the clinical outcome of mTBI is hard to predict, as a proportion of patients continue to suffer life-disrupting cognitive and psychological symptoms (Livingston et al., 2020). A range of factors, not necessarily directly reflecting injury severity, are associated with poor outcome following mTBI, including previous neurological or psychiatric problems and whether the patient had suffered a previous head injury. Indeed, patients with a history of mTBI can experience changes in emotions and behaviour, often expressed as anxiety and depressive-like behaviours, which can lead to diagnostic difficulties regarding the determination of the cause of ongoing symptoms. In many cases the neurological basis of mTBI cognitive impairments can be overshadowed by apparent psychological symptoms of depression and anxiety (Sharp & Jenkins, 2015).

For the clinical neuropsychologist working in traumatic brain injury services, many referrals reference ongoing symptoms following suspected mTBI, with the clinical question often being one of differential diagnosis between neurological injury and psychiatric symptoms. Whilst in clinical practice these diagnostic issues are important, they are not necessarily the forefront of clinical decision making, as applied clinical neuropsychology involves a formulation-driven approach in which the clinical complaints the patient is presenting with are formulated and addressed. However, the differential diagnosis between neurological injury and psychiatric symptoms is of prominent concern to solicitors and claimants within the context of medicolegal practice, as the Guidelines for the Assessment of General Damages in Personal Injury Cases (Judicial College, 2019) specify very different rates of compensation awards for symptoms associated with psychiatric illness versus symptoms associated with traumatic brain injuries, with the latter being associated with a higher rate of financial compensation.

Many neuropsychologists work as expert witnesses for the courts, providing clinical opinions for civil compensation claims either as a claimant or defence expert. However, the origin of the instruction notwithstanding, all expert witnesses are independent (their primary duty is to the court), and there are clear rules set out regarding their conduct (Ministry of Justice, Civil Procedure Rules, updated 2021). The aim of instruction of the neuropsychologist expert witness is to estimate the date of stabilisation of symptoms, and appraise sequelae, which in turn enables the solicitors to evaluate damage suffered and derive financial compensation for the patient. There is a complex relationship between litigation and outcome following TBI, with a vast majority of studies concluding that litigants suffer from greater distress when compared to non-litigants (Bay & Donders, 2008; Kristman et al., 2014; Reynolds et al., 2003). As mTBI is a diagnostically difficult condition, clinical debate often ensues between clinicians regarding diagnosis, treatment, and long-term prognosis. This in itself can lead to increased stress, as in cases of suspected mTBI there can be significant variation amongst opinions regarding the presence of a neurological insult; and, due to the adversarial nature of UK litigation, a dichotomy can be set up between 'sides' (claimant and defence) in which the same clinical data can be interpreted differently, leading to confusion for the claimants and their family regarding what the clinical problem is and the best ways to address it.

The following case illustrates the challenges of diagnosis of cognitive impairment, following suspected mTBI in the context of litigation. The case is from a historic and now settled medicolegal claim. Some features have been amended to protect confidentiality, although all involved have given permission for the clinical material to be presented. The author was one of two neuropsychologists instructed, one for the defence and one for the claimant. As is common in medicolegal cases, there was a difference of opinion regarding the attribution of the symptoms the claimant experienced. The case is presented here with learning points regarding the complexity of assessment of mTBI and highlights how advances in MRI scanning can assist in the resolution of differing opinions and the formulation of a clinical care pathway for these clients.

Case presentation

Thomas was 52 at the time of the assessment; he had been involved in a road traffic accident (RTA) and was referred for neuropsychological assessment as part of a medicolegal claim.

Prior to the RTA, Thomas was fit and well and ran his own chain of retail businesses. He stated that business was good prior to the accident; he manned one shop himself part time, as he enjoyed the 'banter' of being in the shop and chatting to his regular customers. The rest of the time he managed the wider staff team and kept an overview of the accounts and ordering systems for his other shops. Thomas and his wife stated that he was very sociable and outgoing prior to the accident. He was also a keen triathlete and trained as a social pastime, cycling around 60 miles per week and running three times a week with friends. He had no psychiatric or medical history of relevance.

Thomas' account of the accident

Thomas reported that he had no recall of the accident. He recalled that he had been riding his bike with six friends on a social event, he knew they had been to the local café, and remembered having coffee and cake. He remembered getting back on his bike afterwards but from that point on – nothing. Witness statements recorded that Thomas and his friends left the café around 60 minutes before the accident. Thomas was riding at the front of the group, when a car pulled out of a junction directly into his path. Thomas hit the side of the car bonnet with his bike and was thrown over the top of the car bonnet, landing on the road on the other side. He was wearing a helmet and reports documented that immediately after the impact he was 'awake but confused'. Thomas' next recollection was being in the hospital several hours later. He recalled a consultant talking to him about the surgery he required on his wrist and clearly remembered asking the consultant if he would be able to ride his bike later that week. Thomas was in hospital for six days due to his orthopaedic injuries.

Account of index event in NHS medical records

The ambulance report documented an emergency call at 13.17; with arrival on scene at 13.38. Thomas' GCS was 15/15 and there was a query regarding loss of consciousness, with confusion documented. He was given morphine at the roadside and placed on a spinal board. The ambulance records documented a severe obvious wrist injury and queried a spinal injury, later ruled out.

On admission to A&E, neurological assessment recorded Thomas' GCS as being 14 with amnesia and confusion documented; 24-hour neuro-observations were commenced during which GCS fluctuated between 14 and 15. The conversation with the orthopaedic consultant that Thomas recalled was documented in the records as occurring at 16.56 (3 hours after the index event). CT brain scanning was reported as: 'Unenhanced scan. No previous CT head for comparison. No acute intracranial haemorrhage, infarction or space-occupying lesion. The ventricles and CSF spaces are unremarkable. No skull fracture. The visualised paranasal sinuses and mastoid air cells are clear.'

Using the classification systems presented in Table 20.1 Thomas' injury would fall between the no brain injury and the mTBI range as Table 20.2 demonstrates.

As part of the litigation, Thomas had been reviewed by two consultant neurologists who varied in their opinions, with one reporting that Thomas had suffered a mTBI and the other stating there was no brain injury.

Symptoms following the index event

Following the accident, Thomas was initially absent from work for six months whilst his orthopaedic injuries healed. Upon his return to work, he believed

Table 20.2 Severity of head injury as applied to the case study

	GCS*	Loss of consciousness	Length of post traumatic amnesia	Abnormal structural imaging
Mild TBI	13–15[2,3,4,7] 15 13–15 after 30 minutes[5]	<30 minutes[1,2,3,4,5,7] Up to 24 hours[7]**	<30 minutes[1] or <24 hours[2,3,4,5]	Not Present[1,2,3,4,7]
No brain injury	15	None	None	Not present
Thomas	14–15	Unclear	Possibly 3 hours	Not present on initial CT

* without subsequent deterioration
** alteration of mental state
[1] Annegers et al. (1998)
[2] Christensen et al. (2009)
[3] Malec et al. (2007)
[4] ICD-10 (WHO, 1993)
[5] American Congress of Rehabilitation Medicine (1993)
[6] Iverson et al. (2012)
[7] Frieden & Collins (2013)

he was coping well; however, his wife started to get complaints from the staff stating orders were being forgotten, too few or too many staff were scheduled for shifts and Thomas was 'snappy and irritable'. These concerns led to Thomas' wife gradually taking over the admin roles and Thomas stating he was 'relegated' to serving customers. However, Thomas stated that he struggled on the shop floor as he couldn't focus on tasks, struggled with the noise in the shop, and felt exhausted after short three-hour shifts. He stated that he tried to work for around six months but felt that the work was affecting his mood, and 12 months after the index event he stopped going into the shop at all. Following this he experienced a decline in his mood, he struggled to engage in any activities, and reported feeling 'useless'. After 12 months off (24 months post index event), he was encouraged by his wife to return to work again in order to re-establish a structure to his week. He returned to doing 12 hours per week in the shop, split over four days. However, he continued to struggle with the busy environment, describing that when he was alone or with one customer he could manage the work; however, once the shop was fuller with serial conversations he felt overwhelmed and described feeling anxious and as if he needed to escape. At over 24 months since the accident there was no improvement and Thomas described how he felt 'stuck' between feeling 'there was something neurologically wrong' versus 'feeling like he was a failure', and that he should 'just should try harder'. However, Thomas reported that, when he had tried harder in the past (for example, his initial return to work or going out to a pub), he experienced problems with filtering out background noise. As such, busy environments felt overwhelming to him and he would avoid going or if he felt he had to go he would sit in a quiet corner or leave early as he felt his 'brain would explode'.

Neuropsychological assessment

During the course of the litigation process, Thomas was assessed by two independent neuropsychologists. One assessment was completed at 24 months post injury, the other nine months later (33 months post injury). The results are documented in Tables 20.3, 20.4, and 20.5.

Pre-morbid assessment

Thomas completed a formal assessment of his pre-morbid ability using the Test of Premorbid Function (TOPF, Wechsler, 2011). The TOPF indicated Thomas' expected IQ to be in the average range with his estimated full-scale IQ scored at 98; this was considered to be consistent with his reported educational and occupational history and as such was used as a comparison for the assessments.

Wechsler Adult Intelligence Scale – fourth edition (WAIS-IV; Wechsler, 2010)

This assessment is a general intelligence test that measures a number of aspects of global intelligence. As Table 20.3 shows, both neuropsychologists obtained clinically similar results and agreed that there was no evidence of general cognitive decline following the index event.

Wechsler Memory Scale – fourth edition (WMS IV, Wechsler, 2010)

The WMS IV memory assessment focuses upon a range of memory skills including immediate recall, delayed recall, and recognition. As Table 20.4 shows, there was a difference of opinion regarding the interpretation of the assessment results between the two neuropsychologists.

It was neuropsychologist A's opinion that the memory scores obtained on the WMS IV were in line with Thomas' general ability. Whilst there was a general reduction in his memory scores this could be accounted for by low mood and anxiety and was not reflective of an underlying neurological impairment. They cited the average scores on the WAIS IV processing speed and working memory tasks and the normal CT scan data.

Neuropsychologist B gave the opinion that the decline in Thomas' WMS IV scores were reflective of an underlying neurological impairment. They posed the view that Thomas' memory difficulties were most likely to be due to an impairment in attentional processing and not anxiety or mood based. The rationale for this opinion was that, whilst Thomas reported specific anxiety symptoms related to specific contexts (work and social events), he did

Table 20.3 WAIS IV (general ability) scores comparisons

	Neuropsychologist A		Neuropsychologist B		Opinion regarding clinical change from expected score	
	95% Conf. interval	Qualitative descriptor	95% Conf. interval	Qualitative descriptor	Neuropsychologist A	Neuropsychologist B
Verbal comprehension	87–96	Average	91–102	Average	None	None
Perceptual reasoning	87–98	Average	94–106	Average	None	None
Working memory	94–106	Average	90–104	Average	None	None
Processing speed	90–104	Average	77–94	Low average	None	None
Full scale	90–97	Average	90–98	Average	None	None

Table 20.4 WMS IV (memory) comparisons

	Neuropsychologist A		Neuropsychologist B		Opinion regarding clinical change from expected score	
	95% Conf. interval	Qualitative descriptor	95% Conf. interval	Qualitative descriptor	Neuropsychologist A	Neuropsychologist B
Immediate memory	81–97	Low average	75–87	Low average	None	Significant decline (TOPF – 17 points, base rate 7.88%)
Delayed memory	62–76	Borderline	69–82	Borderline	None	Significant decline (TOPF – 35 points, base rate 0.24%)
Auditory memory	72–87	Borderline	73–85	Borderline	None	None
Visual memory	75–85	Low average	77–88	Low average	None	None
Visual working memory	84–99	Average	84–99	Average	None	None

Table 20.5 Executive function measures comparisons

	Neuropsychologist A		Neuropsychologist B		Opinion regarding clinical change from expected score	
	Percentile	Qualitative descriptor	Percentile	Qualitative descriptor	Neuropsychologist A	Neuropsychologist B
Delis Kaplan Executive Function System (DKEFS; Delis, Kaplan, & Kramer, 2001)						
Trail making						
Visual scanning	60th	Average	9th	Low average	None	Slight decline
Number sequencing	60th	Average	37th	Average	None	None
Letter sequencing	84th	Average	63rd	Average	None	None
Switching	2nd	Borderline impaired	2nd	Borderline impaired	None	Decline
Motor speed	75th	Average	63rd	Average	None	None
Verbal fluency						
Letter	37th	Average	25th	Average	None	None
Number	16th	Low average	9th	Low average	None	Decline
Switching	25th	Average	25th	Average	None	None
Switching accuracy	16th	Low average	9th	Low average	None	Decline
Colour word						
Naming	Not administered		16th	Low average		Decline
Reading			37th	Average		
Inhibition			37th	Average		
Inhibition plus switching			16th	Low average		Decline
Brixton (Burgess & Shallice, 1997)						
	Not administered		Scaled score 3	poor		Decline

not report any generalised anxiety symptoms. It was also noted that his mood symptoms appeared to be secondary to his experience when socialising and working, rather than being related to a general depression.

Executive function assessment

Both neuropsychologists completed a series of executive function measures. As Table 20.5 demonstrates, there was a further disagreement regarding the attribution of the scores obtained.

It was neuropsychologist B's opinion that the executive function assessment indicated subtle issues with complex executive processing mainly affecting Thomas' ability to multi-task and switch between two competing stimuli. Neuropsychologist A reported no evidence of any executive decline and attributed reduced scores to Thomas' mental health, recommending psychological therapy to address his anxiety symptoms.

Tests of effort

Both neuropsychologists administered standardised assessments of effort and symptom validity measures. Both agreed that Thomas was co-operative with the testing situation and he passed both the effort and symptom validity testing.

Mood and anxiety screening

Neuropsychologist A completed a mood and anxiety screen using the Hospital Anxiety and Depression scale (Zigmond & Snaith, 1983). Thomas scored 7 for depression and 10 for anxiety, indicating elevated anxiety symptoms.

Neuropsychologist B completed a mood and anxiety screen using Generalised Anxiety Disorder 7 Scale (GAD-7, Spitzer et al., 2006) and the Patient Health Questionnaire (PHQ-9; Kroenke & Spitzer, 2002). Thomas scored 5 on the GAD-7, which was within the mild range and not consistent with clinical levels of generalised anxiety. Thomas scored 8 on PHQ-9, which was within the mild range and not consistent with clinical levels of depression.

Clinical opinions

There was varying neurological opinion between a diagnosis of mTBI and no brain injury. The clinical question was posed to the neuropsychologists to determine whether Thomas had any neurocognitive symptoms that may help differential diagnosis between no TBI and mTBI. Neuropsychologist A was of the opinion that Thomas was suffering from anxiety and depression, which was the cause of his cognitive symptoms, and recommended psychological therapy, expecting no lasting symptoms once treatment was completed.

Neuropsychologist B considered that Thomas was suffering from subtle neurocognitive impairment affecting executive and memory processing and gave the opinion that Thomas' symptoms met the diagnostic criteria for mild neurocognitive disorder (DSM-5 331, APA, 2013) due to mTBI. The situational anxiety and low mood symptoms were viewed as being secondary to his neurocognitive impairment. Neuropsychologist B recommended a series of neuropsychological therapy sessions to help Thomas fully understand and adjust to his neurocognitive processing difficulties, expecting that he would learn to compensate for his cognitive symptoms, thus reducing the impact on his daily functioning.

Treatment

Given the context of the assessments, treatment was determined by the court process. As there were differences of opinions with regard to the aetiology of Thomas' symptoms, the experts were asked to provide a joint statement (this is common in UK law and is part of the Civil Procedure Rules). Whilst both neuropsychologists remained opposed with regard to their opinions, agreement was made that it would benefit Thomas to have treatment regarding anxiety and depression, and then his cognitive symptoms could be reviewed.

At the same time in a joint statement, the expert neurologists agreed that CT was unreliable and recommended enhanced 3T MRI to aid their discussion and differential diagnosis.

In accordance with the experts' recommendations. Thomas was referred for an initial 12 sessions of cognitive-behavioural therapy (CBT). Thomas declined further sessions after session 6; whilst he noted some improvement regarding avoidance, he noted no change in any cognitive symptoms. After session 5, Thomas had the 3T MRI scan results. Clinical review of the 3T MRI reported by a consultant neuro-radiologist documented the following:

> 3 Tesla MRI Head demonstrates presence of multiple microbleeds within the left frontal lobe periventricular white matter as well as a single focus of microbleed within the right frontal lobe periventricular white matter.

The neuroradiologist was of the view that

> In my opinion, the areas of microbleeds are likely due to post traumatic brain injury. Microbleeds cannot be accurately dated. On a balance of probabilities, these areas of brain microbleeds within bilateral frontal lobe white matter are more likely related to the index accident.

This finding led to the neurologists agreeing that Thomas had most likely suffered a mTBI. Following these findings, the two neuropsychologists provided a further joint statement, reviewing the CBT and neurologists' findings. It was agreed that the MRI evidence was consistent with Thomas' self-report and with neuropsychologist B's findings of executive dysfunction. Both agreed that, whilst the CBT was helpful, further sessions were unlikely to be productive and that Thomas would be best supported to understand and manage the mTBI-related cognitive impairments. The court then instructed occupational therapy and neuropsychological therapy to assist Thomas in adjusting to his impairments and the case moved to financial settlement.

Conclusion

mTBI is a difficult clinical diagnosis. In this case, the resources of enhanced MRI scanning were available and aided diagnosis; however, this is not always available in clinical practice. More commonly, patients present with reports of normal CT and 1.5T MRI but ongoing neurocognitive deficits that would indicate neurological insult.

Using a hypothesis-testing approach to neuropsychological assessment can help the clinician understand the clinical presentation. Hypothesis testing allows an exploration of differential diagnosis; in Thomas' case, one hypothesis was that he had neurocognitive impairments affecting his mental health. The alternative hypothesis was that Thomas was anxious and depressed, leading to his experience of cognitive impairment. Whilst both are valid hypotheses, when looking at the neuropsychological test data, all of Thomas' reduced scores were on tasks of dual processing, suggesting subtle but specific impairments in attentional control – these are known effects of frontal lobe damage. In addition, the neuropsychological data was consistent with his experience in loud busy environments, where dual processing and filtering out information would be required.

Whilst patients can present with psychiatric symptoms, it can be helpful for clinicians to identify the context in which psychiatric symptoms occur. In Thomas' case, the triggers for his anxiety were always loud busy environments; there was no evidence of generalised anxiety; and he did not describe any anxious cognitions when at home. His mood decline was secondary to being unable to cope with his work and being unable to cope in social situations. In this context, a clear trigger pattern of increased cognitive demands prior to the psychiatric symptoms occurring can be identified. This hypothesis was further confirmed by Thomas attending CBT, although he did not complete the full course of therapy; after six sessions he was using anxiety management skills but these had no effect on his experience. This would be unsurprising if one accepts that Thomas was experiencing neurocognitive processing impairments due to mTBI; in this context, his experience depends on the external environment rather than his internal mental state. This is a key distinction and a clinical assessment; utilising an ABC (antecedent, behaviour, consequence) analysis can be useful to the clinician when attempting to formulate and understand clinical presentations.

The added dimension of litigation requires further discussion and, whilst a full review of the issues involved in litigation is beyond the scope of this chapter, the clinical context and adversarial nature of the legal process can cause an unconscious filter regarding the interpretation of information. There is always the factor of financial gain to be considered when assessing patients engaged in litigation. As such, it can be suggested that claimants have a 'vested interest' in their symptoms. This issue is less problematic in the context of severe TBI, where there are clear neurological insults identified; however, in cases such as Thomas', whereby the initial CT or 1.5T scanning is reported as normal, the clinical presentation and attribution of symptoms is more difficult. In medicolegal cases there can therefore be an argument for claimants to be referred for enhance scanning techniques, which can add to the overall clinical picture and ensure that all the relevant evidence is considered prior to cases being settled, as the implications for misdiagnosis are likely to be lifelong.

References

American Psychiatric Association (2013). *Diagnostic and Statistical Manual of Mental Disorders* (5th ed.). APA.

American Congress of Rehabilitation Medicine (1993). Definition of mild traumatic brain injury. www.acrm.org/wp-content/uploads/pdf/TBIDef_English_10-10.pdf

Annegers, J. F., Hauser, A., & Rocca, W. A. (1998). A population based study of seizures after traumatic brain injuries. *The New England Journal of Medicine, 338*, 20–24.

Asken, B. M., DeKosky, S. T., Clugston., J. R., Jaffee, M. S., & Bauer, R. M. (2018). Diffusion tensor imaging (DTI) findings in adult civilian, military, and sport-related mild traumatic brain injury (mTBI): A systematic critical review. *Brain Imaging and Behavior, 12*, 585–612.

Bay, E., & Donders, J. (2008). Risk factors for depressive symptoms after mild-to-moderate traumatic brain injury. *Brain Injury, 22*, 233–241.

Biagianti, B., Stocchetti, N., Brambilla, P., Van Vleet, T. (2020). Brain dysfunction underlying prolonged post-concussive syndrome: A systematic review. *Journal of Affective Disorders, 262*, 71–76.

Burgess, P. W., & Shallice, T. (1997). *The Hayling and Brixton tests*. Pearson.

Christensen, J., Pedersen, M. G., Pedersen, C. B., Sidenis, P., Olsen, J., & Vestergaard, M. (2009). Long-term risk of epilepsy after traumatic brain injury in children and young adults: A population-based cohort study. *The Lancet, 373*, 1105–1110.

Delis, D. C., Kaplan, E., & Kramer, J. H. (2001). *Delis-Kaplan Executive Function System D-KEFS*. Pearson.

Dewan, M. C., Rattani, A., Gupta, S., Baticulon, R. E., Hung, Y-C., Punchak, M., Agrawal, A., Adeleye, A. O., Shrime, A. G., Rubiano, A. M., Rosenfeld, J. V., & Park, K. B. (2018). Estimating the global incidence of traumatic brain injury. *Journal of Neurosurgery, 1*, 1–18.

Frieden, T. R., & Collins, F. S. (2013). *Report to Congress on traumatic brain injury in the United States*. www.cdc.gov/traumaticbraininjury/pdf/report_to_congress_on_traumatic_brain_injury_2013-a.pdf

Iverson, G. L., Lange, R. T., Waljas, M., Liimatainen, S., Dastidar, P., Hartikainen, K. M., Soimakallio, S., & Ohman, J. (2012). Outcome from complicated versus uncomplicated mild traumatic brain injury. *Rehabilitation Research and Practice*, 415740.

Jolly, A. E., Balaet, M., Azor, A., Friedland, D., Sandrone, S., & Graham, N. S. N., Zimmerman, K., & Sharp, D. J. (2021) Detecting axonal injury in individual patients after traumatic brain injury. *Brain*, 144, 92–113.

Judicial College (2019). *Guidelines for the assessment of general damages in personal injury cases*. Oxford University Press.

Kristman, V. L., Borg, J, Godbolt, A. K., Salmi, L. R, Cancelliere, C., Carroll, L. J., Holm, L. W., Nygren-de Boussard, C., Hartvigsen, J., Abara, U., Donovan, J., Cassidy, J. D., (2014). Methodological issues and research recommendations for prognosis after mild traumatic brain injury: Results of the International Collaboration on Mild Traumatic Brain Injury Prognosis. *Archives of Physical Medicine and Rehabilitation*, 95, S265–S277.

Kroenke, K., & Spitzer, R. L. (2002). The PHQ-9: A new depression and diagnostic severity measure. *Psychiatric Annals*, 32, 509–521.

Livingston, G., Huntley, J., Sommerlad, A., Ames, D., Ballard, C., Banerjee, S., Brayne, C., Burns, A., Cohen-Mansfield, J., Cooper, C., Costafreda, S.G., Dias, A., Fox, N., Gitlin, L. N., Howard, R., Kales, H. C., Kivimäki, M., Larson, E. B., Ogunniyi, A., Orgeta, V., Ritchie, K., Rockwood, K., Sampson, E. L., Samus, Q., Schneider, L. S., Selbæk, G., Teri, L., & Mukadam, N. (2020). Dementia prevention, intervention, and care: 2020 report of the Lancet Commission. *Lancet*, 396, 413–446.

Malec, J. F., Brown, A. W., Leibson, C. L., Flaada, J. T., Mandrekar, J. N., Diehl, N. N., & Perkins, P. K. (2007). The Mayo classification system for traumatic brain injury severity. *Journal of Neurotrauma*, 24, 1417–1424.

Ponsford, J. (2013). Factors contributing to outcome following traumatic brain injury. *NeuroRehabilitation*, 32, 803–815.

Reynolds, S., Paniak, C., Toller-Lobe, G., & Nagy, J. (2003) A longitudinal study of compensation-seeking and return to work in a treated mild traumatic brain injury sample. *Journal of Head Trauma Rehabilitation*, 18, 139–147.

Rutgers, D. R., Toulgoat, F., Cazejust, J., Fillard, P., Lasjaunias, P., & Ducreux, D. (2018). White matter abnormalities in mild traumatic brain injury: A diffusion tensor imaging study. *American Journal of Neuroradiology*, 29, 514–519.

Scheid, R., Walther, K., Guthke, T., Preul, C., & von Cramon, D. Y. (2006). Cognitive sequelae of diffuse axonal injury. *Archives of Neurology*, 63, 418–424.

Sharp, D. J., & Jenkins, P. O. (2015). Concussion is confusing us all. *Practical Neurology*, 15, 172–186.

Shenton, M. E., Hamoda, H. M, Schneiderman, J. S., Bouix, S., Pasternak, O., Rathi, Y., Vu, M. A., Purohit, M. P., Helmer, K., Koerte, I., Lin, A. P., Westin, C. F., Kikinis, R., Kubicki, M., Stern, R. A., & Zafonte, R. A. (2012). A review of magnetic resonance imaging and diffusion tensor imaging findings in mild traumatic brain injury. *Brain Imaging Behaviour*, 6, 137–192.

Smith, D. H., Nonaka, M., Miller, R., Leoni, M., Chen, X. H., Alsop, D., & Meaney, D. F. 2000). Immediate coma following inertial brain injury dependent on axonal damage in the brainstem. *Jpournal of Neurosurgery*, 93, 315–322.

Spitzer, R. L., Kroenke, K., Williams, J. B., & Lowe, B. (2006). A brief measure for assessing generalized anxiety disorder: the GAD-7. *Archives of Internal Medicine*, *166*(10), 1092–1097.

Wagner, A. K., Sasser, H. C., Hammond, F. M., Wiercisiewski, D., & Alexander, J. (2000). Intentional traumatic brain injury: Epidemiology, risk factors, and associations with injury severity and mortality. *Journal of Trauma Acute Care Surgery*, *49*, 404–410.

Wechsler, D. (2011). *Test of Premorbid Function*. The Psychological Corporation.

Wechsler, D. (2010). *The Wechsler Memory Scale* (4th ed.). The Psychological Corporation.

Wechsler, D. (2010). *The Wechsler Adult Intelligence Scale* (4th ed.). The Psychological Corporation.

World Health Organization (1993). *The ICD-10 classification of mental and behavioural disorders: Diagnostic criteria for research*. World Health Organization: Geneva.

Zigmond, A. S., & Snaith, R. P. (1983). The hospital anxiety and depression scale. *Acta Psychiatrica Scandinavica*, *67*(6), 361–370.

21 Does this man have or not have mental capacity to make decisions about his discharge from hospital?

Leigh Leppard

Introduction

'Does this person have mental capacity?' is a common question for professionals working with people with acquired brain injury (ABI). In the acute and post-acute phases of recovery this question can be particularly pertinent – at a time when an individual's cognitive abilities are the most compromised, major decisions must be made. Should the person undergo a surgical procedure? Should they transfer to a neurorehabilitation unit? Will they need to go to a nursing home? What care package will they require? Such decisions can have lasting impacts on health, well-being, and quality of life.

When an individual's mental capacity is under question, a formal assessment is required. Such assessments are usually conducted through semi-structured interviews. However, accurately assessing mental capacity can be challenging when someone is able to 'say the right things' in conversation, and may even perform well on traditional, highly structured assessments of cognitive function, but fails to put their plans into practice and shows little awareness of this discrepancy. This is known as the 'frontal lobe paradox' (Walsh, 1985; Williams & Wood, 2017). In these cases, it becomes necessary to undertake a more comprehensive assessment, taking into account 'real world' observations and assessments, rather than relying solely on interview. This chapter outlines one challenging case of a man who presented with complex health needs and the frontal lobe paradox, who was an inpatient on a neurorehabilitation unit. This chapter will explore the dilemmas raised and how they were resolved.

Defining mental capacity

Mental capacity can be broadly defined as 'the ability to use information in order to reason and make an informed decision' (Wilkinson, 2020, p. 20). Legal frameworks vary around the world but tend to be underpinned by international conventions such as the Universal Declaration on Human Rights (UDHR; The United Nations, 1948) or the Convention on the Rights of Persons with Disabilities (CRPD; The United Nations, 2006).

DOI: 10.4324/9781003228226-24

In England and Wales, the Mental Capacity Act (2005) states that a the components of decision making are:

- understanding the information relevant to the decision,
- retaining that information,
- using or weighing that information as part of the process of making the decision, and
- communicating the decision (whether verbally, using sign language or any other means).

When, by reason of an impairment of mind or brain, someone lacks capacity to make a decision, it either falls to a legally appointed decision maker (such as someone with power of attorney) to make the decision, or a decision is made in someone's 'best interests', usually by a professional, in consultation with the individual, their loved ones, and other professionals.

Cognitive impairment and mental capacity

A person's mental capacity following an acquired brain injury can be affected for various reasons. A memory impairment, for example, might prevent someone from retaining all of the relevant information, or aphasia might impede someone's ability to communicate their decision. When it comes to weighing up information in the process of decision making, executive functioning plays a key role.

The cognitive factors affecting capacity vary over the course of an individual's recovery. Dreer et al. (2008) found that, whilst verbal memory impairments were the strongest predictor of decision-making capacity at the acute hospitalisation stage, at six-month follow-up executive functioning and working memory were the best predictors. The authors argued this is because memory functions are particularly vulnerable to TBI, and good verbal memory is a prerequisite to more sophisticated executive functions. In other words, one cannot weigh up new information if one does not have prerequisite abilities to encode, retain, and recall it. Such a finding is particularly pertinent to people who have undergone a period of neurorehabilitation because, by the point of discharge, most such patients are several months post-ABI, and executive impairment is likely to be key to their decision-making capacity.

The frontal lobe paradox

As noted above, the frontal lobe paradox refers to circumstances in which someone shows an inconsistency between, for example, their stated intentions and their actions (Teggart & Dimmock, 2020). Wood and Bigler (2017) hypothesise that this reflects an ability to verbalise an intention but a failure to convert this into goal-oriented behaviour. Individuals who demonstrate the frontal lobe paradox can seem to have a superficial understanding of their situation but lack a deeper awareness of how they behave in the moment, and this seems to be a key aspect of this 'good in theory, poor in practice' discrepancy (George & Gilbert, 2018).

Toglia and Kirk's (2000) model of awareness may shed some light on this phenomenon. The model makes a distinction between 'intellectual awareness' (knowledge of one's own cognitive strengths and weaknesses, and one's ability to complete tasks) and 'on-line awareness' (in-the-moment monitoring of one's performance during a task, including noticing errors and adjusting one's approach). People with the frontal lobe paradox may have a degree of intellectual awareness of their difficulties and so can state how to complete a task successfully in principle, yet have poor on-line awareness and so fail to implement those compensatory strategies in practice. Moreover, on-line monitoring impairments can mean the individual fails to notice errors or mismatches between expected and actual task performance (Amanzio et al., 2020), and so is unable to update their intellectual awareness and develop insight into this theory–practice discrepancy. Multiple brain regions are involved in mediating awareness, but the medial prefrontal cortex and cingulate gyrus are thought to have particularly salient roles (Stuss & Anderson, 2004; Johnson et al., 2002; Palermo et al., 2014).

The frontal lobe paradox causes particular challenges in mental capacity assessments, which are typically conducted in an interview format, where stated intention, rather than actual action, is assessed. This structured format, somewhat removed from a person's everyday life, can mean that impairments are masked and the interviewer can fail to draw out whether the individual is accurately appraising the challenges of meeting their care needs, or their ability to put intended plans into practice (Teggart & Dimmock, 2020; George & Gilbert, 2018). There is a risk, therefore, that someone can be incorrectly deemed to have mental capacity to make a decision. This can have important consequences, particularly when the decision to be made carries significant risk.

Case presentation

David[1] was a 56-year-old man who was admitted to a district neurorehabilitation unit following surgical draining of a thoracic epidural abscess, T5/6 laminectomy and a T4–7 fixation and decompression. Although ostensibly admitted for physical rehabilitation following his spinal injury, it quickly became apparent that David also had marked cognitive impairments that warranted further investigation. An MRI identified moderate cortical atrophy, predominantly in the frontal and temporal regions. It emerged that David had had meningitis at the age of five, and also had highly unstable Type 1 diabetes that had been poorly managed for some years.[2] He had poor hypo awareness and his diabetes was highly unstable, so he had several hypoglycaemic episodes per week. He had cataracts in both eyes and diabetic retinopathy, which meant his vision was markedly impaired. He also had diabetic peripheral neuropathy, causing problems with sensation and movement. This, coupled with his spinal injury, made him vulnerable to pressure sores.

History

David was the youngest of four children. He was largely raised by his older sister, as his father died when David was around ten years old and his mother worked long hours and had significant physical health problems. In childhood, he struggled to relate with his peers and left school without qualifications. He worked for some time in low-skilled employment such as cleaning but had not worked since his twenties. He had very limited contact with his siblings.

David lived alone in a small, ground floor flat. He reported that he had had one long-term partner who had died unexpectedly around ten years prior, but no other friends. Whilst they had never lived together, his partner provided him with emotional, practical, and financial support. David struggled with low mood and suicidal ideation following this loss. It was also evident that David had struggled to care for himself independently, since his diabetes had been managed poorly for some years and there was some suggestion of self-neglect.

Presentation on unit

David had several months of intensive input from the neurorehabilitation team but had made few improvements. He was unable to sit unsupported, could not stand or propel his wheelchair independently, and required a hoist for all transfers. He was doubly incontinent and required an indwelling catheter. He required assistance with much of his personal care and was unable to make meals independently.

David also required significant nursing input to meet his daily needs, and to address his complex health issues. Nurses needed to attend to all of his diabetes management, particularly as he was not hypo-aware. They often needed to remind David to adjust his position, and checked and treated pressure sores when required.

Initial mental capacity assessment

David's clinical team were of the view that his health needs were too complex to be met at home, even with carers, and he would need to be discharged to a nursing home. David, however, frequently expressed his desire to be discharged home without care so that he could be alone. He explained that he had previously been in a care home and found the experience to be objectionable as he reported that staff had read his post and rifled through his possessions. In conversations about potential discharge to a care home, David would become angry, verbally abusive and threatening towards staff, and said that he would end his life if he were to be discharged to a nursing home.

Given the high risks, the complexity of the decision, and David's cognitive impairments, the author carried out a mental capacity assessment jointly with one of the senior nurses on the ward, who knew David well.

David presented well in this mental capacity assessment. He plausibly explained how he would be able to meet some of his basic care needs (e.g. asking a neighbour to buy him microwave meals, having his medication delivered by the pharmacy), while acknowledging that there were things he would struggle to do safely, such as transferring in and out of bed, changing his pad, or washing and dressing. He could explain clearly the procedure of checking his blood–glucose levels, the optimal blood glucose level range, how much insulin to administer and what he could do in an emergency (e.g. having a chocolate bar beside his bedside in case of a hypoglycaemic episode, calling an ambulance). David said that he recognised that discharge home carried significant risks, including risk of death, but said that, in his view, this risk was preferable to going into a nursing home.

On the basis of this assessment alone, then, David seemed to be making a capacitous, if unwise, decision, as he had demonstrated an understanding of the relevant information and seemed to have weighed up costs and benefits. However, there were some inconsistencies between his account and how he presented on the ward, and the assessors had doubts as to whether his interview accurately reflected his mental capacity. Given the gravity of the decision to be made and the potential for serious untoward consequences, it was agreed that David should undergo formal neuropsychological assessment to better understand the nature of his cognitive impairments, and then the capacity assessment should be repeated.

Neuropsychological assessment

David engaged well in formal testing, though tests had to be chosen carefully to circumvent his comorbidities, such as avoiding tests that involved hand dexterity or good visual acuity. A magnifying sheet was also employed to ensure that he could see any visual aspects of tests.

General intellectual skills

David's premorbid functioning was found to be in the *borderline impairment* range. His global functioning was also in the *borderline impairment* range, based on subtests from the Wechsler Adult Intelligence Scale, 4th edition (WAIS-IV), though he could not complete the full assessment.

Memory

David's memory was assessed using verbal subtests (List Learning and Story Memory) from the Repeatable Battery for the Assessment of Neurological Status (RBANS).

He scored in the *impaired* range on immediate recall, indicating that he had significant difficulties encoding newly presented information. He had additional difficulties with delayed recall and recognition, even for information that he had successfully encoded. David also showed a limited learning curve with repetition, and he showed a marked primacy and recency effect, suggesting that he quickly became overwhelmed by large volumes of information.

Working memory was assessed using subtests from the WAIS-IV and was found to be in the *impaired* range.

Attention

David's attention was assessed using subtests from the Test of Everyday Attention (TEA). David performed in the *low average* range on a test of selective attention and in the *borderline impairment* range on a test of sustained attention. This was not consistent with his performance on everyday tasks that required him to attend to and retain/learn new verbal information, such as list learning (see 'Memory', below) or when engaging in conversation, and so it was hypothesised that the relatively brief test duration might not have captured his true level of impairment in these areas, which might become more pronounced as task demands or environmental stimulation increased.

Executive functioning

The following areas were assessed:

- *Cognitive flexibility*: David performed in the *impaired* range on both the Verbal Fluency test of the Delis-Kaplan Executive Function System (D-KEFS) and the Brixton Spatial Anticipation Test. His performance in the Brixton Test was particularly noteworthy, as it was evident that he could not adjust his approach in response to feedback that he was making errors.
- *Inhibition and strategy development*: On the Hayling test, David made a high number of errors, and did not develop a strategy to overcome this. As with the Brixton, he also appeared unable to adjust his behaviour when given feedback that he was incorrect.
- *Problem solving*: On the Key Search and Action Programme subtests from the Behavioural Assessment of Dysexecutive Syndrome (BADS), David performed relatively well, indicating relative strengths in developing efficient and effective solutions to novel problems. However, it is noteworthy that he took a considerable time to complete each task, and that in the Action Programme task David was unable to find an effective solution until he was shown the first step.
- *Initiation*: Observations from nursing staff indicated that he had difficulties initiating behaviours, in that he presented as generally passive.

David did not engage readily in leisure activities, rarely interacted with other patients, and required prompting to attend to many aspects of daily living.

Formulation

David's global cognitive abilities were marginally above the range at which learning disabilities would be considered, but he had additional impairments that prevented him from fully utilising his cognitive resources. Based on pen-and-paper assessment, he had impairments of working memory and memory. Executive functioning assessment indicated that he had deficits in inhibiting his initial responses, thinking flexibly and adjusting strategies based on feedback. In other words, he could come up with a 'Plan A', but struggled to identify when it was ineffective and to implement a 'Plan B'.

Whilst David could remember the gist of information provided (primarily information at the beginning and end or a conversation/event), he struggled to recall the detail. He tended to mask the extent of this memory impairment by smiling and nodding appropriately when he had not fully understood all of the information. He also seemed to have learnt responses to commonly asked questions by rote, which further masked his poor memory.

David had limited insight into his impairments, and dismissed the findings of the assessment when they were fed back to him. For instance, he maintained that if his eyesight were restored he would have no difficulties managing his diabetes, and showed no awareness of other barriers (e.g. cognitive impairments, hand dexterity). Moreover, because David found it difficult to form trusting relationships with others, he often dismissed feedback as others' attempts to obstruct or control him, and this presented a further barrier to his developing awareness.

Second mental capacity assessment

Neuropsychological assessment greatly enriched the team's understanding of David's ability to understand and weigh up information. A second capacity assessment was undertaken by a neuropsychologist and a clinical psychologist. His responses in the second assessment were much the same as in the first. However, the assessors were aware that David's relatively stronger verbal abilities meant that he could give verbal responses to create an impression that he has understood something when he had not. The assessors therefore asked more probing follow-up questions, and asked questions on a broader range of relevant topics to reduce the likelihood that he was giving a rote response.

A lack of understanding of the relevant information was discovered. For instance, it was evident that David had learnt key information about his diabetes management as he had lived with diabetes since an early age. He could therefore speak fluently about all aspects of diabetes management. However, when the assessors intentionally asked questions about pressure sore management (a health topic that was equally important but less familiar to him), he was not able to provide any information. David also maintained that he had no cognitive impairments and could not describe how they might impact on his ability to meet his care needs. This provided some evidence of poor understanding and weighing up of relevant information.

Evidence of the frontal lobe paradox also became more apparent in this assessment. For example, David said that he could manage hypoglycaemic episodes by placing a chocolate bar by his bedside if he was home alone. He was, however, unable to recognise that in practice this would be challenging because he would be unable to go to the shops to buy chocolate; he might forget to place a chocolate bar by his bedside; or that he might not think to eat it during a hypoglycaemic episode. It was also demonstrable on the ward that David was not hypo-aware and did not take any independent action during a hypoglycaemic episode, highlighting that his performance in practice was incongruent with what he was suggesting.

Based on this assessment, the assessors determined that David lacked mental capacity to make decisions about his discharge, and so a decision needed to be made by the professionals in David's best interests.

Challenges

Disagreements over capacity

Once the clinical team were satisfied that David lacked mental capacity, a referral was made to the local authority to start the discharge process. A case manager was allocated. A referral was also made for an Independent Mental Capacity Advocate (IMCA) to ensure that David's voice was heard, given his vociferous opposition to discharge to a nursing home and the fact that he had no close family who could advocate on his behalf. Both the case manager and IMCA visited David and conducted their own informal capacity assessments in interview. As ever, David was able to demonstrate an apparent insight into his disabilities and care needs and gave the impression that he had carefully weighed up the decision to go home. On the basis of this, both the case manager and IMCA disputed the team's capacity assessment and took the view that David should be supported in his choice to return home, despite the serious risks.

The clinical team were also required to seek authorisation for a Deprivation of Liberty Safeguards (DoLS). This is a requirement in law for anyone held in a hospital or care home where they lack capacity, are under 'continuous supervision and control', and are not free to leave.[3] Authorisation was initially declined, however, because the Best Interests Assessor also took the view that David had capacity to choose to leave hospital, however unwise this might be. This caused a difficult situation in which David could self-discharge from the ward and the staff would have no legal framework to prevent him. By this point, David had been in hospital for eight months, and was becoming understandably frustrated at his length of stay, so the risk of self-discharge was high.

Evidencing the frontal lobe paradox

The clinical team needed to ensure that other professionals were aware that David lacked the mental capacity to make decisions about discharge so that he could be placed under a DoLS and so that his discharge planning could progress.

It was agreed that this could be best evidenced by demonstrating that he presented with the frontal lobe paradox, so his presentation in interview was not an accurate representation of his abilities. His diabetes management was chosen to illustrate this. This was specifically chosen because diabetes management was essential for his survival, and a mental capacity assessment hinged on whether he was adequately appraising the risks around this when considering his discharge options. Moreover, David had consistently maintained that he could manage his diabetes entirely independently at home, yet this had thus far been managed by the medical and nursing team.

The neuropsychologist devised a practical assessment in which David was asked to manage his own diabetes for two weeks. The practical assessment was designed to ascertain whether David could put his plans into practice, whilst also looking at his emergent awareness of any challenges and whether he could adjust his behaviour or perceptions of his needs in response to errors.

David was told that all responsibility for managing his diabetes would be handed over to him over the trial period. He would be expected to check his blood glucose levels and administer his insulin independently. The equipment would be stored in the medication cabinet, so he needed to push the call button to request his glucose monitor and insulin whenever necessary. He was also told that he would need to look out for any hypo- or hyperglycaemic episodes. If this happened, he should use the call bell to summon the nurses, and to tell them what remedial action he would like to take. Finally, David was told that meals would no longer be given to him unless he asked, and the domestic staff were instructed the same. David readily accepted this plan and predicted that he would have no difficulties. As in previous conversations, he believed he could successfully attend to this independently, and was able to explain all of the steps that he would need to take to manage his diabetes in detail, including his insulin regimen and the processes of checking his blood-glucose levels. He also described the warning signs of a hypo- or hyperglycaemic episode, and the action he would need to take if this were to happen (e.g. having a sugary drink or using glucogel).

The task was intentionally left unstructured so that David himself needed to generate strategies to maximise his success. Nurses were asked to record his performance on a monitoring form. Without David's knowledge, nurses also implemented a monitoring procedure and contingency plans to ensure David's safety throughout this trial. If David did not ask for his meal, blood glucose monitor, or insulin independently within 15 minutes of his usual time, nursing staff prompted him, and then at 30 minutes, nurses intervened directly. Nurses were also surreptitiously monitoring David for symptoms of a hypoglycaemic episode.

The results of the trial were stark. David was physically able to use his blood glucose monitor and insulin pen despite his visual impairments and difficulties with hand dexterity, but his cognitive impairments presented as a significant barrier. In the trial, he omitted half of his insulin doses. He was generally able to remember his insulin or blood glucose monitoring when prompted, but on four occasions took no action even after a prompt. His performance and approach to the task showed no improvement over time, and he did not introduce any compensatory strategies, even when it was apparent that he was missing doses.

David's performance on this task was indicative of difficulties with prospective memory, and provided further evidence of poor cognitive flexibility and self-monitoring. It also demonstrated that David had limited self-awareness or insight into his impairments and his level of care needs in day-to-day life, and if he were to be discharged without any support then he would inevitably miss insulin doses and enter a diabetic coma. Moreover, when this was fed back to him at the end of the task, David downplayed the errors, and maintained that he would be able to manage his diabetes independently, and with complete accuracy, at home.

This trial demonstrated that although David could accurately describe his diabetes management plan and express his intention to follow it, he was unable to put this into practice. It also demonstrated that David was unaware of this discrepancy. The team successfully argued that this showed that, despite presenting well in capacity assessments, David lacked mental capacity because he was not adequately weighing up the information relating to discharge.

Resolution

Following this trial, a third mental capacity assessment took place, this time jointly with the case manager. She was satisfied that David lacked mental capacity to make decisions about discharge, and the Best Interests Assessor and IMCA agreed. He was placed under a DoLS and a best interests meeting took place in relation to his discharge. It was agreed that it would not be in David's best interests to return home without support, but the multi-agency team could not agree on an appropriate discharge destination. David, on the other hand, remained of the view that he could manage his diabetes at home without care, and was becoming increasingly verbally abusive whenever anyone attempted to talk to him about discharge to anywhere else. Because of this, the Best Interests Assessor determined that the case should be passed to the Court of Protection for consideration. By this stage, he had been in hospital for a year, but David was required to remain in hospital until the judge heard the case and made a decision.

The court process lasted for another year. As part of the judge's deliber-ations, an independent psychiatrist was employed to assess David's mental capacity. They considered all evidence, including the assessments that had been completed by the team, and agreed that David lacked mental capacity. All options were explored, but ultimately the judge deemed that it would be in David's best interests to be discharged to a supported living service with an extensive care package. Understandably, David resisted this plan and the staff team worked with him to help him see the positives of the care home that had been chosen. The team showed David photographs and videos of the service, introduced him to his new care team, and arranged a visit to the new flat. Whilst David was initially hostile to any mention of the discharge plan, over time he became more positive. Careful contingency plans were made for the day of discharge in case he changed his mind or became aggressive during transit, but ultimately this went smoothly.

At the time of writing, David remains at the supported living service. He appears settled and content but remains angry at the hospital for perceived injustices. This is perhaps understandable when one considers the distress caused over the course of the discharge process, and the fact that his admis-sion was planned as ten 10 weeks but lasted over two years.

Discussion

The significant disagreements over David's mental capacity greatly length-ened his admission and caused unnecessary distress and frustration to David, and had significant financial implications for the health service. The learning from his case therefore centres around how consensus among professionals could be reached more quickly.

David's case highlights the limitations of relying solely on interviews to conduct mental capacity assessments, particularly in individuals who present with the frontal lobe paradox. Timely and comprehensive cognitive assess-ment, direct observation, or experiments to directly test out a person's verbal report can often inform mental capacity assessments, particularly where exec-utive dysfunction is identified or suspected and/or where there is a suspicion of confabulation, anosognosia, or the frontal lobe paradox.

Effective communication and joint working between professionals in-volved is essential in these particularly complex cases. George and Gilbert (2018) point out that professionals from local authorities and advocacy ser-vices do not always have specialist knowledge of brain injury and are trained to take a strength-based approach, focused on empowering individuals to make their own decisions. As such, it can be seen as controlling, paternalis-tic, or risk averse to suggest that a patient's self-report should not be taken at face-value, and that the person making a risky decision lacks capacity despite apparently being aware of the risk. Open and respectful discussions about differing ideologies or perspectives were crucial in bridging these gaps in

David's case, but this can be challenging when encounters between professionals are time-pressured, as is often the case when social workers visit inpatient wards. Joint mental capacity assessments from the outset may also have reduced the disagreements between different professionals.[4]

David's case required an unusually high degree of multidisciplinary and multi-agency working, particularly once the case was taken to the Court of Protection. By this stage, solicitors became involved, and David's case had become sufficiently complex so as to require the direct involvement of senior managers and directors from both health and social care services. One particularly memorable discharge planning meeting, ordered by the judge, was attended by David's clinical team, his case manager, an IMCA, members of the safeguarding teams from both the hospital trust and social services senior managers, matrons, and directors from the hospital and social care services, and representatives from three law firms (acting for David, social services, and the hospital). This totalled 20 people. Although such broad involvement was often necessary, it raised logistical complications and often slowed decision-making processes. The psychologist took on a central role in this, acting as a liaison between agencies and co-ordinating meetings. However, this was time consuming and there could perhaps have been alternative ways of handling this (e.g. through allocating a named representative from each agency; allocating an administrator to act as a co-ordinator). It also highlights the need for effective case management in negotiating in complex brain injury cases, as case managers have a central role in facilitating transitions between establishments (Cornforth & Varley, 2006), though it should be noted that there is at present a need for further research into the effectiveness of case management (Lannin et al., 2014).

Notes

1 All names and identifiable information changed.
2 Even well-managed diabetes has been found to cause a deterioration in cognitive functioning over time, particularly executive dysfunction, processing speed, and working memory. Repeated hypo- and hyperglycaemic episodes are known to exacerbate this cognitive decline (Brands et al., 2005; Broadley et al., 2017).
3 Depriving someone of their freedom is potentially a breach of their human rights, so this process is to ensure that any such restrictions are lawful. Making an application means that two assessors visit the patient: one, usually a psychiatrist, confirms that they have a mental disorder that limits capacity. The second assessor, called a 'Best Interests Assessor', determines whether the individual lacks capacity to consent to their current admission, and whether it is in the individual's best interests to be deprived of their liberty. In the UK, new legislation has been drafted to replace the the cumbersome DoLS process with a more streamlined one, the Liberty Protection Safeguards. It is anticipated that this change will happen in 2023 or 2024.
4 Indeed, joint assessments are recommended in the Mental Capacity Act Code of Practice (Office of the Public Guardian, 2007) but this particular recommendation is not always adhered to in busy clinical environments, where pinning down a clinician can be difficult.

References

Amanzio, M., Bartoli, M., Cipriani, G. E., & Palermo, S. (2020). Executive dysfunction and reduced self-awareness in patients with neurological disorders: A mini-review. *Frontiers in Psychology*, *11*(1697), https://doi.org/10.3389/fpsyg.2020.0169

Brands, A. M., Biessels, G. J., de Haan, E. H. F., Kappelle, L. J., & Kessels, R. P. C. (2005). The effects of type 1 diabetes on cognitive performance: A meta-analysis. *Diabetes Care*, *28*(3), 726–735. https://doi.org/10.2337/diacare.28.3.726

Broadley, M. M., White, M. J., & Andrew, B. (2017). A systematic review and meta-analysis of executive function performance in type 1 diabetes mellitus. *Psychosomatic Medicine*, *79*(6), 684–696. https://doi.org/10.1097/PSY.00000000 00000460

Cornforth, E., & Varley, C. (2006). The role of the case manager in supporting the brain injured person during transition. In J. Parker (Ed.), *Good practice in brain injury case management* (pp. 109–121). Jessica Kingsley.

Dreer, L. E., DeVivo, M. J., Novack, T. A., Krzywanski, M. S., & Marson, J. D. (2008). Cognitive predictors of medical decision-making capacity in traumatic brain injury. *Rehabilitation Psychology*, *53*(4), 486–497. https://doi.org/10.1037/a0013798

George, M., & Gilbert, S. (2018). Mental Capacity Act (2005) assessments: Why everyone needs to know about the frontal lobe paradox. *The Neuropsychologist*, *5*, 59–66.

Johnson, S. C., Baxter, L. C., Wilder, L. S., Pipe, J. G., Heiserman, J. E., & Prigatano, G. P. (2002). Neural correlates of self-reflection. *Brain*, *125*(8) 1808–1814. https://doi.org/10.1093/brain/awf181

Lannin, N. A., Laver, K., Kareena, H., Turnbull, M., Elder, M., Campisi, J. Schmidt, J., & Schneider, E. (2014). Effects of case management after brain injury: A systematic review. *Neurorehabilitation*, *35*(4), 635–641. https://doi.org/10.3233/NRE-141161

Office of the Public Guardian (2007). *Mental Capacity Act Code of Practice*. The Stationery Office.

Palermo, S., Leotta, D., Bongioanni, M. R., & Amanzio, M. (2014). Unawareness of deficits in ischemic injury: Role of the cingulate cortex. *Neurocase*, *20*(5), 540–555. https://doi.org/10.1080/13554794.2013.826686

Stuss, D. T., & Anderson, V. (2004). The frontal lobes and theory of mind: Developmental concepts from adult focal lesion research. *Brain Cognition*, *55*, 69–83. https://doi.org/10.1016/S0278-2626(03)00271-9

Teggart, V., & Dimmock, K. (2020). What to do when someone says one thing but does another: Capacity to make a decision and put it into practice. In J. A. Mackenzie & K. E. Wilkinson (Eds.), *Assessing mental capacity: A handbook to guide professionals from basic to advanced practice* (pp. 241–254) Routledge.

Toglia, J., & Kirk, U. (2000). Understanding awareness deficits following brain injury. *NeuroRehabilitation*, *15*(1), 57–70. https://doi.org/ 10.3233/NRE-2000–15104

United Nations Convention on the Rights of Persons with Disabilities (2006, December 13). www.un.org/development/desa/disabilities/convention-on-the-rights-of-persons-with-disabilities/convention-on-the-rights-of-persons-with-disabilities-2.html

United Nations Universal Declaration of Human Rights (1948, December 10). www.un.org/sites/un2.un.org/files/udhr.pdf

Walsh, K. W. (1985). *Understanding brain damage: A primer of neuropsychological evaluation*. Longman Group.

Wilkinson, K. (2020). Some basic concepts of the Mental Capacity Act (2005). In J. A. Mackenzie & K. E. Wilkinson (Eds.), *Assessing mental capacity: A handbook to guide professionals from basic to advanced practice* (pp. 20–29). Routledge.

Williams, C., & Wood, R. L. I. (2017). Disorders of emotion recognition and expression. In T. M. McMillan & R. L. I. Wood (Eds.), *Neurobehavioural disability and social handicap following traumatic brain injury* (pp. 30–42). Routledge.

Wood., L. I., & Bigler, E. (2017). Problems assessing executive dysfunction in neurobehavioural disability. In T. M McMillan & R. L. I. Wood (Eds.), *Neurobehavioural disability and social handicap following traumatic brain injury* (pp. 88–100). Routledge.

22 The importance of accuracy when diagnosing locked-in-syndrome (LIS)

Sarah Crawford, Sal Connolly, and Alexandra E. Rose

Introduction

Locked-in-syndrome (LIS) is a rare condition where individuals are fully conscious but unable to speak or display voluntary movement other than eye movement. The nature of this syndrome includes the diagnostic feature that the individual is cognitively intact; this is because it is caused by damage to the brain stem, usually a lesion in the pontine region, and the higher cortical functions remain unaffected (Smith & Delargey, 2005). Since people with LIS have tetraparesis and are unable to speak, they have limited means of demonstrating their largely intact cognition.

The diagnosis of LIS can be challenging initially due to multifactorial issues such as medical instability, patient fatigue, and clinician inexperience in assessing patients with limited communication ability. There is an established literature of cases where people with LIS have been misdiagnosed as being in a prolonged disorder of consciousness (PDOC), often on the basis of incomplete assessments – essentially where their intact eye-movement control has been missed (Laureys et al., 2005; Vanhaudenhuyse et al., 2018). Minimally conscious patients with severe cognitive difficulties but visible eye movements may also appear to be locked-in; however, they would not be able to consistently respond to questions due to their reduced awareness. A thorough neuropsychological assessment using tasks with yes/no or forced-choice responses can be undertaken with such patients in order to demonstrate their cognitive strengths and ensure that they are diagnosed correctly as being in LIS rather than PDOC. However, this assessment is also vital for avoiding the opposite diagnostic error, i.e. describing a patient as being in LIS when their cognitive functioning is, in fact, severely impaired.

The current authors have extensive clinical experience of working with patients with severe to profound cognitive impairment (including PDOC), and also patients with LIS. Collectively, we have encountered a range of cases where the patient has tetraparesis, inability to speak, *and* severe cognitive impairment such that they are unable to perform basic cognitive tasks, but clinicians working with the patient have described them as having LIS. This is in spite of the patients' inability to make basic choices, and in the context

DOI: 10.4324/9781003228226-25

of them invariably having damage to areas of the brain beyond the pons. We contend that using the label 'locked-in-syndrome' (LIS) to describe patients with severe cognitive impairments is clinically misleading and carries significant risks that patients' families will develop expectations for recovery and quality of life that simply will not be realised. This chapter describes what the neuropsychologist and broader multidisciplinary team (MDT) can do to assess cognition and optimise the presentation of these complex patients to ensure an accurate understanding of their cognitive strengths and weaknesses. Illustrative case examples are used to demonstrate the techniques. The reasons for choosing illustrative cases rather than presenting a real case are outlined in the discussion.

Clinical features

LIS is a specific syndrome characterised by tetraparesis (inability to move any of the four limbs) and anarthria (the inability to produce sound or speak). Anarthria is due to paralysis of the muscles and is distinct from an inability to produce sound due to cognitive impairments. Paralysis of the muscles in the face and neck also result in dysphagia (impaired swallow), and flat, unchanging facial expression that does not reflect the person's emotional state. In contrast, eye-lid control and vertical eye movement tends to be spared as the area used to control this, the mid-brain tectum, is not damaged in 'classic' LIS (see below). Hearing is generally well preserved but visual difficulties may be present. The damage is centralised to the brain stem region, most commonly damage to the pons. Given that the cortex is intact, the patient is assumed to be fully aware with no change in cognition (Smith & Delargey, 2005).

LIS has been classified into three categories (Bauer et al., 1979):

1. Classic/Classical LIS: tetraparesis and anarthria with preserved consciousness and vertical eye movement.
2. Incomplete or partial LIS: the same as classic LIS but with some limited additional voluntary movements other than vertical eye movement, e.g. some mouth or finger movements.
3. Total LIS: total immobility including absence of voluntary eye movements, but with presumed full consciousness – these patients can currently only be identified using EEG or functional imaging techniques (see e.g. Smith & Delargy, 2005; Schnakers et al., 2009).

A survey of 44 LIS patients (Leon-Carrion et al., 2002) reported the main cause of LIS to be stroke (86.4%), followed by traumatic brain injury (13.6%). The authors found that diagnosis was challenging for clinicians unfamiliar with the syndrome, and that family and friends were more likely than clinicians to be first to notice that patients were trying to purposefully communicate with eye movements (55% family/friends, as opposed to 23% being recognised by physicians); this contributed to the mean time to reach a diagnosis of LIS being longer than two months (mean of 78.6 days).

Prognosis

In terms of prognosis, a review by Halan et al. (2021) found that the prognosis for full recovery was poor, with most patients remaining in LIS. Due to the associated medical complexities, death within the first year is common; however, if patients survive the first year the authors reported that the five-year survival rate can reach 86%, with the 10-year survival rate being 80%. The review highlighted that mood disorders and poor perceptions of quality of life were more common in people with LIS than in healthy controls. Nevertheless, a study examining self-reported well-being in a group of patients with chronic LIS found that most reported being 'happy' rather than 'unhappy', and that happiness correlated with the length of time since LIS diagnosis, suggesting that many of these individuals adapt to their disabilities over time (Bruno et al., 2011).

Assessment

When considering whether a diagnosis of LIS is appropriate, clinicians must first establish the patient's awareness and level of consciousness. When it has been established that the patient is aware, it is necessary for clinicians to establish a method for communicating as a first step. It is suggested that basic functional ability to make use of the eye movement is optimised, i.e. using the patient's better eye and manually opening eyelids if ptosis (a droop in the upper eyelid) is present. As Wilson et al. (2011) point out, these patients are not easy to assess and questions and assessments need to be adapted to ensure accuracy. People with classic LIS are restricted to blinking or looking up/down to communicate and thus are initially limited to binary questions (i.e. yes/no) or binary forced-choices. These responses can be used to ask them a series of closed questions, on different occasions and at different times of day, to explore their reliability and consistency in responses (Laureys et al., 2005). With support, patients can potentially make further use of their eye blinks or up/down eye movements to spell words out using a communication board with a communication partner, or even learn to use high-tech aids such as eye-gaze (Lugo et al., 2015). However, they can tire easily which impacts their ability to use these eye movements to communicate.

Evidence for broad preservation of cognitive functioning has been found in several studies. For example, in a study of two chronic LIS cases, cognitive abilities on the measures administered (see Table 22.1) were found to be preserved (Allain et al., 1998). In a survey of 44 people with LIS, Leon-Carrion et al. (2002) found that the majority reported being orientated to time (86%) and having good levels of attention (97.6%); only a minority (18.6%) of those surveyed reported having memory problems and those that reported memory difficulties had traumatic aetiology.

Table 22.1 Tests used to assess cognitive functioning in LIS
(Allain et al., 1998)

Verbal abilities	Verbal comprehension (BDAE)
	Written comprehension (BDAE)
Intelligence	Verbal WAIS-R subtests
	Raven Coloured Progressive Matrices
Memory	Digit Forward and Backward (WAIS-R)
	Rey's 15 words
	Paired associate learnings (WMS-R)
	Delayed recognition (BEM 144)

BDAE = Boston Diagnostic Aphasia Examination, WAIS-R = Wechsler Adult
Intelligence Scale Revised, WMS-R = Wechsler Memory Scale Revised,
BEM 144 = Batterie d'efficience mnésique

More detailed neuropsychological assessments have been completed with
LIS patients, despite the limitations of using yes/no responses and communication boards. For example, Schnakers et al. (2008) demonstrated that a
battery of tests could be administered to patients in LIS. Their battery con-
sisted of the Doors subtest of The Doors and People for non-verbal episodic
memory, a shortened Wisconsin card sorting test for executive functioning,
and a modified digit span using yes/no responses for working memory. They
also included a word-picture naming task and a picture vocabulary test to
assess language and a bespoke auditory attention task. Although their study
showed that their sample of LIS patients had largely intact cognitive function,
they also found that some presented with cognitive impairments, which were
typically associated with additional organic damage beyond the brainstem.

A more thorough battery of neuropsychological tests was carried out in
a single case study reported by Wilson and colleagues (Wilson et al., 2011),
which included tests using forced-choice responding (e.g. Spot the Word,
Matrix Reasoning), tests using yes/no responses (e.g. face and picture recognition from the Rivermead Behavioural Memory Test version 3), and tests in
which the patient was asked to spell words using her communication chart
(e.g. California Verbal Learning Test). Their patient scored within the average or above average range on most of the tests administered, consistent with
people in LIS having largely preserved cognitive functioning. Nevertheless,
she scored below expectations on several tests, which the authors concluded
was likely to be due primarily to visual processing difficulties secondary to
diplopia and blurred vision.

Whilst the studies described above demonstrate that neuropsychological
assessments can be used with people who are in LIS, they do not tell us what
approach should be taken when patients cannot participate with these tests
and potentially have more severe cognitive impairments. Formal measures of
awareness, which are used to diagnose disorders of consciousness, may be of
some use with those who are most severely impaired, but caution must be ex-
ercised given these patients' profound motor impairments. For example, the

most widely used measure, the Coma Recovery Scale-revised (Giacino et al., 2004) has several hierarchical scales, but some of these, e.g. the Motor Function Scale, are not suitable for use with patients with tetraparesis who cannot hold and manipulate objects because of their physical disabilities. Similar challenges affect interpretation of the Wessex Head Injury Matrix (Shiel et al., 2000), on which a patient in classic LIS will potentially pass items towards the end of the scale (e.g. item 56: 'Knows the name of one member of staff' or item 61: 'Remembers something from earlier in the day'), but will fail items much earlier in the hierarchy such as item 10: 'Expletive utterance' or item 19 'Speaks in whispered tones'. This means that for patients with tetraparesis, the number of the most advanced behaviour observed will hold much greater meaning than the total number of behaviours observed, and that assessors should potentially examine some of the higher behaviours rather than following the instruction to stop after ten consecutive failures.

As described above, Wilson et al. (2011) showed that three different formats could be used to assess their patient in LIS, i.e. forced-choice responding, yes/no responding, and spelling out words letter-by-letter. The first two of these can be used with patients with profound physical impairments to explore cognitive functioning when it has either been established that formal neuropsychological tests are too challenging, or the assessor has judged that the informal evidence of cognitive impairment is sufficient that establishing whether the patient can answer simple questions is indicated before attempting more complex assessment.

Yes/no responding can be explored using the method described by McMillan (1997), in which a series of counterbalanced yes/no questions are constructed, and binominal statistics used to establish whether or not responding is above chance. When this method is employed, it is particularly important to avoid assuming that a patient's ability to answer some questions correctly means that they can answer all questions correctly. Thus, a patient who can answer biographical questions correctly may not be able to answer situational questions, and a patient who can answer both of these may be unable to answer abstract questions. Examples of counterbalanced questions of different types can be found in Annex 1a of the RCP (2020) guidelines, and the Putney PDOC Toolkit (Wilford et al., 2019), both of which are available as free downloads.

Forced-choice responding can be explored using the method described by Murphy (2018), in which patients are presented with two stimuli and asked to identify one of them. For example, the patient may be shown a spoon and a ball and asked to look at the ball. The strength of Murphy's approach was to design a paradigm in which counterbalanced targets could be presented in a sufficient number of trials that, like McMillan's method, binomial statistics could be used to determine whether responding was above chance. Murphy's study looked at patients' abilities to discriminate between six basic stimuli (objects, pictures, words, letters, numbers, and colours); in our clinical practice, once patients have demonstrated this ability, we expand the methodology to assess more complex questions, for which examples are given below.

Crucial to both methods is that there must be sufficient trials in order to determine whether the person is responding correctly at a probability significantly greater than chance, and that correct responses are counterbalanced with incorrect responses in order to avoid drawing false conclusions if the person has, for example, a 'yes' response-bias. Murphy's paradigm used ten questions for each type of stimulus, for which a score of 8/10 or above can be judged to be significantly higher than chance using binomial statistics. The RCP guidelines (RCP, 2020) currently recommend six trials for yes/no questions, with 6/6 needing to be correct in order for the patient to be judged to have passed the test; however, this approach has been criticised as insufficiently evidence-based (Pundole & Crawford, 2017), and we generally apply Murphy's criteria of ten trials when we use yes/no closed questions in our clinical practice.

Illustrative case studies

In order to illustrate how to differentiate between LIS as defined in the literature (i.e. with largely intact cognition), and conditions in which patients with profound physical disability also present with significant cognitive impairment, we have outlined some illustrative case studies below. These cases are fictitious and are intended to demonstrate the techniques involved. Because of this, details about pathology and medical history have not been included. Readers should assume that symptoms had sudden onset necessitating acute hospital admission and that, prior to admission to post-acute level 1 services, the patients underwent detailed medical evaluation from appropriately qualified specialists who concluded that there was clear evidence of a non-reversible organic basis for their physical disabilities. It should also be assumed that limited information was available about any brain scans that were undertaken, as is often the case in clinical practice. The reasons for choosing illustrative rather than real case examples are described in more detail in the Discussion section.

Case 1: Steve

On admission, Steve's family expressed how happy they were that Steve had been admitted for level 1 neurorehabilitation. They said that the team in the referring hospital had told them that Steve had LIS and had recommended the family read 'The Diving Bell and the Butterfly'. They were delighted to read Jean-Dominique Bauby's autobiographical account of living with LIS; they realised that Steve was unlikely to recover any speech but were excited that he would soon have support to learn to spell out words and sentences. They were aware that we had a specialist in-house assistive technology service and were hopeful that Steve would be set up with an eye-gaze system as soon as possible.

On initial assessments, Steve was able to look up and down to command. He was also able to look at 'Yes' and 'No' cards presented in the vertical plane, and to look at 'Yes' when asked if his name was Steve and 'No' when asked if his name was Peter. A preliminary assessment of Steve's ability to discriminate between two stimuli was completed (Murphy, 2018). Steve passed 3/6 subtests, scoring 10/10 for pictures and colours and 9/10 for real objects. His scores were below the cut-off score of 8/10 on the other three subtests, scoring 4/10 for words, 5/10 for letters, and 6/10 for numbers. Informally, it was observed that Steve's responses were often unclear on his weaker subtests, with him tending to switch his gaze between both items rather than selecting the target. He required a large amount of encouragement to clearly select an answer on these subtests, adding informal evidence to the formulation that he was guessing.

For the three subtests he passed he was subsequently asked semantic questions using the same forced-choice paradigm, e.g. 'which one do you eat with?', 'which one is the colour of grass?'. Steve passed semantic questions relating to colours (9/10), but scored below the cut-off for both pictures (5/10) and real objects (4/10). Further exploration of his abilities showed that he could correctly answer colour-related questions about the real objects (8/10), but he remained unable to correctly answer questions about their function. When asked yes/no questions, Steve was consistently able to answer simple biographical questions – e.g. about his own name, or whether or not he had a brother (9/10), and questions relating to identifying objects (e.g. 'is this a toothbrush?') and colours (e.g. 'is this red?') and met criteria for emergence from a disorder of consciousness on this basis. However, he scored below chance on situational questions (4/10) and more complex biographical questions (5/10).

Because Steve could identify pictures, an equivalent paradigm was designed using emojis for emotions – e.g. 'which one is happy?', 'which one is sad?', etc. Steve scored 5/10, showing that he could not reliably distinguish between these emotions above chance levels. This was also true when simple line drawings were used (4/10). A similar paradigm was designed using words associated with the same emotions, although the working hypothesis was that Steve would fail this trial given his difficulties with the initial words task; indeed, Steve's score was at chance levels of responding (6/10). The team was informed that there was no reliable and valid method to assess Steve's ability to self-report mood. Behaviourally, Steve engaged well with therapy sessions, showed no differences in engagement between family and staff and showed no signs of tearfulness – there was therefore no indication of major concern about his emotional well-being.

His recognition memory was assessed using the pictures and faces subtests of the Rivermead Behavioural Memory Test, third edition. However, Steve's scores were impaired on both measures. His memory for words was not assessed, given that Steve had failed the simple word discrimination tasks.

Consistent with these findings, assessments with the occupational therapist (OT) showed that Steve could discern between a toothbrush and a comb, but was inconsistent when asked questions like 'which one is for brushing teeth?' Due to his tetraplegia, his ability to use the objects in function could not be assessed. The speech and language therapist (SLT) worked with Steve and his family to establish what methods of communication Steve could use. Despite a large amount of prompting and support, Steve was not able to learn to consistently use an alphabet chart or other methods such as an e-tran or eye-gaze system. He remained limited to simple, concrete yes/no or force-choice binary responses.

Following these assessments, the MDT conclusion was that Steve presented with significant cognitive impairments that precluded him from a diagnosis of 'classic locked in syndrome' and the formulation was explained to the family as tetraplegia with severe cognitive impairment. The team focused interventions aimed at disability management and maximising Steve's quality of life. Psychology support was provided to the family alongside education sessions with the SLT to explain why Steve was not able to spell out his thoughts or needs and that he was unfortunately not in the same situation as Jean-Dominque Bauby. This was challenging for the family to accept, given the high expectations they had prior to Steve's admission. While they were given support to manage their expectations and plan for the future, his closest family members remained convinced at the point of discharge that Steve's cognition was fully intact and that he understood everything that was said to him.

Case 2: Antoine

Antoine was referred to the rehabilitation ward following a severe stroke. On assessment, he was able to pass all six of the simple forced-choice stimulus identification subtests and also scored above chance when semantic questions were asked about the same items. Further cognitive assessments showed that Antoine scored in the impaired range on all recognition memory tests attempted (RBMT-III for faces and pictures; Camden Memory Tests for words) and that he was effectively 'living in the moment'. This limited his progression and ability to use an alphabet board or eye-gaze functionally. In SLT sessions, Antoine was able to look at a letter when asked to do so using an eye-gaze system. If Antoine was asked to spell a word, e.g. his name, he could look at the first and sometimes the second letter but would then seemingly choose letters at random, even with reminders about the purpose of the task. This remained the case when the assessor used an AEIOU alphabet chart with Antoine and wrote the letters he chose on a whiteboard that remained in front of him during the task – thus although this potentially reduced the memory demands of the task, Antoine was either unable to sustain his attention or was unable to remember the instruction part-way through. When asked open questions, he would randomly look at letters but was unable to spell out any words. This was trialled in English, in French (his first language), and was attempted both with a range of clinicians, and with family members supporting him, but no difference in his performance was observed. It was not possible to tell if Antoine had thought of a word but was unable to spell it, and/or forgot his word mid-way through the task, or if he was unable to generate a response at all. Regardless, Antoine was unable to use any method to communicate functionally and he therefore presented with tetraparesis plus severe cognitive impairment rather than classic LIS.

It was observed that Antoine could differentiate people since his reactions (e.g. eyes widening, tears) to family members were clearly different to staff members; he was also able to discriminate between different family members when shown two photographs in a personalised adaptation of the forced-choice paradigm (e.g. 'Look at the picture of Simone'). Antoine frequently displayed tearfulness when family arrived or when shown pictures of his family. He did not show this response toward staff or pictures of strangers. Antoine engaged well throughout family visits but would cry when his family left, although tears did not occur in other settings. Antoine was able to discriminate between different emojis, line drawings, and emotion-related words. However, when a set of counterbalanced yes/no questions was developed to ask Antoine about his own mood, his responses across several sessions were contradictory (e.g. giving a 'yes' response to both 'sad' and 'happy'). It was concluded that although Antoine was able to discriminate between the stimuli, he was unable to reflect on and communicate about his own internal mood-state. Although it was not possible to elicit self-report from Antoine, the observations described above suggested that he did not have a mood disorder, but had normal emotional reactions to familiar people. Via yes/no responses, Antoine tended to communicate that he liked TV and radio programmes in French rather than English, and that he liked hearing people speaking French. Thus, although Antoine was unable to communicate in either language, there was evidence that his first language was more familiar to him. Interventions moved away from a focus on communication methods to supporting him to spend time with his family. Recommendations for discharge were for Antoine to be with or near to his family, to have carers who spoke his first language whenever possible, and for Antoine's daily routine to contain opportunities for him to listen to and watch programmes in French.

Case 3: Susan

On admission, Susan presented with anarthria and tetraparesis with the ability to use her eyes to look up and down. Communication was explored using this eye movement. Susan was able to successfully discern between two stimuli to command on all the discrimination subtests and was also able to correctly answer both biographical and situational questions reliably. SLT sessions established that Susan could spell simple words using an alphabet chart and trials using an eye-gaze system began. More in-depth neuropsychological assessments were commenced when the SLT was satisfied that a communication method had been established and the MDT priorities of optimising medical stability, increasing seating tolerance, and attempting to reduce her levels of fatigue were managed. The choice of tests was influenced by balancing the need to understand Susan's cognitive profile with conserving her windows of responsiveness to be able to interact with family and use her environmental controls (e.g. to access the BBC website, YouTube etc.), given that Susan continued to fatigue quickly when using her eye-gaze.

Susan was able to correctly answer forced-choice semantic questions in all modalities. The Spot the Word test (version 2) was used to establish an estimate of her premorbid cognitive abilities and Susan scored within the average range. Memory was assessed via the RMBT-III faces and pictures subtests, the Camden words for verbal memory, and the Doors subtest of the Doors and People. Susan scored in the average range or above on all of these recognition memory tests. Recall tests were not administered as Susan's letter-by-letter spelling was judged to be too substantial a deviation from the standardised instructions for a valid interpretation of her performance to be made. Her basic visuo-perceptual and visuo-spatial abilities were assessed using subtests from the VOSP with minimal response–demands and Susan passed all subtests administered. Since Susan's basic visual processing skills were intact, the Matrix Reasoning subtest from the WAIS-IV was completed to assess current non-verbal abilities and Susan scored within the high average range. Susan's semantic memory processing ability was assessed using the three picture Pyramids and Palm Trees test, which she passed. Her language ability was assessed in function in that she was able to spell words and communicate effectively using alphabet charts and her eye-gaze. Executive functioning was assessed using the Brixton test. The test was adapted by asking her to select the number the pattern was moving to rather than pointing. Susan took longer than expected to recognise changes in pattern and showed a tendency to perseverate, scoring in the 'below average' range; however, fatigue potentially affected her performance, given the length of the task. Mood was assessed using open questions and Susan initiated spelling words such as 'OK' and 'fine' using her eye-gaze communication system indicating no significant concerns regarding her mood or anxiety levels.

Although the tests showed a profile that suggested that Susan's cognitive abilities were largely intact, only one test of executive functioning was carried out, since most executive tests are not suitable for patients with anarthria and tetraparesis, and Susan's weakest score was on this task. Informal observations of executive functioning are also extremely limited when assessing patients in LIS due to the extensive motor impairments that constrain their ability to demonstrate behaviour. However, there was informal evidence of rigidity and perseveration when Susan was using her eye-gaze. This impacted some of her complex decision-making ability and the MDT focus moved to assessing which decisions she was able to make independently and which required support (e.g. prompts, visual aids, simplified information) in order for Susan to have as much autonomy as possible. Guidelines were created to advise others on how to support her, and for her family to understand how to interact with her when executive difficulties impacted upon their interactions.

Discussion

The aim of this chapter is to highlight the diagnostic challenges surrounding LIS and the central role that the clinical psychologist can play in elucidating patients' cognitive profile. We hope to have raised awareness of the need for the psychologist and wider MDT to have an open mind about cognitive impairment in patients with suspected LIS and to approach assessment using a hierarchical hypothesis-testing approach. The illustrative case studies are designed to show how the methodology described by Murphy (2018) and McMillan (1997) can be applied to these cases to explore cognition when a patient is either failing simple standardised tests or it is obvious to the clinical team that formal testing is the wrong starting point. It must be emphasised that, whilst the focus of this chapter is on the role that the clinical neuropsychologist can play, collaborative team-working is essential in order to pool the findings from SLT, OT, psychology, and the wider MDT to arrive at a shared formulation. The role of the SLT in particular is crucial in exploring optimal methods of communication, and OTs and technicians who are specialist in assistive technology are likely to be vital in setting up equipment such as eye-gaze systems for those patients who have the cognitive abilities to learn to use these.

For more able patients such as 'Susan', a range of standardised neuropsychological instruments can be used, albeit usually with some adaptations that necessitate a degree of caution in interpreting the findings. Test choice is therefore constrained by clinical priorities, fatigue levels, and methods of responding that the patient can access. Other tests that may be useful for assessing these patients have been described elsewhere, as summarised in the introduction to this chapter (e.g. Wilson et al., 2011; Schnakers et al., 2008). However, our key recommendation is to avoid a rigid 'LIS battery' approach in favour of an individual formulation-driven assessment in collaboration with the patient and team. This will ensure that testing focuses on answering key clinical questions rather than necessarily administering all tests that can be utilised. We emphasised this approach with 'Susan', our most cognitively able illustrative case, to highlight that Susan's priorities were about family/quality of life and we consequently needed to strike the right balance – focusing on what we felt we 'should' do, not just what we 'could' do. Nevertheless, some patients in LIS are keen to explore their cognitive functioning in depth, and we have certainly encountered patients who become very engaged with testing and feel empowered to demonstrate their intact skills, similar to the case described by Wilson and colleagues (2011), and again highlighting the importance of a person-centred approach.

Also in Susan's case study, we addressed the challenge of assessing executive functions in a patient group in which both the range of tests and the scope for informal behavioural observations are curtailed by the patients' physical disabilities. Informally, in our clinical practice, we have observed that patterns of rigid thinking and difficulties with problem-solving are relatively common in patients with LIS even when scores on those tests that can be administered are within normal limits. It is beyond the scope of the current chapter to address possible reasons for this in detail, although factors such as organic dysfunction beyond the brainstem, mood factors, personality traits, and the possible role of 'use it or lose it' in maintaining cognitive skills in the context of severe disability are all factors that we have considered within our formulations. The message to psychologists working with patients with LIS is to be aware of this possibility and to be ready to support patients, teams, and families if such features become evident, since many of the strategies that can be helpful can be used regardless of the underlying cause(s).

Another challenge that arises with this patient group is around the assessment of potential mood disorders. In clinical practice, we firstly recommend exploring the reasons why concerns about mood have been raised. Patients with classic LIS will have very little movement of the facial muscles and the facial expression can therefore appear flat due to physiological factors, which can be misinterpreted as low mood. For patients with cognitive impairments, we have tried to illustrate how binary methodologies can be adapted to ask emotion-related questions. However, we would advise caution in interpreting results from such assessments, given the abstract reasoning required to introspect about one's own mood-state and respond accordingly. Similarly, we would advise caution in using standardised mood questionnaires with patients with memory difficulties as these patients are highly unlikely to be able to recollect how they have been feeling over periods of time such as a week or two weeks and the evidence suggests that there are no self-report measures that are valid with patients with severe cognitive impairments (Rose et al., 2022). We suggest that potentially more valid data can be obtained from a combination of direct and informant-observations, open questions, and monitoring of behaviours such as whether patients engage in activities with families, carers, or therapists.

As described in the introduction and in our case study about 'Steve', inaccurate descriptors of LIS for patients with severe cognitive impairments can create false hopes and unrealistic expectations that can be difficult for clinical teams to unpick. There are similar challenges with using terms such as 'partially locked in' or 'incomplete locked in syndrome' for these patients, since these terms describe those with additional motor movements, not cognitive impairments (Bauer et al., 1979). The risks associated with overestimating patients' cognitive abilities include poor clinical decision making, misjudgements about mental capacity and vulnerability, and compromised best interests decision making due to reasoning being based on incorrect information. There are a range of reasons why this mislabelling might occur. Firstly, some clinicians may mistakenly believe that tetraparesis and LIS are interchangeable terms. Secondly, clinicians may be so keen to avoid the other diagnostic error – i.e. underestimating patients' cognitive abilities – that they may have a bias towards overestimation. This can be linked with family beliefs and expectations, and also with an understandable desire to ensure no option is left unexplored in determining patients' levels of responsiveness. Thirdly, if a diagnosis has been written in a report by a senior clinician, there could be an assumption from less experienced clinicians that it must be correct; in this scenario it is important for the team to fact-check the history and review the diagnostic labelling if assessments indicate that the term was mis-applied. In all these scenarios, robust assessment and information gathering is important. In the exceptionally rare case that 'complete' LIS is hypothesised (Schnakers et al., 2009), then a referral for EEG and/or functional imaging may be indicated.

There is a fourth potential reason why the term LIS might be applied to patients with significant cognitive impairments. As described above, the concept that patients with LIS have *no* cognitive difficulties has been challenged in a number of studies (Schnakers et al., 2008; Wilson et al., 2011). There could potentially be an assumption on the part of some clinicians that this means that *all* patients with the physical presentation of LIS have some level of cognitive impairment and the term 'LIS' therefore captures their physical disabilities plus cognitive dysfunction of a greater or less extent. However, the participants in the studies cited above scored within normal limits on most tests administered and their deficits were focal rather than global, similar to our fictional case 'Susan'. Thus, while there might be evidence of some cognitive dysfunction in most, or even potentially all, people with classic or incomplete LIS, we contend that the key question is whether difficulties are focal or global. When patients have focal deficits, this means that they will perform within normal limits on a range of cognitive tests, and will therefore also have the potential to communicate functionally and apply their preserved cognitive skills – provided they have specialist support to do so. This might include emailing friends or turning a television on and off using an eye-gaze system, operating a powered wheelchair using a head or chin switch (for those with incomplete LIS who have some limited head movements), or using up/down eye movements to make a range of everyday choices with a communication partner. We have known patients who have written poetry and songs, DJ'd, and kept in touch with friends around the globe, because they have sufficiently intact cognitive abilities to learn to use the tools that enable these activities, and to initiate using them. Our suggestion is that these patients are correctly classified as having LIS. In contrast, those with global deficits that severely constrain any functional ability such as 'Steve' or 'Antoine' are more accurately described as having severe global cognitive impairments. For these patients, the task of the psychologist and MDT is to look for any 'islets' of intact ability within a context of profound impairment, rather than the usual neuropsychological approach of looking for 'deficits' within a pattern of normal functioning (Beaumont, 2008).

Our desire to highlight the challenges that arise when families have high expectations based on misapplication of the term 'LIS' is the reason why we used illustrative rather than real cases. It will be obvious to the reader that any patients with similar cognitive profiles to 'Steve' and 'Antoine' would be unable to give informed consent for their information to be published. However, we did not feel it appropriate to approach families of real-life case examples due to the potential ongoing differences of opinion about formulation and the risk of causing additional distress. Whilst a detailed discussion of the psycho-therapeutic work we undertake with such patients and their families, regardless of the extent of cognitive impairment, is beyond the scope of the current chapter, this is also an essential part of the clinical psychologist's role. We hope to have illustrated why accurate diagnosis of the range and extent of cognitive difficulties should inform the approach taken to education, adjustment, and other therapeutic interventions.

In summary, it is important for psychologists and neuropsychologists to explore patients' cognitive abilities in conjunction with the MDT and to provide psycho-education for patients and families. A thorough understanding of their neuropsychological strengths and weaknesses should support expectation management and enable patients, families, and teams to target their focus on enhancing quality of life.

References

Allain, P., Joseph, P. A., Isambert, J. L., Le Gall, D., & Emile, J. (1998). Cognitive functions in chronic locked-in syndrome: A report of two cases. *Cortex, 34*, 629–34.

Bauer, G., Gerstenbrand, F., & Rumpl, E. (1979). *Varieties of the locked-in syndrome. Journal of Neurology, 221*, 77–91.

Beaumont, J. G. (2008). *An introduction to neuropsychology* (2nd ed). Guilford Press.

Bruno, M-A., Bernheim, J. L., Ledoux, D., Pallas, F., Demertzi, A., & Laureys, S. (2011). A survey on self-assessed well-being in a cohort of chronic locked-in syndrome patients: happy majority, miserable minority. *British Medical Journal Open, 1.* https://doi.org/10.1136/bmjopen-2010-000039

Giacino, J. T., Kalmar, K., & Whyte, J. (2004). The JFK Coma Recovery Scale-revised: Measurement characteristics and diagnostic utility. *Archives of Physical Medicine and Rehabilitation, 85*(12), 2020–2029. Retrieved from www.ncbi.nlm.nih.gov/pubmed/15605342

Halan, T., Ortiz, J., Reddy, D., Altamimi, A., Ajibowo, A., & Fabara, S. P. (2021). Locked-in syndrome: A systematic review of long-term management and prognosis. *Cureus, 13*(7), e16727. https://doi.org/10.7759/cureus.16727

Laureys, S., Pellas, F., Van Eeckhout, P., Ghorbel, S., Schnakers, C., Perrin, F., Berré, J., Faymonville, M., Pantke, K., Damas, F., Lamy, M., Moonen, G., & Goldman, S. (2005). The locked-in syndrome: What is it like to be conscious but paralyzed and voiceless? *Progress in Brain Research, 150*, 495–611.

Leon-Carrion, J., van Eeckhout, P., Dominguez-Morales Mdel, R., & Perez Santamaria, F. J. (2002) The locked-in syndrome: A syndrome looking for a therapy. *Brain Injury, 16*, 571–82.

Lugo, Z., Bruno, M-A., Gosseries, O., Demertizi, A, Heine, L., Thonnard, M., Blandin, V., Pellas, F., & Laureys, S. (2015). Beyond the gaze: Communicating in chronic locked-in syndrome. *Brain Injury, 29*, 1056–1061.

McMillan, T. (1997). Neuropsychological assessment after extremely severe head injury in a case of life or death. *Brain Injury, 11*(7), 483–490.

Murphy, L. (2018). The Cognitive Assessment by Visual Election (CAVE): A pilot study to develop a cognitive assessment tool for people emerging from disorders of consciousness. *Neuropsychological Rehabilitation, 8*, 1275–1284.

Pundole A., & Crawford S. (2017). The assessment of language and the emergence from disorders of consciousness. *Neuropsychological Rehabilitation*, https://doi.org/1 0.1080/09602011.2017.1307766

Rose, A. E., Cullen. B., Crawford, S., & Evans J. J. (2022). A systematic review of mood and depression measures in people with severe cognitive and communication impairments following acquired brain injury. *Clinical Rehabilitation, 15*, 2692155221139023. https://doi.org/10.1177/02692155221139023. Epub ahead of print. PMID: 36380679.

Royal College of Physicians (2020). Prolonged disorders of consciousness following sudden onset brain injury: national clinical guidelines Annex 1a: Assessing for emergence from MCS. www.rcplondon.ac.uk/guidelines-policy/prolonged-disorders-consciousness-following-sudden-onset-brain-injury-national-clinical-guidelines

Schnakers, C., Majerus, S., Goldman, S., Boly, M., Van Eeckhout, P., Gay, S., Pellas, F., Bartsch, V., Peigneux, P., Moonen, G., & Laureys, S. (2008). Cognitive function in the locked-in syndrome. *Journal of Neurology, 255*, 323–330.

Schnakers, C., Perrin, F., Schabus, M., Hustinx, R., Majerus, S., Moonen, G., Boly, M., Vanhaudenhuyse, M.A., & Laureys, S. (2009). Detecting consciousness in a total locked-in syndrome: an active event-related paradigm. *Neurocase, 15*, 271–277. https://doi.org/10.1080/13554790902724904

Shiel, A., Horn, S. A., Wilson, B., Watson, M. J., Campbell, M. J., & McClellan, D. L. (2000). The Wessex Head Injury Matrix (WHIM) main scale: A preliminary report on a scale to assess and monitor patient recovery after severe head injury. *Clinical Rehabilitation, 14*(4), 408–416.

Smith, E., & Delargy, M. (2005). Locked-in syndrome. *British Medical Journal (Clinical research ed.), 330* (7488), 406–409. https://doi.org/10.1136/bmj.330.7488.406

Vanhaudenhuyse A., Charland-Verville V., Thibaut, A., Chatelle, C., Tshiband J-F., Maudoux, A., Faymonville, M-E., Laureys, S., & Gosseries, O. (2018). Conscious while being considered in an unresponsive wakefulness syndrome for 20 years. *Frontiers of Neurology, 9*, 671. https://doi.org/10.3389/fneur.2018.00671

Wilford, S., Pundole, A., Crawford, S., & Hanrahan, A. (2019). The Putney Prolonged Disorders of Consciousness Toolkit. www.rhn.org.uk/content/uploads/2019/05/Putney-PDoC-toolkit-v1.0-WEB.pdf

Wilson, BA., Hinchcliffe, A., Okines, T., Florschutz, G. & Fish, J. (2011) A case study of locked-in-syndrome: Psychological and personal perspectives. *Brain Injury, 25*(5), 526–538. https://doi.org/10.3109/02699052.2011.568034

23 Ethical and practical issues for the psychologist working with patients in a disorder of consciousness

Elena Olgiati, Jonathan Hinchliffe, Andrew Hanrahan, Paolo Mantovani, and Sarah Crawford

Introduction

Prolonged disorders of consciousness (PDOC, a DOC lasting longer than 28 days) are a rare consequence of sudden onset global, catastrophic acquired brain injury. Note that, although similar states can result in other circumstances, such as the late stages of dementia, the term PDOC is not typically applied in those circumstances. With recent advances in emergency trauma care and intensive care, survival rates for people who have suffered the most catastrophic brain injuries have increased (Moran et al., 2018). After such profound global brain damage, individuals may present in a state of coma, where there is no evidence of wakefulness or awareness as outlined by the Royal College of Physicians in their most recent clinical guidelines (RCP, 2020). A subset of coma survivors may then recover reflexive functions such as eye opening and sleep and wake cycles, either without any evidence of awareness of themselves, others, or their environment (vegetative state; VS), or with limited and inconsistent evidence of awareness (minimally conscious state (MCS)) (RCP, 2020). [Those who remain in VS/MCS for longer than four weeks are described as being in a prolonged disorder of consciousness (PDOC).] Many of these patients will regain some awareness over time, for example move from VS to MCS, or emerge from MCS into a state of more consistent awareness. However, even those who emerge from PDOC, over time will typically continue to present with significant cognitive and physical sequelae and dependence upon others for all daily tasks (RCP, 2020). Other patients in PDOC do not show any discernible *trajectory* of change over time, and for these individuals it becomes a chronic, and potentially permanent, condition requiring round-the-clock care for the duration of life. A recent review of international studies estimated the incidence of PDOC to be around five in every 100,000 people per year (Wade et al., 2022). It follows that thousands of people in the UK will present in low awareness states, and it is therefore important for neuropsychologists and clinical psychologists working in neuropsychology to have an understanding of these conditions and of how to support patients, their families, and their clinical teams. The term 'clinical psychologists' is used throughout the chapter in recognition

DOI: 10.4324/9781003228226-26

that not everyone working in these settings will be on the British Psychological Society's specialist register of clinical neuropsychologists. This chapter highlights some of the ethical and practical issues that clinicians encounter in this field, presents an illustrative case study, and describes implications for clinical practice.

Clinical psychologists work as part of the clinical team to support the person in PDOC and their wider system. In an acute or post-acute setting, the clinical team assesses the person's behaviour in order to infer awareness and responsiveness and diagnose their condition. Diagnosis is a complex process involving background information such as aetiology, neuroimaging, electrophysiology, and medical history, combined with a range of behavioural data. Behavioural information is obtained longitudinally using formal measures of awareness such as the Coma Recovery Scale-revised (CRS-R) (Giacino et al., 2004), Wessex Head Injury Matrix (WHIM) (Shiel et al., 2000), and Sensory Modality Assessment and Rehabilitation Technique (SMART) (Gill-Thwaites & Munday, 2004), alongside informal behavioural observations, and collaborative working with families (RCP, 2020). Psychological skills in handling and interpreting complex multi-modal data are highly valuable in this process, and neuropsychology is acknowledged to be a key discipline in the multidisciplinary team (MDT) (RCP, 2020).

Beyond diagnosis, the MDT works with the patient to manage complex disability, including management of medical complications, optimising medications and posture, and delivering specialist care around basic needs such as breathing, nutrition, incontinence, skin care, etc. (Wade, 2014). The clinical psychologist often works with the patient, team, and family to understand and manage behaviours that challenge, such as tube-dislodging, accidental self-harm, or repetitive movements or vocalisations. They will also assess any emotion-related behaviours such as tears, smiling, and grimacing and formulate these in the context of the profound cognitive impairment associated with a disorder of consciousness. When present, these behaviours may be misinterpreted by families and members of the MDT as indicative of self-awareness and emotional experience, for example depression or elation (Crawford & Beaumont, 2005). In such cases, a psychology-led systematic assessment and formulation of the behavioural evidence is indicated, with ongoing bespoke behavioural monitoring and outcome measurement in cases where medication such as anti-depressants are trialled (e.g., Wilford et al., 2019).

One aim is for the MDT and family/friends of the person to work together to arrive at a shared formulation of the level of awareness and prognosis to support decision making about the person's care. However, although providing families with clear and honest information about the patient's condition, prognosis, and degree of uncertainty around these is integral to best practice (RCP, 2020), it can be challenging to initiate such difficult conversations and share distressing information with families who may be already experiencing significant distress about their relative's condition. A recent systematic review showed that family members of people in PDOC report high levels of loss and grief, carer burden, depression and anxiety, and difficulties with coping (Soeterik et al., 2017). It has also been acknowledged that providing psychological support to these families requires considerable skills in order to judge the most appropriate timing and avoid family members feeling that their emotional responses are being pathologised (Kitzinger & Kitzinger, 2014). In our experience, families may sometimes disagree about the diagnosis, believing the patient to be much more aware relative to the team formulation (Crawford & Beaumont, 2005), may have high expectations for recovery, and/or appear inconsistent in their views about the patient's diagnosis and prognosis. Many team members do not feel that they have had sufficient training in managing these difficult conversations (Logeswaren et al., 2018). As team members who have had such training, it is often appropriate for clinical psychologists to explore the similarities and differences in MDT and family views and develop a formulation to understand any incongruence. This formulation then informs interventions, which may include further psycho education sessions, joint sessions between families and the team, and psychological intervention sessions, e.g. drawing on non-linear models of grief such as ambiguous loss (Boss, 2000), in addition to supporting staff to understand apparent contradictions such as family members reporting giving up hope of recovery on one day, whilst expressing high expectations the next (e.g., Illman & Crawford, 2018).

The importance of this collaborative work with families is vital when working with people in PDOC because, if the diagnosis is correct, the person in PDOC will lack the mental capacity to make any decisions for themselves. This is because this level of profound cognitive impairment is incompatible with the patient having any ability to comprehend even the most basic information, and/or having any reliable method of communication – which in turn renders the question of retention or weighing up/use of information redundant. An individual in PDOC will therefore fail all four steps of the functional assessment of mental capacity as outlined in the Mental Capacity Act (Department of Health, 2005) and its Code of Practice (Office of the Public Guardian, 2007) in relation to any decision. This in turn means that patients in PDOC cannot give informed consent to any aspect of their care or treatment and third parties must therefore make decisions on their behalf. Further guidance on application of the MCA is available from the British Psychological Society (BPS, 2021) and, specifically in relation to PDOC, the Royal College of Physicians (RCP, 2020). However, it has to be acknowledged that this is an ethically complex area where different principles underpinning medical ethics may conflict with each other and/or prove inadequate (RCP, 2020).

The principles of best interests decision making apply to all interventions, from routine day-to-day care (e.g. showering, clothing choices, medication administration) to non-routine treatments or investigations (e.g. X-rays, vaccinations), and life-sustaining treatments such as clinically assisted nutrition and hydration (CANH). It is important for all clinicians working with patients in PDOC to be aware that best interests decision making is not solely about interventions to improve the person's physical presentation, but it is a much broader concept encompassing their past wishes and beliefs, their current condition, and their prognosis. The opinions of family and friends are usually (in the absence of a valid advance directive/decision) the primary sources of information about the patient's subjective views and values.

While ethical dilemmas may arise around many aspects of best-interests decision making, one of the most sensitive areas in this field is discontinuation of life-sustaining treatment, and particularly discontinuation of CANH. The vast majority of patients in PDOC are unable to eat food or drink fluids due to a combination of profound cognitive impairments and physical difficulties such as dysphagia. A detailed history of the case law relating to this issue is beyond the scope of the current chapter, but the key points are: (1) providing nutrition and hydration via a feeding tube is considered to be a medical treatment, (2) any medical treatment must only be given with consent and, in its absence, if it is the patient's best interests, (3) the potential for some improvement in the patient's awareness does not automatically mean that treatment is in their best interests – the key question, as determined in case law, is whether the prognosis is for a quality of life that the patient would personally have valued (see RCP, 2020 for a detailed overview). The MDT must therefore work with the family to determine whether ongoing treatments such as CANH are in the patient's best interests, and, if it is concluded that they are not, guidelines for discontinuing the treatment should be followed (BMA/RCP, 2018). Inevitably, once CANH has been discontinued, the patient will die within a few days or weeks (RCP, 2020). As would be expected, this process can present ethical dilemmas to those involved. While CANH has a settled clinical and legal status as a treatment in the UK, it is by no means a settled moral, religious, or social question. It is important to be aware that the cause of death in such cases is attributed to the catastrophic brain injury that caused the person to be in PDOC, and not to the action of discontinuing treatment. Nevertheless, because the process of discontinuing CANH is different to that of discontinuing other life-sustaining treatments, it is understandably an emotive situation, and clinical psychologists can play a key role in supporting families and team members.

Below we present a case study in which one of the authors (JH) was the clinical neuropsychologist within the specialist MDT, and another of the authors (AH) was the medical consultant. Our aim is to illustrate some of the ethical issues described above, and to portray the role of the clinical psychologist in working with the patient, family, and team. Personal identifiers have been removed.

Case presentation

Jane was living an active and sociable life before her brain injury. She was in her fifties, and lived with her husband Tony, their children, and pets. Jane was devoted to her family and her large group of friends, and enjoyed many different outdoor passions including long-distance running and cycling. She worked in advertising and marketing and had previously worked as a photographer. She also provided care for her mother, who had, with Jane's support, made a good recovery from a severe stroke.

Jane was hit by a car whilst training for a long-distance charity bike ride. Her GCS at the scene was 3/15 (i.e. she was completely unresponsive). She was airlifted to the nearest major trauma centre where a CT scan showed a right traumatic subarachnoid haemorrhage, a right subdural haematoma, and multiple parenchymal haemorrhages which were managed conservatively (i.e., there were no neurosurgical interventions). Jane remained unresponsive. She had further neurological complications including autonomic dysfunction and a seizure, for which anti-epileptic medications were prescribed. She was unable to eat or drink, and a gastrostomy tube was inserted for life-sustaining administration of nutrition, hydration, and medications. She additionally had a tracheostomy inserted to maintain and protect her airway. During her acute hospital admission, she was observed to have a sleep–wake cycle, but there was no behavioural evidence of awareness of herself, others, or her environment, and initial CRS-R scores were 0/23.

When Jane's physical presentation was stable, she was admitted to our Level 1 service at the Royal Hospital for Neuro-disability. This unit specialises in assessment and disability management for people with severe brain injury, including those in PDOC. Jane presented as profoundly cognitively and physically impaired and she was fully dependent on others for all of her needs. She lacked the mental capacity to make any decisions about her care, and was unable to express any preferences of any kind. As such, a care plan was created in her best interests by the specialist MDT in conjunction with her family. She had complex 24-hour care requirements in relation to medical treatment, postural management, incontinence management, and skin care. She was unable to swallow, hence all of her nutrition and hydration continued to be provided via the gastrostomy tube, as prescribed by the dietitian; her medication was given in liquid or crushed form via the same tube. The MDT worked to optimise her physical and medical presentation; interventions included weaning medications that could reduce alertness (including opiate and anti-epileptic medications), and successfully removing the tracheostomy tube.

Jane's family had their first meeting with the MDT shortly after admission. They were given information about PDOC and the multifaceted means of assessment that the team were conducting with Jane, caring for her body whilst looking for evidence of awareness or communication. The medical team outlined Jane's treatment escalation plan, which specified that she would not be actively resuscitated in the unlikely event of cardiac arrest, but she would be transferred to an acute hospital if other emergency treatments were indicated, such as intravenous antibiotics or blood transfusions. Tony asked about the possibility of improvement in Jane's condition and about how long this might take. It was explained that prognosis is unclear so soon after a traumatic brain injury, but it was possible that Jane might show more awareness over time. Tony expressed some concerns about how Jane would have viewed her current quality of life, and was anxious that intensive rehabilitation efforts might leave her aware of her catastrophic predicament, with no means to understand it or express herself. He sought assurances that all efforts undertaken would not in fact leave her 'worse off'. The team validated this important point, which indicated that Tony was considering Jane's sense of identity and wishes, and reassured him that they would monitor Jane closely for awareness levels as well as for any signs that might indicate distress.

The emotional impact for families who have a relative in PDOC was also explored with Tony, and the concept of ambiguous loss (i.e. the loss experienced by others when the body of the person they love is present but their personality is absent) was introduced. Family support was offered by clinical psychology and welcomed by the family. This input included (1) the exploration of different family members' experience of grief and loss with concurrent emotional support; (2) psycho-education to increase familial understanding of the injury and sequelae; (3) considering ways in which the family could manage their own self-care and support as a pre-requisite for supporting Jane.

Assessment of awareness

During her admission, Jane underwent a range of assessments to help establish a diagnosis and inform prognosis. Her evoked potentials, which measure electrical activity in response to stimulation, showed that the primary visual, auditory, and somatosensory pathways were intact. This implied that any absence of meaningful behavioural responses in any domain must be attributable to higher-order cortical areas being damaged. While reassuring for a diagnostic formulation, it did mean that the focus of severe brain damage was indeed profound cortical dysfunction and not a peripheral sensory cause.

Behavioural assessments of awareness were conducted longitudinally using the CRS-R and WHIM, alongside informal observations and bespoke assessments. The findings were discussed weekly in MDT case reviews to examine whether there was evidence of a trajectory of change and to formalise a diagnosis in line with professional practice guidelines (RCP, 2020).

The CRS-R was used in ten sessions over two months. Jane's scores ranged between 5–8 out of 23 with no evidence of consistent trajectory of change. The highest level of behaviours observed were in the visual function scale, as Jane was able to fix her gaze on a brightly coloured object in her left visual field in several sessions. Less consistently, she was able to demonstrate some awareness of a moving object by tracking the movement of a mirror with her eyes, although she was not able to maintain this for the 45 degrees needed to obtain a full score. There was no evidence of any higher level behaviours. For example, Jane was not able to localise and reach for objects such as a comb or a toothbrush when these were presented in front of her and she was not able to use these objects functionally. On other scales of the CRS-R, she showed very little evidence of responding to auditory stimuli, showing a threat response (blinking) in response to a loud noise in only one of the ten assessments, and no other auditory responses.

The WHIM (score 0–62) was completed across 24 assessment sessions, with Jane's highest behaviour ranging between 4 and 28. Although the range of scores may suggest a change in trajectory over time, the chronology of her profile of scores indicated a scattered rather than linear picture. In addition, it has been argued that some of the highest-scoring behaviours Jane showed (looking at an object when requested and grimacing) should actually be placed lower in the hierarchy, at positions 22 and 8 respectively, rather than their original placings of 28 and 26 (Turner-Stokes et al., 2015).

Overall, Jane's behavioural repertoire was restricted to brief and inconsistent visual tracking and maintaining some visual contact with people, indicative of a diagnosis of low level minimally conscious state (i.e. 'MCS minus'; MCS–). Beyond this, Jane showed some emotion-related behaviours that are typically associated with discomfort, including groaning and grimacing. Jane was unable to provide any self-report about mood, comfort, or pain. Assessments showed that these behaviours appeared to arise spontaneously at times, but were associated with specific stimuli at other times. These associative links, combined with evidence of some, albeit very limited, evidence of awareness, meant that it was conceptually possible that Jane might have had some conscious experience of distress as opposed to indicating entirely 'physiological' (i.e. autonomically and spinally mediated) reflexive distress.

Traumatic brain injuries are typically associated with a longer potential window for recovery than non-traumatic injuries (e.g. hypoxia). However, Jane's trajectory of behavioural change was indicative of a plateau despite the multitude of specialist MDT interventions to optimise her condition. A diagnosis of VS or MCS– (as opposed to MCS+), and a lack of evidence of change in awareness over time, are both associated with poor prognosis for functional change (RCP, 2020; Turner-Stokes et al., 2015; Whyte et al., 2013). It was therefore highly likely that Jane would have significant residual cognitive and physical disability for the rest of her life and would be unable to return to the rich and active lifestyle that she had previously led. Once this lack of trajectory was clear and Jane's physical condition was stable, she was transferred from the level 1 service to a nursing home ward within the same organisation, but with ongoing specialist consultancy from members of the level 1 MDT, including the consultant in rehabilitation medicine and the clinical neuropsychologist.

Discontinuation of life-sustaining treatment

In this context, the existential question was whether Jane would have accepted her current and future state as being worth living. The clinical question was whether, in the clear absence of consent to ongoing treatment, it was lawful to continue to do so in her best interests. The ethical question was whether the perceived beneficence of continuing treatment conflicted with the need to respect Jane's autonomy. Current clinical guidelines are explicit that treatment decisions should not be delayed until the diagnosis is 'permanent' but should be made whenever a treatment is needed (RCP, 2020). Under the MCA, if Jane had made a valid and relevant advance decision to refuse treatment (ADRT), then actions would lawfully need to be consistent with this. However, Jane had not made an ADRT and it was therefore necessary to determine what decision she would have made for herself in this situation (i.e. her best interests). Jane did not have a lasting power of attorney or court appointed deputy for decisions relating to her health and welfare, and the doctor responsible for her care (a GP) was appointed as the decision maker for this decision.

As part of the best interests process, in addition to the evidence about Jane's diagnosis and prognosis, it was necessary to consider what Jane herself would say if she had the requisite cognition to participate. Given that no one other than Jane could state this with absolute certainty, it was necessary for the team to seek the views of others who knew Jane well. The MCA is clear that it is not sufficient to ask just one spokesperson or 'next of kin' (a term which has no legal standing in terms of decision making); instead, anyone in the person's family or friendship group who has involvement in caring for them and/or an interest in their welfare, should be consulted. The aim was to explore what Jane would have said before her brain injury, but within the context of her current presentation. This is a caveat that clinicians should be aware of, since it is possible for a person's perspective on quality of life to change after brain injury.[1] However, in Jane's case, she was unable to express a preference of any kind, and her behavioural presentation was more consistent with discomfort than contentment.

In order to explore the views of all of the relevant people in Jane's close social network, six further family meetings were conducted with different members of the family. In addition to Tony's view, opinions were sought from Jane's four adult children, her sibling, her mother, her aunt, and her closest friend. The MDT provided detailed information relating to diagnosis, biopsychosocial prognosis and lack of trajectory of change. Participants were invited to ask any questions they may have and share their views about what Jane would say if she could let us know her views on discontinuation of CANH. Following these meetings, the family were also invited to write statements to submit privately to the MDT. This enabled them to collect their thoughts, and reduced the possibility of people hiding their views (e.g. via conformity bias, leading to acquiescence to more vocal or dominant others within a meeting).

The views expressed by the family portrayed a vivid, powerful picture of a woman who lived her life fully by the motto 'do one thing every day that scares you'. Jane's youngest son eloquently explained that Jane had taught her children to accept risks as a necessary part of life. He stated 'had you told her over 25 years ago, just when she started cycling, that it was eventually going to be the death of her, I don't think she would have stopped', and stated 'she would be so scared if she knew what was going to happen, but I think she would be more scared if she knew that she would spend the rest of her life as she is now'. Her family strongly felt that she would have never wanted to face the prospect of living in a care home or being a burden to others, with a family member adding that Jane had said that, in that eventuality, she would want someone to 'put me on a bike and push me off a cliff'. They provided vivid examples of Jane watching medical documentaries of patients with less severe disabilities and stating: 'if I am ever in that situation, let me die'. They strongly believed that her current quality of life was 'not one that she would have accepted'. Tony's view was that Jane 'would want to make this courageous decision [to no-longer be sustained by CANH] rather than live a life so significantly compromised' and 'ask that we live her values and celebrate the joy that she would always bring'.

It proved to be particularly important to support Jane's mother in this process, considering her specific experience as a brain injury survivor herself. Jane's mother made an extremely good post-stroke recovery, and initially expressed that she would not 'give up' on Jane as Jane 'did not give up on me'. Psychological work focused on psychoeducation around different types of brain injuries leading to different outcomes, and discussions around the importance, in the best interests process, of separating one's own views from Jane's views (i.e., mentalising). The 'empty chair technique' (Perls et al., 1951), a key method in Gestalt therapy where you imagine your loved one in the room, sitting on the empty chair across from you and able to share their view and wishes, was used to support Jane's mother with mentalising. This technique can be particularly helpful in bringing the patient's perspective to life. In our experience, this exercise aids family members to separate their own thoughts and feelings from the patient's, a process which can be particularly difficult for families of people in PDOC, given the inability of the patient to communicate on their own behalf. Neuropsychologically informed supportive counselling was employed to explore experiences of loss, grief, and the perception of 'recovery'. Jane's mother recognised that Jane's current quality of life would be intolerable to her and was supported to understand the unfavourable prognosis for significant change. What looked like an initial disagreement on what constituted Jane's best interests was therefore resolved.

Following the process of family and team consultations, a best interests meeting was convened. The meeting was chaired by the clinical neuropsychologist, with the GP as the decision maker. The entire process was supported by the consultant lead for end of life care. By the time of the meeting there was a settled view that Jane would not wish to continue to receive CANH. A best interests decision to discontinue CANH was made. At this point, Jane's husband noted that the sun had come through the clouds, and reflected that he felt that this was an apt metaphor for Jane's views finally being realised.

The BMA/RCP guidelines, which reflect the Supreme Court judgment in *An NHS Trust v Y* (2018), were carefully followed in this process. They provide a 5-point checklist for such decisions (Appendix 2, BMA/RCP 2018). In circumstances such as Jane's where she remains in PDOC, and there are no disagreements about what constitutes the patient's best interests, it is not necessary to bring an application before the Court of Protection. In these cases, an extensive and robust process of documentation and external scrutiny is mandatory, including an external second opinion from an expert PDOC physician. Once this was done, the hospital Ethics Committee was consulted, as required by hospital policy. This was to independently verify at Board and Executive level that due diligence had been applied and that the process had been carried out fully in line with national guidelines.

Once a decision around CANH discontinuation was made, the clinical team worked with Jane's family to create a personalised end of life care plan. Her family felt that Jane would not want to die in hospital and so a home discharge was arranged with support from a local hospice. Jane's CANH was discontinued and she died peacefully five weeks later in her second home, where she had planned to retire, surrounded by her family and pets.

In summary, the clinical neuropsychologist working with this case was able to incorporate neuropsychology into the formulation, including assessment of awareness and psychological distress, and providing brain injury psychoeducation to family, drawing on specialist neuro-rehabilitation and neuro-palliative input and experience from the wider team. They were able to use core therapeutic skills including active listening when exploring views from relevant family members and friends. They supported family, and particularly Jane's mother, to mentalise, i.e., making sense of others' thought processes and separate them from our own. For this aim, the Gestalt 'empty chair technique' proved to be particularly helpful. Psychotherapeutic skills to support sharing of emotional content were used throughout the process. It was indeed acknowledged by Jane's family that the process was incredibly difficult, as the 'stakes are so high'. Psychology in this context is, however, well placed to support family and MDT with such difficult but essential conversations, whilst supporting their understanding and emotional responses.

Discussion

This chapter aimed to outline the role of clinical psychologists working in this ethically complex field. We aimed to highlight how we draw upon both neuropsychology skills and core clinical psychology techniques in supporting effective systemic work in often emotive situations. It is worth noting, however, that this does not necessarily mean that the psychologist must be centrally involved in supporting families in such cases: similar to other areas of work in neuro-rehabilitation, there is overlap between the role of the psychologist and that of other disciplines (Wade, 2020) and there may be situations in which an experienced MDT would be able to support these conversations without direct input from psychology. Nevertheless, our view is that the psychologist should make the team aware of their willingness to support these families since our core training equips us with extensive relevant theoretical knowledge and practical expertise in psychological interventions.

Best interests process

Beyond mastering core psychological skills, it is crucial for clinical psychologists working in this field to have a good understanding of the MCA and best interests decision making. It is key to adopt a strong person-centred approach, such that each patient's individual beliefs and culture are of paramount importance in determining what quality of life they personally would have valued. In the case example illustrated here, Jane's beliefs and values led to life-sustaining treatment being discontinued in her best interests, but there are other cases where life-sustaining treatment has been continued for many years because it has been concluded that this is what the person would have wanted. Clinicians need to ensure that families are empowered to speak honestly about the patient's values, beliefs, and culture, and that each member of the family system is given the opportunity to do so. This may entail separate discussions with different family members if there are tensions within families, or when one person is particularly vocal, e.g. due to strength of opinion or to traditional roles. These best interests conversations with family potentially include complex medical and prognostic information that must always be delivered in a clear and compassionate way. Our experience is that when these conversations are competently raised, the benefits are significant and help to establish an enduring relationship worthy of mutual trust.

Psychologists trained in working with clients from a wide range of diverse backgrounds are likely to be invaluable in making sure that all families are supported to understand the relevant information and advocate for the patient's best interests. Clinicians need to be respectful of cultural differences and recognise that some families may find it difficult to trust what the team are saying to them for a wide range of reasons. In addition, careful use of skilled interpreters is likely to be necessary when family members do not have English as a first language. It is important to note that when a patient was known to hold strong cultural and religious beliefs before their injury, it should not be assumed that they would inevitably have held a particular view on a medical treatment. For instance, according to case law, the emphasis must still be on the person's 'own religious views and practices ... not the received doctrine of the faith to which he subscribes' (EWCOP 59, 2021).

Professionals working in this ethically complex field should also reflect on their own beliefs and values and how these impact upon their practice, whether overtly or even subconsciously. Discontinuing CANH is not a form of euthanasia (which is illegal in the UK); nevertheless, there is potential for clinicians to experience considerable discomfort with the best interests process if it conflicts with their personal views. If the psychologist experiences cognitive dissonance due to incompatibility between the beliefs expressed by the family on behalf of the patient and their own personal beliefs, then it is important to reflect on how this may affect their professional decision making. A psychologist who believes that in potential cases of discontinuing CANH, their personal values would bias their views on the patient's best interests in either direction – i.e. towards either continuing or discontinuing treatment, they should then consider whether this field of practice is best suited to them. For those who do choose to work in this area, effective use of clinical supervision is vital.

Timing of discussions about ongoing CANH

Determining timing of best interests conversations with the family can be challenging. In the case described above, Tony raised questions about Jane's quality of life early in the admission which led naturally into these conversations. However, many families and friends of people in PDOC attend these initial family meetings with a focus on hope for recovery; it is not uncommon for family members to be vehemently against discussing ceilings of treatment of any kind, interpreting these as 'giving up' on their loved one. Our clinical experience suggests that these conversations can be particularly hard for families when the brain-injured person is young and/or when the brain injury has occurred in unexpected circumstances (e.g. a road traffic accident) or as a consequence of a suicide attempt.

One potential solution would be for clinicians to avoid discussing these questions until the family is 'ready'. However, although this sounds intuitively appealing, it carries several challenges. These include the problem of how 'readiness' is defined or judged, the potential risk of clinicians using the family's supposed lack of readiness as a screen to avoid (deliberately or otherwise) their own lack of confidence in approaching these conversations, and the central problem that neglecting these discussions removes the patient themselves from being at the centre of decision making. Finally, waiting for family to raise discussions may also impart a psychological burden, as the family member may feel a greater degree of responsibility for the eventual outcome.

In general, clinical teams should strive to be proactive in initiating best interest conversations in an effort to make the whole process as short as possible, while following all necessary steps. This is both in the patient's best interests and likely to reduce unnecessary familial distress. It also has broader societal/ethical implications, given the enormous costs involved in caring for patients who would not have agreed to life-sustaining treatment. In Jane's case, a settled view was reached relatively early between the family and the clinical team that ongoing treatment was not in Jane's best interests – and, as such, the case did not need to be referred to the Court of Protection, and relevant guidelines were instead followed closely (BMA/RCP, 2018). Even so, the process lasted for 11 months. Whilst this length of time can be stressful for family members and should ideally be reduced, it is considerably shorter than taking an application before the Court (Kitzinger & Kitzinger, 2017). However, when there are disagreements about the best interests decision, the matter should be referred to the court. Whilst waiting for the court hearing, it is good practice for clinicians to continue to consult with the family and potentially seek external support and/or mediation in the hope of arriving at a settled view.

Challenges around diagnosis and prognosis

A further area of epistemological and ethical complexity lies in the limitations of determining diagnosis and prognosis. Clinical guidelines provide clear operational definitions about diagnosing PDOC, which involve inferring consciousness from behaviour. However, there is evidence from functional MRI and EEG studies that a subset of patients who show no behavioural evidence of awareness can show neural evidence of command following (Kondziella et al., 2016; Pan et al., 2020), and that a small proportion of these patients can use these responses to demonstrate a basic level of yes/no communication (Monti et al., 2010). This has been referred to as cognitive motor dissociation or non-behavioural MCS. This presents a clinical and ethical dilemma for clinicians working with these patients as it introduces the idea of there being covert awareness that cannot be detected by behavioural assessments. However, it should be noted that, in the most recent EEG study, the vast majority of patients who showed these responses went on to show clear behavioural evidence of awareness within three months (Pan et al., 2020); indeed, imaging and electrophysiology are not currently included in UK clinical practice guidelines due in part to doubts about whether they add anything to clinical/behavioural observations over time (RCP, 2020). It is also important to recognise that a limited increase in awareness should not necessarily be framed as 'improvement'. This was an issue highlighted by Tony in relation to Jane, but it has also been raised in court settings (EWCOP13, 2022).

Clinical guidelines also specify when a label of 'permanent' VS or MCS can be applied (RCP, 2020). However, a range of cases have been described in which patients emerged from PDOC after considerable periods of time with changes in levels of awareness and cognition ranging from relatively subtle (e.g. Yelden et al., 2018) to more substantial changes (e.g. Dhamapurkar et al., 2016; Illman & Crawford, 2018). Although cases showing significant late change are relatively rare, the evidence suggests that it is more likely for a traumatic versus non-traumatic aetiology, and for patients in MCS+ rather than VS or MCS−. Other potentially relevant prognostic factors for significant changes following late emergence include age at the time of injury and optimal management of neurological complications and neuro-stimulants (Illman & Crawford, 2018; Sancisi et al., 2009; Wilson et al., 2016).

The challenge facing both clinicians and families is that there is no definitive test that can determine the prognosis for each individual patient with certainty. Nevertheless, factors such as those described above are relevant in considering the formulation, as is the trajectory of any change in presentation. These features are embedded in current practice guidelines about when a label of 'permanence' can be made, ranging from a minimum of six months post-injury for non-traumatic VS/MCS– to a minimum of two years post-injury for traumatic MCS+, within the context of an absence of change on CRS-R scores for six months (RCP, 2020). However, this does not mean that clinicians can avoid best interests decisions until criteria for permanence are reached. The legal framework is explicitly clear that the patient must always be at the centre of decision making and that delays in making best interests decisions are not acceptable. This is true not just for ongoing CANH but for all life-sustaining treatments (RCP, 2020), and there is evidence from in-depth qualitative interviews with families that if a 'window of opportunity' to allow the patient to die is missed then this can lead to what the families describe as a 'fate worse than death' (Kitzinger & Kitzinger, 2013). Part of the challenge for the team is therefore to weigh up the likelihood of positive change in terms of a quality of life the patient would value, against the probability of no change or a worsening of quality of life. We contend that clinical psychologists within these teams should be aware of all of these factors and ready to support both families and teams with the ethical dilemmas they pose in the context of keeping the individual patient at the centre.

Additional resources

For any psychologists interested in learning more about this area of work, in addition to the references included in this chapter, there are a range of training programmes available at organisations such as ours (www.rhn.org.uk), and online (e.g. via the Coma and Disorders of Consciousness Research Centre (CDOC) at Cardiff University: https://cdoc.org.uk). There is also a useful resource collated by the CDOC team of their interviews with family members with experience of having a relative in a disorder of consciousness, which can be of value for both clinicians and for families in a similar situation (https://healthtalk.org/family-experiences-vegetative-and-minimally-conscious-states).

Acknowledgements

The authors would like to thank Jane's family for giving their consent to us sharing her story. We are grateful for the opportunity to honour her memory. We thank Jane and her family for giving us the opportunity to work closely as a team, and develop our skills and experience that will invariably help others. We thank all staff at the RHN who have helped.

Note

1 See e.g. McMillan for a case in which a patient with severe disability disagreed with the views she had previously expressed in a verbal advance directive
(McMillan, 1997), and Bruno and colleagues for a description of the views of
people in locked-in-syndrome on their quality of life in the context of profound
physical disability (Bruno et al., 2011).

References

BMA/RCP. (2018). Clinically-assisted nutrition and hydration (CANH) and adults
who lack the capacity to consent: Guidance for decision-making in England and
Wales. www.bma.org.uk/media/1161/bma-clinically-assisted-nutrition-hydration-
canh-full-guidance.pdf

Boss, P. G. (2000). *Ambiguous loss. Learning to live with unresolved grief.* Harvard University Press.

British Psychological Society. (2021). Supporting people who lack mental capacity:
A guide to best interests decision making. www.bps.org.uk/news-and-policy/sup-
porting-people-who-lack-mental-capacity-guide-best-interests-decision-making

Bruno, M. A., Bernheim, J. L., Ledoux, D., Pellas, F., Demertzi, A., & Laureys, S.
(2011). A survey on self-assessed well-being in a cohort of chronic locked-in syndrome patients: Happy majority, miserable minority. *British Medical Journal Open,*
1(1), e000039. https://doi.org/10.1136/bmjopen-2010-000039

Crawford, S., & Beaumont, J. G. (2005). Psychological needs of patients in low
awareness states, their families, and health professionals. *Neuropsychological Rehabilitation, 15*(3–4), 548–555. https://doi.org/10.1080/09602010543000082

Department of Health. (2005). Mental Capacity Act. www.nhs.uk/condi-
tions/social-care-and-support-guide/making-decisions-for-someone-else/
mental-capacity-act/

Dhamapurkar, S. K., Rose, A., Florschutz, G., & Wilson, B. A. (2016). The natural
history of continuing improvement in an individual after a long period of impaired
consciousness: The story of I.J. *Brain Injury, 30*(2), 230–236. https://doi.org/10.31
09/02699052.2015.1094132

EWCOP13. (2022). www.bailii.org/ew/cases/EWCOP/2022/13.html

EWCOP 59. (2021). www.bailii.org/ew/cases/EWCOP/2021/59.html

Giacino, J. T., Kalmar, K., & Whyte, J. (2004). The JFK Coma Recovery Scale-
Revised: Measurement characteristics and diagnostic utility. *Archives of Physical Medicine and Rehabilitation, 85*(12), 2020–2029. https://doi.org/10.1016/j.apmr.2004.02.033

Gill-Thwaites, H., & Munday, R. (2004). The Sensory Modality Assessment and
Rehabilitation Technique (SMART): A valid and reliable assessment for vegetative state and minimally conscious state patients. *Brain Injury, 18*(12), 1255–1269.
https://doi.org/10.1080/02699050410001719952

Illman, N. A., & Crawford, S. (2018). Late-recovery from 'permanent' vegetative
state in the context of severe traumatic brain injury: A case report exploring objective and subjective aspects of recovery and rehabilitation. *Neuropsychological Rehabilitation, 28*(8), 1360–1374. https://doi.org/10.1080/09602011.2017.1313167

Kitzinger, C., & Kitzinger, J. (2014). Grief, anger and despair in relatives of severely
brain injured patients: Responding without pathologising. *Clinical Rehabilitation,*
28(7), 627–631. https://doi.org/10.1177/0269215514527844

Kitzinger, J., & Kitzinger, C. (2017). Causes and consequences of delays in treatment-withdrawal from PVS patients: A case study of *Cumbria NHS Clinical Commissioning Group v Miss S and Ors* [2016] EWCOP 32. *Journal of Medical Ethics, 43*(7), 459–468. https://doi.org/10.1136/medethics-2016-103853

Kitzinger, J., & Kitzinger, C. (2013). The 'window of opportunity' for death after severe brain injury: Family experiences. *Sociology of Health and Illness, 35*(7), 1095–1112. https://doi.org/10.1111/1467-9566.12020

Kondziella, D., Friberg, C. K., Frokjaer, V. G., Fabricius, M., & Moller, K. (2016). Preserved consciousness in vegetative and minimal conscious states: systematic review and meta-analysis. *Journal of Neurology, Neurosurgery, and Psychiatry, 87*(5), 485–492. https://doi.org/10.1136/jnnp-2015-310958

Logeswaren, S., Papps, B., & Turner-Stokes, L. (2018). Staff experiences of working with patients with prolonged disorders of consciousness: A focus group analysis. *International Journal of Therapy and Rehabilitation, 25*(11), 602–612.

McMillan, T. M. (1997). Neuropsychological assessment after extremely severe head injury in a case of life or death. *Brain Injury, 11*(7), 483–490. www.ncbi.nlm.nih.gov/pubmed/9210985

Monti, M. M., Vanhaudenhuyse, A., Coleman, M. R., Boly, M., Pickard, J. D., Tshibanda, L., Owen, A. M., & Laureys, S. (2010). Willful modulation of brain activity in disorders of consciousness. *The New England Journal of Medicine, 362*(7), 579–589. https://doi.org/10.1056/NEJMoa0905370

Moran, C. G., Lecky, F., Bouamra, O., Lawrence, T., Edwards, A., Woodford, M., Willetts, K., & Coats, T. J. (2018). Changing the System: Major trauma patients and their outcomes in the NHS (England) 2008–17. *EClinicalMedicine, 2–3*, 13–21. https://doi.org/10.1016/j.eclinm.2018.07.001

Office of the Public Guardian. (2007). Mental Capacity Act Code of Practice. www.gov.uk/government/publications/mental-capacity-act-code-of-practice

Pan, J., Xie, Q., Qin, P., Chen, Y., He, Y., Huang, H., Wang, F., Ni, X., Cichocki, A., YU, R., & Li, Y. (2020). Prognosis for patients with cognitive motor dissociation identified by brain–computer interface. *Brain, 143*(4), 1177–1189. https://doi.org/10.1093/brain/awaa026

Perls, F. S., Hefferline, R.F., & Goodman, P. (1951). *Gestalt therapy*: Julian Press.

Royal College of Physicians. (2020). *Prolonged disorders of consciousness following sudden onset brain injury: National clinical guidelines*. RCP.

Sancisi, E., Battistini, A., Di Stefano, C., Simoncini, L., Simoncini, L., Montagna, P., & Piperno, R. (2009). Late recovery from post-traumatic vegetative state. *Brain Injury, 23*(2), 163–166. https://doi.org/10.1080/02699050802660446

Shiel, A., Horn, S. A., Wilson, B. A., Watson, M. J., Campbell, M. J., & McLellan, D. L. (2000). The Wessex Head Injury Matrix (WHIM) main scale: A preliminary report on a scale to assess and monitor patient recovery after severe head injury. *Clinical Rehabilitation, 14*(4), 408–416. https://doi.org/10.1191/0269215500cr326oa

Soeterik, S. M., Connolly, S., Playford, E. D., Duport, S., & Riazi, A. (2017). The psychological impact of prolonged disorders of consciousness on caregivers: A systematic review of quantitative studies. *Clinical Rehabilitation, 31*(10), 1374–1385. https://doi.org/10.1177/0269215517695372

Turner-Stokes, L., Bassett, P., Rose, H., Ashford, S., & Thu, A. (2015). Serial measurement of Wessex Head Injury Matrix in the diagnosis of patients in vegetative and minimally conscious states: a cohort analysis. *British Medical Journal Open, 5*(4), e006051. https://doi.org/10.1136/bmjopen-2014-006051

Wade, D. T. (2014). Managing prolonged disorders of consciousness. *Practitioner*, *258*(1769), 25–30, 23. www.ncbi.nlm.nih.gov/pubmed/24791408

Wade, D. T. (2020). A teamwork approach to neurological rehabilitation. In *Oxford Textbook of Neurorehabilitation* (2nd ed.). Oxford University Press.

Wade, D. T., Turner-Stokes, L., Playford, E. D., Allanson, J., & Pickard, J. (2022). Prolonged disorders of consciousness: A response to a critical evaluation of the new UK guidelines. *Clinical Rehabilitation*, 2692155221099704. https://doi.org/10.1177/02692155221099704

Whyte, J., Nakase-Richardson, R., Hammond, F. M., McNamee, S., Giacino, J. T., Kalmar, K., Greenwald, B. D., Yablon, S. A., & Horn, L. J. (2013). Functional outcomes in traumatic disorders of consciousness: 5-year outcomes from the National Institute on Disability and Rehabilitation Research Traumatic Brain Injury Model Systems. *Archives of Physical Medicine and Rehabilitation*, *94*(10), 1855–1860. https://doi.org/10.1016/j.apmr.2012.10.041

Wilford, S., Pundole, A., Crawford, S., Hanrahan, A. (2019). *The Putney Prolonged Disorders of Consciousness Toolkit*. www.rhn.org.uk/content/uploads/2019/05/Putney-PDOC-toolkit-v1.0-WEB.pdf

Wilson, B. A., Dhamapurkar, S. K., & Rose, A. (2016). *Surviving brain damage after assault: From vegetative state to meaningful life*. Psychology Press.

Yelden, K., Duport, S., James, L. M., Kempny, A., Farmer, S. F., Leff, A. P., & Playford, E. D. (2018). Late recovery of awareness in prolonged disorders of consciousness -a cross-sectional cohort study. *Disability Rehabilitation*, *40*(20), 2433–2438. https://doi.org/10.1080/09638288.2017.1339209

24 Losing memories overnight

A unique form of human amnesia or life imitating art?

Shai Betteridge and Priyanka Pradhan

Introduction

Current clinical neuropsychological practice is informed by theories and models of memory that have changed little since the early 1990s (Squire & Knowlton, 1995). In fact, seminal work from the 1950's which shone a light on how bilateral damage to the hippocampus causes anterograde amnesia has meant the hippocampus has been the primary focus of research into episodic memory; however, to the exclusion of other connected brain regions (Milner and Scoville, 1957). Based on assumptions drawn from the existing evidence base, clinical neuropsychologists usually purport that amnesia caused by organic factors (i.e. detectable physical and/or biochemical changes within the cells, tissues, or organs of the body) will have a specific profile on formal neuropsychological tests. The profile is characterised (e.g. see Wilson, 2009) by the inability to freely recall or recognise newly presented episodic information after a delay of a few minutes, and retrograde amnesia from the date of the index event, with a temporal gradient of autobiographical memory loss that correlates with the severity of the organic damage. Implicit memory is usually intact, and neuroanatomical memory research suggests this is because explicit and implicit memory rely on structurally different brain regions. For instance, it is widely accepted that explicit memory is associated with the medial temporal lobes and midline diencephalon, whereas implicit memory is associated with the basal ganglia, cerebellum, and limbic system (Camina & Güell, 2017). Organic anterograde amnesia is frequently diagnosed by clinical neuropsychologists based on the cognitive profile described above and triangulation with evidence of organic factors that can explain the profile. In contrast, profiles that do not conform with this pattern are usually considered to be functional in origin (i.e. caused by changes to the functioning of the systems of the body rather than its structure).

This chapter describes the ongoing and unresolved diagnostic conundrum of Lizzie, a young woman who presented to neurosciences services following a traumatic brain injury, and whose memory profile was similar to that depicted in the fictional film '50 First Dates' (Segal, 2004). A memory profile in which new information is learned during the day but lost after a night of sleep has always been understood by the professional community to be unrealistic, as it cannot be explained by our existing theories of memory and had never

DOI: 10.4324/9781003228226-27

been reported in the clinical literature. However, it is noteworthy that in the London Science Museum it is documented that many of our scientific developments were first depicted in the arts. This phenomenon of 'life imitating art' in science has been attributed to scientists who grew up reading fiction being inspired to design and develop the fictional objects from their childhood that were depicted in the comics and books they read. Given this evidence, it is reasonable to assume that people's knowledge of memory impairments might be constructed via their exposure to representations of this disability in the media. Consequently, they might hold overvalued and fixed beliefs that are inaccurate but might shape the lens with which they view and report their condition.

This construct of 'life imitating art' was used to formulate the first published case of the '50 First Dates' memory profile by Smith and colleagues (2010). They describe the case of FL, who was involved in a car accident in which she hit the left side of her head and suffered a brief loss of consciousness. She was treated and discharged from the emergency room, but on waking the next morning she had no memory for the previous day and thought the accident had just occurred. Every morning thereafter she awoke feeling anxious, believing the accident had just occurred, and with no memory for anything that had happened since the accident. She was typically orientated to the relevant information by her husband prompting her to refer to a journal where all salient information is recorded. She reported her memory as 'normal' during the day but stated that memory for each day is lost at night during sleep. Her husband reported that she did not lose any memory if she took a nap during the day. FL's husband described her condition as being like the memory impairment depicted in the film *50 First Dates*, but FL stated that she had not seen the film before the accident.

High-resolution anatomical MRI brain scans were considered normal; although FL's hippocampal volume bilaterally was 6.8% below the mean of four age-matched controls, and the volume of her parahippocampal gyrus was 1.8% below the control mean, both values were within the SD of the control mean. Independent review by a neurologist and psychiatrist concluded the diagnosis was psychogenic amnesia secondary to trauma related to the car accident. There was no past psychiatric or mental health history.

FL was treated for depression with increasing doses of escitalopram to a final dose of 30mg daily and with a sleep training programme. The latter involved sleep deprivation for 36 hours followed by a programme of being woken after longer and longer periods of sleep each night. The treating team found that FL retained all memories after 1, 2, 3, or 4 hours of sleep, but recurrence of memory loss occurred after 6 hours of sleep. At 12-month follow-up she had been able to retain memories for successive days by maintaining a sleep regime of being woken after 3.5 hours of sleep a night.

It is noteworthy that on formal cognitive assessment, despite FL reporting good memory for information learnt each day, her cognitive profile did not support this. Her profile was characterised by decrements in free recall and recognition of auditory and visual information at delayed recall compared to three controls and two simulators (i.e. volunteers who were asked to simulate

FL's pattern of memory impairment). It is noteworthy that her delayed free recall on an incidental visual memory measure (i.e. Rey Complex Figure) was fractionally better than simulators but not as good as the controls. Furthermore, on measures of implicit memory and motor skills (i.e. mirror drawing task), FL was observed to demonstrate some new learning on the same day (i.e. decrease in performance time across the ten administration trials) but no carry over to the following day. In contrast, controls and simulators demonstrated a pattern of implicit learning. Smith et al. (2010) argue that this finding supports the assumption widely accepted in clinical practice that implicit memory and motor skills learning is intact in organic amnesia; therefore, it follows that impairments in these areas indicate functional amnesia.

In contrast, Burgess and Chadalavada (2016) present five case examples of patients with impaired implicit learning on a motor skills task, and argue that these cases demonstrate an organic amnesia caused by the breakdown of intermediate-to-late-stage consolidation that does not depend on the structural integrity of the hippocampi. A recent review highlights the essential role of the fornix (an axonal tract of the hippocampus) in memory formation, given it serves as a conduit for theta rhythms and acetylcholine to the hippocampus, and provides mnemonic representation to deep brain structures that guide motivated behaviour (Benear et al., 2020). Further evidence that supports an organic explanation for the profile of impaired implicit memory secondary to a breakdown in consolidation of memories during sleep is the work of Gyorgy Buzsáki, who in 2011 won the Brain prize for establishing the important role of hippocampal sharp wave ripples (SWR) in the two stage model of memory. He found that lesions in the fornix of rats resulted in them presenting with a '50 First Dates' memory profile. During the day the rats could learn a route around a maze to find food, getting quicker on each trial, but after a night of sleep the rats' performance returned to baseline. Usually when a mammal sleeps the brain is active, consolidating the memories from that day via SWR. If memories are not consolidated, the knowledge acquired from the day will not be recalled on waking (see Watson & Buzsáki, 2015). This work, which shows that lesions to the fornix as a subcortical tract can result in anterograde amnesia, was very influential in our formulation of Lizzie's case.

Case presentation

Foreword

Before describing this case, it is important to highlight that the information reported here took several months to collate and was only pieced together after Dr Pradhan conducted a rigorous analysis of all the biopsychosocial sources of evidence, in accordance with a clinical neuropsychological formulation approach (cf. Sunak, 2019). This involved obtaining original ambulance records and hospital discharge reports in addition to detailed analysis of collateral informants' accounts and the patient's personal notes and memory aids. Much of the information Dr Pradhan obtained had not been available and/or viewed at the consultations by the original neurologists and neuropsychiatrist who saw and diagnosed Lizzie. It is testament to the diligence of Dr Pradhan, the support of Lizzie's parents, and the therapeutic relationship Dr Pradhan built with this family that enabled the formulation that follows to be constructed. However, in the interests of brevity the full case history is reported in chronological order, rather than the order in which information was discovered.

Case history

Lizzie first presented to neurosciences services two months following a traumatic brain injury (TBI) secondary to a fall from a horse. The witness accounts of the accident, detailed in the ambulance records, report that her horse became 'out of control' and she was thrown off the left side of the horse at speed, landing directly onto the left side of her head. She was unconscious with 'abnormal/noisy breathing' when the 999 call was made. The ambulance arrived 30 minutes later at which point her Glasgow Coma Scale (GCS) was recorded as 14/15 and her loss of consciousness was estimated to have lasted for five minutes. Minor swelling was noted over the left frontal bone where she hit the floor but with minimal damage observed to her riding helmet. However, it was later found that the inside of the helmet was severely cracked.

She was observed to be 'slightly confused and suffering with amnesia'. She was unable to speak in full sentences and unable to recall events, names, or her home address. Her temperature was noted to increase during the period in which her vital signs were monitored, and her level of confusion fluctuated resulting in her GCS being recorded as ranging between 13/15 and 15/15. She was observed to start using incomprehensible words and become very repetitive, continually asking the same questions and telling the paramedics she had 'hurt her head'. She was noted to become combative and agitated during the journey by ambulance to hospital. She was very nauseated, with five episodes of vomiting haemoptysis (i.e. bloody mucus).

On admission to hospital her GCS was 12/15, and a CT brain scan was conducted but reported to be 'normal'. According to the Accident and Emergency (A&E) junior doctor, Lizzie noted that she 'remembered the accident'. She recalled that the horse had bolted and was at full gallop, so she made the decision to jump off as it would be a safer option than being thrown off. As such, Lizzie recalls removing her feet from the stirrups, shifting her balance, rolling off to the left and curling her body to try and 'break the fall'. Lizzie explained later to the authors that controlled falls in such circumstances are an essential technique that proficient riders use for safety. Approximately six hours later another medic examined her and reported she 'cannot remember the accident'.

Interviews with her parents corroborated this change in her memory recall during her admission. They described that, on the day of the accident, when they went to see their daughter in hospital, she was *'very groggy'* but recounted the accident in great detail and clarity – but only until the point she rolled off the horse. She did not recall the fall or the impact. She recalled *'snatches'* of being on the ground and of lots of people around her. She did not recall how long it was before the ambulance arrived, and only had a patchy memory of the journey in the ambulance. She did not recall arriving at the hospital. After speaking to her parents for about 15 minutes she felt tired and went to sleep. Her parents reported that she was drifting in and out of sleep while she was awaiting a bed on the Surgical Ward. When more alert, she would ask where she was. Later on, when she woke up in hospital that evening, she had no recollection of anything from the moment she arrived at work that morning, which was around 45 minutes prior to the accident, and was completely disorientated.

Lizzie was admitted overnight for observation, and discharged to the care of her parents the following day with a diagnosis of concussion. She was advised that her memory difficulties should resolve in a few days. On discharge, her parents observed she was very tired, easily confused, and at times easily worried. Her memory was erratic, with patchy memories of the previous few days. Sometimes she recalled she had been in hospital and sometimes she did not. However, as time progressed, she was no longer able to recall any details of the day of the accident or any anterograde memories acquired since that day. However, with the exception of the day of the accident, her retrograde memory for events and important issues seemed to be largely intact.

Due to Lizzie's ongoing anterograde amnesia she was referred by her GP to neurology and seen in an outpatient clinic at her local hospital. At that time her presenting symptomatology included dense anterograde amnesia (with her last memory being 45 minutes before the accident), fatigue, poor concentration, generalised weakness, slight dizziness with blurred vision on standing quickly, and some stabbing headaches. Review of the CT brain scan undertaken in A&E on the day of the accident revealed some hyperdense acute blood on the original trauma sequence. An MRI brain scan revealed a small focal area of damage and microhaemorrhage in the splenium of the corpus callosum, left fornix, and left thalamus. The neurologist diagnosed a traumatic brain injury (TBI) and referred her to the TBI specialist clinic at the regional neurosciences centre for advice regarding treatment options.

Diagnosis of dissociative amnesia

Lizzie was subsequently seen by a consultant neurologist and neuropsychiatrist who specialise in TBI. Due to the COVID-19 pandemic the assessment was conducted virtually. They reviewed the letter from the referring consultant and considered the collateral information provided by Lizzie's parents, who reported that she wakes up everyday believing it is the date of the accident and then becomes confused and frustrated. She uses a diary and notes by her bedside to orientate herself. Lizzie and her parents were very clear that 'for the day she is in, she has no real significant memory problems'. However, after a night of sleep she cannot recall anything of the previous day. Her notes orientate her but she cannot recall any explicit memories for the events recorded. It was noted that she experiences difficulty sleeping, and had initially suffered from vivid dreams but now does not recall any dreams at all. Sometimes she finds it harder to concentrate and multitask. She is easily fatigued and simple tasks take longer. However, she was able to drive and had returned to work, conducting basic office tasks she had been familiar with prior to the accident. She had not been able to return to horse-riding due to poor coordination with fine motor tasks, such as plaiting hair and using cutlery. She described feeling like her limbs are 'full of lead' and having difficulty coordinating movement on stairs. She suffers from headaches, described as a 'dull frontal ache' most days. Her mood was described as low at times but at other times her mood can be good.

A full account of her past medical and mental health history was taken, and it was noted that she had experienced significant physical disability in childhood (e.g. a congenital problem that required her to use a prosthesis, and orthopaedic and hearing difficulties that required her to undergo multiple surgeries). In her early adulthood she suffered a back injury that prohibited her from completing her university studies. As a result, she had spent large amounts of time in hospitals feeling powerless, which she had found highly distressing. These experiences, together with the experience of being bullied at school, have triggered episodes of low mood and anxiety throughout her life. In particular, it is noteworthy that she expressed having learnt to use dissociation as a coping strategy at school because she found if she expressed her emotions about the bullying it resulted in more intense bullying. Prior to the TBI, she subsequently used dissociation to good effect to cope with the pain and physically invasive procedures she was required to undergo throughout her life.

Having reviewed the correspondence available, and on the basis of the parents' collateral information, the TBI specialists concluded that the severity and nature of her amnesia (i.e. reported difficulties of amnesia induced following sleep) were inconsistent with the severity of the injury, area of structural brain damage, and the established theories of memory. Based on her reported psychiatric history (e.g. experience of being bullied and having to suppress her feelings about this, together with her experience of depression and anxiety as a young adult), they hypothesised that the severity of her memory impairment was due to 'dissociative amnesia'. They recommended psychological intervention.

Psychological treatment

Lizzie reported a history of psychological trauma (e.g. bullying at school and multiple physical health problems growing up that required regular contact with hospitals, which she had experienced as traumatic). Lizzie described learning to use dissociation to cope with bullying at school because if distress was expressed it incited increased intensity of bullying behaviour. Once dissociation was learnt as a coping strategy Lizzie used it to good effect to cope with the extensive operations and other physically painful procedures required during the many years of interventions for complex physical health problems.

On standardised assessments of mood Lizzie endorsed high levels of emotional distress (i.e. consistent with clinical depression). She reported her low mood as being a response to having read the notes in the morning regarding her day-to-day challenges as a result of her cognitive and physical difficulties since the accident over 12 months ago, and the hopelessness she felt regarding a recovery, given the length of time the condition had persisted for. Her parents reported that they had noticed that her mood has been gradually deteriorating over time and she appeared to be exhibiting behavioural signs of depression, such as flat affect, difficulty getting out of bed in the morning, and not sleeping at night (although she reported to her parents that the latter was due to the fear of going to sleep and losing her memory). Her parents described observing increasing apathy and loss of interest and motivation for tasks she used to enjoy.

Lizzie was seen by a clinical psychologist who provided 14 sessions, which included treatment with eye movement desensitisation and reprocessing (EMDR), as well as a narrative exercise (co-created life story) to help Lizzie integrate the past with the present. While Lizzie did not recall her therapist from session to session, there were no issues in building rapport. Lizzie did not recall the session content but was encouraged to write notes after each one, and in her notes there is an indication that she liked being able to talk with someone objectively and have a space to reflect on her feelings. Unfortunately, trauma focused work did not have the expected outcome. It was noted by the treating therapist that, unlike other patients treated for functional cognitive disorders, Lizzie did not demonstrate reduced distress in subsequent sessions after processing early trauma memories. The therapist noticed that Lizzie's presentation was often like 'groundhog day', with her language, comments, and emotional responses being identical to the previous session as though she was experiencing the trauma memory for the first time. There was also no change in Lizzie's daily episodic amnesia, whereas when working clinically with functional cognitive disorders there are often improvements in function that correlate with the reduction in distress in EMDR sessions. Therefore, the therapist referred Lizzie for comprehensive neuropsychological assessment.

Lizzie was also reviewed in a Sleep Disturbance Clinic to establish whether or not the physiology of her sleep was abnormal. The physiologist concluded that Lizzie's pre-existing tendency to have difficulty initiating sleep was exacerbated by her current situation. He acknowledged that cognitive behaviour therapy for insomnia is unlikely to be effective, given Lizzie's inability to retain information. As such, he suggested that she and her family avoid detailing her sleep problems in the notes she keeps, as this would likely exacerbate them. Instead, he suggested writing down a simple sleep regime, whereby she has a regular bedtime to allow herself seven hours in bed before the alarm goes off. The physiologist declined to conduct a polysomnogram in the sleep laboratory (i.e. to allow a closer look at Lizzie's sleep) because he was concerned that it may be distressing for her to wake in a strange environment.

Neuropsychological assessment and interpretation

Dr Pradhan conducted a comprehensive battery of cognitive assessments with Lizzie at 12 months post-injury after she was referred to the neuropsychology diagnostic assessment service at the regional neurosciences centre. The battery of tests was administered in one day, as per the service's standard assessment model. However, given Lizzie's reported global amnesia after a night of sleep, some additional testing was administered the following day. After viewing the empirical literature described in the introduction, Dr Pradhan hypothesised that the damage to Lizzie's fornix may be causing a failure of sharp wave ripples during slow wave sleep and producing the observed memory profile. Hence, she also reviewed Lizzie at 16 months post-injury and the assessment battery was repeated the following day to qualitatively examine Lizzie's level of amnesia for the material and to establish whether there was any evidence of implicit learning, as would usually be observed in a person with anterograde amnesia.

Lizzie passed stand-alone and embedded performance validity measures. Her performance on tests of general intellectual functioning indicated a mild degree of downgrading compared to her High Average premorbid ability, specifically her verbal abstract reasoning (i.e. Similarities) and ability to perform motor manipulation of visuoconstructional material under timed conditions (i.e. Block Design).

Of note, immediate and delayed memory were significantly impaired, contrary to Lizzie and her family's assertion that she has no memory problems within the day. Her verbal recall was more impaired than her visual recall, consistent with the lesion in the left fornix, which is known to primarily carry verbal memory information (Raslau et al., 2015).

She also presented with executive dysfunction affecting predominantly verbal tasks and those that require mental flexibility. Her working memory, attention (sustained and divided), and processing speed (cognitive and motor) were impaired compared to premorbid estimates.

Tests of implicit and procedural memory demonstrated her inability to recall any new information from one day to the next. This is on the backdrop of intact visuospatial and perceptual processing and only relatively weak visual memory and language skills.

Dr Pradhan concluded that Lizzie's neuropsychological profile was consistent with anterograde amnesia affecting fronto-temporal regions with evidence of subcortical involvement, including the corpus callosum. Furthermore, there is strong evidence of lateralisation to the dominant (left) hemisphere. This profile is consistent with the location of the brain injury reported by the neuroradiologist (i.e. the left fornix and thalamus). The test results are also consistent with what Lizzie and her family report her day-to-day post-injury changes and challenges to be.

Comprehensive holistic neuropsychological rehabilitation

Following cognitive assessment, Lizzie was referred to the local NHS day patient holistic neuropsychological rehabilitation programme, and to date has attended a 12-week group therapy programme but is still receiving individual day patient treatment to help her achieve her goals of returning to horse-riding and independent living. Behavioural observation of Lizzie during her admission has revealed that she does not display retention of new learning during the day, as she or her family described, but in fact presents as a typical TBI amnesic, with patchy retrieval in the moment triggered by environmental stimuli that enables retrieval but an inability to freely recall information on demand. From the assessments and interventions delivered to date, it has been established that Lizzie does demonstrate some evidence of implicit learning consistent with anterograde amnesic patients (e.g. finding her way to the toilets in the centre independently and without signage). Lizzie has also demonstrated very subtle signs of implicit new learning, largely related to emotionally salient information. For instance, she was able to acknowledge that she felt 'safe' visiting a new livery yard where her horse is kept because she felt 'the people there are nice'. At the point that this information was retrieved there was no evidence of this information being recorded in her notes. Lizzie found the feedback about the evidence of new learning encouraging and uplifting because prior to this she feared that she would never be able to progress in her career if she cannot learn new information. Since then there is evidence that her confidence has grown and she has been engaging in increasingly more adventurous activities with good success (e.g. going on holiday to a novel environment with peers). In many ways Lizzie presents with a classic severe anterograde memory impairment after TBI. If sufficient detail is not recorded in her notes then she struggles to maintain motivation to engage in rehabilitation interventions. The treating team observed that her family were significantly scaffolding her, but when this support was removed it exposed the fact that her cognitive compensatory strategies were insufficient, in keeping with the classic presentation of someone with anterograde amnesia after TBI. Lizzie continues to receive cognitive rehabilitation currently and the treating team are working with the formulation that her presentation is fundamentally organic with psychological factors causing some variability in her behavioural presentation that can be understood as a direct consequence of the psychological sequelae of the TBI. It is important to highlight here the inevitable interaction between her acquired cognitive impairments secondary to TBI and her premorbid personality, values, and belief systems. It would be impossible to separate these things into a primary diagnosis of organic or functional aetiology as the functional symptoms would not exist if the organic impairment had not occurred. Therefore, the importance of formulating the symbiotic relationship between these factors is key to any treatment plan. The psychological impact of the associated losses caused by the cognitive impairments for Lizzie are huge, as all of her personal strengths were perceived to be related to her academic and cognitive abilities. Loss of these on a background of multiple other physical disabilities historically has inevitably impacted her self-confidence and mood, and need to be formulated as the psychological sequelae of the accident rather than a trigger to a functional overlay.

Discussion and conclusions

There remain many more questions than there are answers surrounding this case, and we continue to work with our multidisciplinary colleagues to achieve a consensus. Our work particularly highlights the importance of obtaining extensive behavioural observations rather than just relying on collateral information, as narratives of presenting difficulties can skew the presenting picture. Despite the ongoing debate in this case, we all agree that the functional–organic distinction that is inherent in the empirical literature, public service delivery models, and, consequently, professional opinion is detrimental to the well-being of patients with multimorbidity and is hampering the evolution of our professions. This dichotomised thinking perpetuates the 17th-century concept of body–mind dualism which, though long outmoded, has driven the lack of integrated physical and mental health services in the UK. Instead, attention needs to be placed on understanding how the body and mind interact from a biopsychosocial perspective to account for the cognitive and behavioural profile observed. We argue that our professions should stop trying to differentially diagnose cases with multimorbidity as *either* organic *or* functional, and instead seek to formulate the symbiotic process by which the organic and functional symptomatology are generated and perpetuate each other.

However, this case also highlights the challenges that busy NHS clinicians face when treating complex cases. Firstly, the clinic structures imposed on them by the organisation, which are driven by the perverse incentives of face-to-face activity, means that clinicians' job plans often have clinics scheduled with no time allocated to review records extensively and/or appointments set-up with no access to past records from other hospitals. Clinicians often only have informant accounts in consultations, and are required to dictate letters on completion of the consultation without adequate time for interdisciplinary formulation. This often leads to information being recounted between health professionals as fact when it is actually erroneous. In the author's experience, such documentation can cause patients significant harm, especially those involved in litigation after TBI, as erroneous accounts reported in NHS clinic letters are used as evidence of inconsistency in the patients' presentation when in fact it illustrates differences in the clinicians' access to information and/or approaches to assessment rather than hard evidence of the patients' condition. We argue it would be best practice for clinicians to caveat the pitfalls and limitations of clinical opinion after a single consultation so that lay readers can understand the validity of the clinical opinion; for example, articulating potential diagnoses as working hypotheses, deferring an opinion until consultation is obtained from multidisciplinary colleagues. This creates space for interdisciplinary formulation and would improve the patient experience. In Lizzie's case, she and her parents were left feeling confused and frustrated by the multiple diagnoses health professionals provided without any attempt to bring this information into a holistic formulation.

This case is ongoing and, sadly for Lizzie, the diagnostic conundrum is not yet fully resolved; nevertheless, it has been established that there is a primary organic deficit that underlies her cognitive presentation. Lizzie has been supported to identify holistic value-based goals, which she feels motivated to engage in, and she is now making important gains in rehabilitation incorporating the principles of Empowerment-based Behaviour Management Approach (Betteridge et al., 2017). Therefore, the learning from this case so far is important to share.

We hope that clinicians will be inspired to change their practice when confronted with complex cases and consider trying to facilitate interdisciplinary holistic formulations by postulating hypotheses and deferring for multidisciplinary opinions before articulating diagnoses. The patient should be empowered by being involved in the diagnostic uncertainty and the process of investigation rather than confused by conflicting diagnoses.

The inadequacy of current NHS stepped care service design for the assessment and treatment of patients with multimorbidity is highlighted by the failings in the timely delivery of assessment and treatment in this case. While the current treating tier 4 specialist cognitive rehabilitation service is seeking to rectify this, the negative impact on the patients' mental health, their trust of health professionals, and motivation to engage with rehabilitation services is palpable. In our experience, the patients' resulting reluctant behavioural presentation is often a significant barrier to progress in cognitive rehabilitation and extends the duration of rehabilitation required and increases the overall cost to the health economy. Access to early specialist holistic interdisciplinary assessment for these patients could help improve triage into specialist services, thereby reducing overall costs. Furthermore, reflective practice, in accordance with the principles of systemic therapy (e.g. Stedmon & Dallos, 2009) for neurosciences professions, needs to be incorporated into everyday practice more consistently. Too often health professions fail to take into account the dynamic role they play in the development of the patients' reluctance to engage in health care services. All too easily, patients' behaviour and ways of responding are labelled or pathologised as 'functional overlay' or 'poor motivation to change', when in fact health professionals and services need to reflect on their own practice and what they might need to change to facilitate the patient's engagement.

References

Benear, S. L., Ngo, C. T., & Olson, I. R. (2020). Dissecting the Fornix in Basic Memory Processes and Neuropsychiatric Disease: A Review. *Brain Connectivity*; 10 (7): 331–354.

Betteridge, S., Cotterill, E., & Murphy, P. (2017). Rehabilitation of challenging behaviour in community settings: The Empowerment Behavioural Management Approach (EBMA). In B. A. Wilson, J. Winegardner, C. van Heugten, & T. Ownsworth (Eds.), *Neuropsychological rehabilitation: The international handbook* (pp. 298–310). Psychology Press.

Burgess, G. H., & Chadalavada, B. (2016). Profound anterograde amnesia following routine anesthetic and dental procedure: A new classification of amnesia characterized by intermediate-to-late-stage consolidation failure?. *Neurocase, 22*(1), 84–94.

Camina, E., & Güell, F. (2017). The neuroanatomical, neurophysiological and psychological basis of memory: Current models and their origins. *Frontiers in Pharmacology, 8*, 438.

Raslau, F. D., Augustinack, J. C., Klein, A. P., Ulmer, J. L., Mathews, V. P., & Mark, L. P. (2015). Memory part 3: The role of the fornix and clinical cases. *American Journal of Neuroradiology, 36*(9), 1604–1608.

Scoville, W. B., & Milner, B. (1957). Loss of recent memory after bilateral hippocampal lesions. *Journal of neurology, neurosurgery, and psychiatry, 20*(1), 11.

Segal, P. (Director). (2004) *50 First Dates* [Film]. Columbia Tristar/Sony Pictures USA.

Smith, C. N., Frascino, J. C., Kripke, D. L., McHugh, P. R., Treisman, G. J., & Squire, L. R. (2010). Losing memories overnight: A unique form of human amnesia. *Neuropsychologia, 48*(10), 2833–2840.

Squire, L. R., & Knowlton, B. J. (1995). Memory, hippocampus, and brain systems. In M. S. Gazzaniga (Ed.), *The cognitive neurosciences* (pp. 825–837). The MIT Press.

Stedmon, J., & Dallos, R. (2009). *Reflective practice in psychotherapy and counselling.* McGraw-Hill Education.

Sunak, S. (2019). Appropriate assessment and formulation for neuropsychological rehabilitation. In B. A., Wilson, & S. Betteridge (Eds.). *Essentials of neuropsychological rehabilitation.* Guilford Press.

Watson, B. O., & Buzsáki, G. (2015). Sleep, memory & brain rhythms. *Daedalus, 144*(1), 67–82.

Wilson, B. A. (2009). *Memory rehabilitation: Integrating theory and practice.* Guilford Press.

25 Learning from experience

How can we best help people with rare, difficult to diagnose, or controversial conditions?

Jessica Fish, Shai Betteridge, and Barbara A. Wilson

In the 23 chapters that make up this volume (excluding our introductory and concluding chapters), we have heard from a group of clinicians across many different areas of practice: those who specialise in working with children and young people, adults of working age, and older people respectively; those who work in the UK National Health Service, those who work in third sector organisations, those who work in independent practice and/or as expert witnesses; and those who work in very different health systems overseas. Contributors include those working in specialised services and those working in more general services, and cases range from those with conditions that are fairly typical for the specialist services they were seen within to those with conditions so extraordinarily rare that the clinicians are unlikely to see anyone similar again. What can we learn from these disparate cases so as to serve people with such conditions better in future? Obviously, each case has unique features and it would be unwise to extrapolate based on the specifics of any one piece of work to other cases with similar presentations that may be encountered. However, taken collectively, we think there are important transferable learning points, and have summarised these as follows.

Learning points for individual practitioners and clinical teams

1. *Allow time to prepare and to do one's homework*: ensure that you are familiar with the pathology associated with the condition, its diagnostic criteria if relevant, any documented neuropsychological consequences, and the availability of specialist services including those in the third sector. This will, of course, involve searching the literature but equally don't be afraid to reach out to specialists for additional consultation. Most are passionate about their areas of expertise and would be only too willing to share their knowledge. Use continuing professional development time and resources to skill up on emerging areas of knowledge. For complex cases, where there might be several working hypotheses about the diagnosis, it is often necessary to simultaneously explore the clinical and empirical evidence

DOI: 10.4324/9781003228226-28

base for each hypothesis. It may help to compile the evidence 'for' and 'against' each hypothesis in a spreadsheet. This will allow you to evaluate the strength of the evidence for each hypothesis methodically over time as you collect your assessment data. Gather as much information from as many sources as possible. For instance, narratives from friends, family and work colleagues, neuroimaging reports, previous cognitive assessments, and medical, mental health, school, and police records. Seek out correspondence from original sources; in our experience, self-reported diagnoses, such as traumatic brain injury, can be recounted for years in medical records but on obtaining the original ambulance and hospital discharge report, it is established that no brain injury occurred. While listening to the reported narratives of clients and their significant others is obviously important, it is equally important to verify this information. Often diagnostic labels are adopted by clients or their support systems to aid access to services in an attempt to address an unmet need. Where discrepancies arise, consider and work with the systems of which the client is a part to help reach a collaborative formulation of the client's needs. However, be aware of the psychological impact of a lengthy and/or contested diagnostic process and prolonged period of uncertainty, and the potentially suboptimal experience of health and care services that may make a client's engagement with you and/or your service more threatening or challenging for them.

2. *Remain person-centred*: regardless of the condition and the nature of the work, the patient's values and long-term objectives should be kept at its centre. In our clinical experience, often external factors, such as discipline-specific preferences for assessment tools or organisational protocols, drive assessments and intervention plans. This results in repetition of assessment in some domains and gaps in others. Often there is no formal process of integrating all the information obtained from the multi-disciplinary assessments. Consequently, intervention is delivered in silos with no holistic framework to help the patient understand its worth. In contrast, the contributors have demonstrated that if you take the time to find out about the person's identity, values, and personal circumstances, this is likely to be as good a start as any driven from a specific profession or organisation's perspective. Reaching an understanding of the *person in context* will rarely send an assessment awry. Keeping the person's interests at heart means you are more likely to focus on what's most relevant for a successful intervention, more likely to encourage your team to 'pull together' in their assistance, and more likely to be aware when things are going off track. Maintaining a person-centred focus is more likely to enable you and your team to achieve a meaningful outcome for the patient and/or their support systems.

3. *Put your scientist–practitioner training into practice by taking a flexible approach and customising your cognitive assessment*: a rigid battery of tests is unlikely to provide all the data you require in an economical way. Our contributors

have conducted assessments that deftly incorporated standardised clinical measures, measures drawn from the scientific literature, and bespoke procedures (including functional and/or observation-based approaches). These have been tailored to the case based on what is known of the person, their context and their clinical needs, alongside what is known of the likely condition(s) and their features. The chapters demonstrate that taking this approach has (i) enabled accurate identification of syndromes, (ii) helped the patient and family to make sense of their experiences, (iii) not just informed but *transformed* approaches to management and rehabilitation, (iv) expanded our scientific understanding of a syndrome, (v) served to test theory and challenge the status quo, and (vi) modelled good practice for others to learn from and build upon.

4. *When formulating, keep an open mind, adopt a broad holistic lens, take the long view, and incorporate reflective practice*: formulate as an interdisciplinary team if you can, through assessment, diagnosis, intervention, and management. Think of intersectionality and be aware of how experiences of disability, disadvantage, or difference might obscure or otherwise influence your understanding of the person and their presentation. Consider the purpose of a diagnosis and its implications for the person's life and care. Be sensitive to developmental factors and think about the ways in which the passage of time may influence the presentation and the person's clinical needs. Continue to formulate over time, particularly when changes in circumstances or symptoms occur. Be careful not to become too wedded to your initial formulation. Be open to reformulating and seeking new explanations when contradictions arise. Engage in a process of triangulation to identify consistencies and inconsistencies between information arising from different sources (e.g. are the results from testing consistent with what is known from neuroimaging and from informant reports? If not, why not, and how might you gain clarification? Is the person responding to treatment in the manner expected, given the formulation? If not, what might explain this, and how might you reconsider your formulation and intervention approach?). This process will help to refine and test your hypotheses and improve the overall accuracy of your formulation and, in turn, allow you to provide a better service.

5. *Share your formulation with all stakeholders – knowledge (and narrative) is power*: A 'good' formulation has been described as 'one that works'. Once you have a sufficient formulation, its impact can be far-reaching. As well as enabling you to optimally direct treatment, it should provide a clear narrative for the person and/or those around them (including family, social groups and healthcare teams as relevant) to understand their circumstances, and especially to appreciate the biopsychosocial interactions that are important in beginning to adapt to new and often challenging aspects of those circumstances. The process of sharing a formulation can also serve as a powerful tool to engage various stakeholders in the process of intervention. However, care should be taken to avoid oversimplification

of the material communicated and attention should be given to setting up accurate expectations in terms of future prognosis.

6. *Apply the scientist practitioner model by continuously evaluating your intervention*: if the formulation is not yet conclusive, or there is no relevant evidence base for treatment, hypothesis-driven interventions may still be identified. Careful experimentation here can help to clarify any inconsistencies in the formulation, as well as make progress towards clinical goals. Several chapters document this approach. Our contributors have reflected on the value of essential therapeutic skills (e.g. unconditional positive regard, validation of the person's perspectives and rights, empowering people to be involved in decision making, ensuring that interventions support the person's identity). Of course, in such cases it is imperative to measure and document progress towards goals and/or other relevant clinical outcomes carefully so as to establish progress or lack of it, and reformulate and adjust the approach as necessary. This is always important because if we don't measure outcomes formally, we run the risk of obtaining only a partial picture of the effects of our work. However, a fuller picture is of particular value when working with 'new', 'rare', or 'uncertain' circumstances.

7. *Ensure your intervention offers an integrated approach for multimorbidity*: multimorbidity is common – NICE (2016) estimated that 23–27% of people have two or more long-term health conditions and prevalence is higher in older adults and people living in socioeconomic deprivation. In some cases there is no single diagnosis to explain the client's presentation, nor any firm conclusions to be drawn. Neuropsychological phenomena are often complex and our scientific knowledge of cognitive function is far from complete. If we only view clients through our narrow professional lens it enforces immediate limits on the precision of our diagnoses and formulations. Several cases in this collection represent people who have more than one neurological condition and some of the most complex cases have combined 'functional' and 'organic' aspects to their presentation, which were challenging for individuals and teams to work with. These chapters emphasise the need for (i) close teamwork as well as multiagency working, (ii) a scientific approach with both assessment and intervention based on the current best evidence, (iii) sustained involvement over time, and (iv) the involvement of specialist services where possible. They also highlight the importance of (i) essential therapeutic skills, (ii) clear and sensitive communication in relation to what is known and what is not known, and (iii) reflection on the case and its implications. As Worthington and Soeterik note in their chapters, even in the absence of complete answers, much useful information can be obtained, and progress is possible, nonetheless.

Many of these learning points reiterate what we are taught in our basic clinical psychology training. Stating them here could seem fatuous, but we actually find it rather reassuring – it means clinical neuropsychologists already possess many necessary skills to forge ahead and work productively with people with rare disorders and unusual or complex presentations. We hope that this book and these learning points inspire individual clinicians to confront their understanding of clients presenting with unusual conditions rather than shying away from them. By formulating these rare presentations holistically we will aid not only our own profession's evolution of knowledge, skills, and practice but also those of the wider community of healthcare professions.

Learning points for our broader professional communities

The cases in this book raise important broader implications. We encourage clinical neuropsychologists to use the following learning points when opportunities arise to influence public health, research, and/or commissioners.

1. *Highlight the 'invisible' nature of most neuropsychological impairments* – to work to improve their identification, increase our understanding of them, and advocate for people experiencing them. This is not specific to working with rare or unusual cases but is at least as important here as it is in relation to the more common neuropsychological conditions.

2. *Raise awareness of preventable causes of neuropsychological disability.* This stems particularly from Urvashi Shah's chapter (Chapter 2), and brings to mind work cited by Winegardner (2022) documenting Morales Bonilla and Mauss' (1998) community-based project to identify suspected lead poisoning (which has documented neurotoxic effects) from a car battery factory in an impoverished neighbourhood in post-revolutionary Nicaragua. This project involved measuring blood lead levels in local children living in demographically and environmentally similar areas either close to or more distant from the factory. Concerning levels were identified in 80% of those living near the factory, and only 30% of those living further away. With this evidence, residents garnered sufficient publicity to force the factory to close. The project's success was considered a result of strong and sustained community engagement from the outset and there is much to be learned from this approach.

3. *Foster a holistic and integrative understanding of the relationship between mind and brain.* Rose and Dilley (Chapter 10) provide an eloquent overview of the negative impacts of the societal dualist understanding of disorders of mind and brain (i.e. that they are distinct), and the divisions within the health system that serve to perpetuate this perspective (e.g. in the existence of separately commissioned neurology and psychiatry services). Our ability to progress holistic models of mind and brain and address the stigma associated with mental illness will only occur with the provision of integrated and jointly commissioned physical and mental health

services; therefore, commissioning and evaluation of holistic services should be a matter of priority for public health research.

4. *Stress that services need to be adequately resourced to enable appropriate assessment and management of 'complex' cases.* Providing good care in this area of practice takes considerable time, and non-patient-facing time is in increasingly short supply in the public sector. Service delivery models and clinicians' job plans both need to account for this, but public health services are often designed and funded based on face-to-face activity for the 'average patient' or the most common patient presentation. This results in clinicians having insufficient time to address the needs of patients with multimorbidity. Consequently, this client group end up accessing multiple services, receiving contradictory advice, and having no overarching clinician to coordinate their care and treatment. Evaluation of the costs associated with the inefficiencies in traditional service delivery models would help inform commissioning priorities, which are often driven by the need to improve health economics.

5. *Know that we need to do more to demonstrate our professional worth and to integrate research and practice.* Mental health is high on the national policy agenda in the UK, as is brain health. Clinical psychology has in recent years advocated very successfully for itself including rigorous and coordinated evaluation of mental health services (e.g. in improving access to psychological therapies (IAPT) services, and early intervention for psychosis). The profession has as a consequence seen much expansion. The field of clinical neuropsychology is much smaller and though there are excellent examples of progress made (e.g. in policy developments in stroke and functional neurological disorders in the UK over the past decade or more), we feel there is considerable room for improvement in the ways we demonstrate the impact of good clinical neuropsychology input in general, and particularly in relation to rare disorders where specialist services need to be advocated for. If we don't evidence how our input improves the care people receive, we are at risk of posts being downbanded or lost, services being decommissioned (or not commissioned in the first place), or commissioned without adequate neuropsychology input. Improvements in routine outcome monitoring and harmonisation of this to enable pooling of data and larger scale evaluation of services is one approach, though one fraught with difficulty, given the unsatisfactory nature of a one-size fits all approach. However, similar comments were likely made about other fields of work that have much more united approaches (e.g. IAPT, neurorehabilitation). Better integration between research and practice is highly likely to be helpful in this regard.

We are not the only people interested in rare disorders; recent years have seen a number of important policy developments in this domain. In 2021, the UK Government's Department of Health and Social Care (2021) published a *Rare Diseases Framework* calling for improved care for people with such conditions.

The framework notes that although a condition is considered rare if it affects fewer than one in 2,000 people, because there are more than 7,000 rare disorders, at some point in their lives, one in 17 people will have one. The framework highlighted four priority areas for improvement over the subsequent five years:

1. Decreasing time to diagnosis
2. Increasing healthcare professionals' awareness
3. Improving coordination of care
4. Widening access to specialist services and treatments.

Underpinning these priorities are five themes: (i) the patient voice, with an emphasis on diverse representation; (ii) national and international collaboration, given the small numbers of people experiencing specific conditions; (iii) research, including new funding streams targeted to rare conditions; (iv) digital data and technology, to be used to improve services and facilitate research; and (v) policy alignment. A phased plan was set out to achieve those aims, with the Rare Diseases Framework being the first phase, and the development of a set of action plans for each of the devolved nations the second.

The Neurological Alliance (2019) published a report finding that relative to those with more common neurological conditions, people with rare neurological conditions are less likely to understand their condition, less likely to receive either written information about their condition or signposting towards this information, less likely to receive a care plan, less likely to see a specialist nurse, less likely to be asked about their mental health, and more likely to experience poor transmission of information between professionals and to have a poor experience of social care. They argue for similar improvements to those identified in the 2021 framework, alongside the need for improved care pathways and commissioning arrangements, informational resources, and information sharing, but also emphasise the mental health needs of people with rare conditions, as well as needs at times of transition between services.

Hence, it seems there is reason to be optimistic that significant developments will be seen in the coming years. It will be important for neuropsychology as a profession to be involved in shaping these developments.

We recognise that there are gaps in the areas covered by this book; you may have been reading this thinking 'my case on topic X should be in there' or 'what about condition Y, or controversy Z'! If so, do get in touch. If we receive enough such approaches, we might be persuaded to produce a second volume.

If you have read this far, we thank you very much for your interest and attention. We hope you have found the cases informative and instructive and that you will take something from this book forward into your practice.

References

Department of Health & Social Care (2021). *UK Rare Diseases Framework.* www.gov.uk/government/publications/uk-rare-diseases-framework

Morales Bonilla, C., & Mauss, E. A. (1998). A community-initiated study of blood lead levels of Nicaraguan children living near a battery factory. *American Journal of Public Health, 88*(12), 1843–1845.

Neurological Alliance. (2019). *Out of the shadows: What needs to change for people with rare neurological conditions.* The Neurological Alliance. www.neural.org.uk/wp-content/uploads/2021/07/neurological-alliance-out-of-the-shadows-2020.pdf

NICE. (2016). *Multimorbidity: Clinical assessment and management.* National Institute for Health and Care Excellence. www.nice.org.uk [Free full-text]

Winegardner, J. (2022). Neuropsychological rehabilitation: Perspectives based on cultural experience. In A. L. Fernandez & J. Evans (Eds.), *Understanding cross-cultural neuropsychology: Science, testing and challenges* (pp.161–173). Taylor & Francis Group.

Index

Note: Locators in *italic* indicate figures and in **bold** tables and page numbers followed by "n" refer to end notes.

Printed in Great Britain
by Amazon

27305358R00218